STUDY GUIDE TO GERIATRIC PSYCHIATRY

A Companion to
The American Psychiatric Publishing Textbook of Geriatric Psychiatry,
Fifth Edition

STUDY GUIDE TO GERIATRIC PSYCHIATRY

A Companion to *The American Psychiatric Publishing Textbook of Geriatric Psychiatry,* Fifth Edition

Edited by

Philip R. Muskin, M.D.
Anna L. Dickerman, M.D.

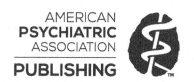

AMERICAN
PSYCHIATRIC
ASSOCIATION
PUBLISHING

If you wish to buy 50 or more copies of the same title, please go to www.appi.org/special discounts for more information.

Copyright © 2017 American Psychiatric Association Publishing

ALL RIGHTS RESERVED

Manufactured in the United States of America on acid-free paper
20   19   18   17   16   5   4   3   2   1
First Edition

American Psychiatric Association Publishing
1000 Wilson Boulevard
Arlington, VA 22209-3901
www.appi.org

Typeset in Palatino LT Std and Helvetica Neue LT Std

Contents

Contributors

Ali Abbas Asghar-Ali, M.D.
Associate Director for Education, South Central MIRECC; Director, Geriatric Psychiatry Fellowship and Associate Professor, Baylor College of Medicine; Geriatric Psychiatrist, Michael E. DeBakey VA Medical Center, Houston, Texas

Jimmy N. Avari, M.D.
Instructor in Psychiatry and Assistant Attending, Department of Psychiatry, Payne Whitney Westchester of New York-Presbyterian Hospital, Weill Medical College of Cornell University, New York, New York

Arnabh Basu, M.B., B.S.
Clinical Fellow, Division of Geriatric Psychiatry, Columbia University, New York, New York

James G. Bouknight, M.D., Ph.D.
Professor of Clinical Neuropsychiatry, University of South Carolina School of Medicine, Columbia, South Carolina

Lisa L. Boyle, M.D., M.P.H.
Clinical Associate Professor of Psychiatry, University of Wisconsin School of Medicine and Public Health, William S. Middleton Memorial Veteran's Hospital, Madison, Wisconsin

Johanna A. Cabassa, M.D.
Attending Geriatric Psychiatrist, Montefiore Medical Center, Montefiore Medical Group, Bronx, New York

Jack Castro, M.D.
Consultation and Liaison and Geriatric Psychiatrist, Montefiore Medical Group, Bronx, New York

Adam Critchfield, M.D.
Fellow, Psychosomatic Medicine, Columbia University Medical Center and New York State Psychiatric Institute, New York, New York

Karina Davis, M.D.
PGY 4 Psychiatry Resident, University of Michigan Department of Psychiatry, Ann Arbor, Michigan

Anna L. Dickerman, M.D.
Assistant Professor of Psychiatry, Department of Psychiatry, Weill Cornell Medical College; Assistant Attending Psychiatrist, Psychiatry Consultation-Liaison Service, New York-Presbyterian Hospital/Weill Cornell Medical Center, New York, New York

Nanette M. Dowling, D.O., M.H.P.A.
Director of Geriatric Psychiatry and Assistant Professor, Department of Psychiatry, SUNY Upstate Medical University, Syracuse, New York

Diana Feldman, M.D.
Assistant Professor of Psychiatry, Weill Cornell Medical College; Attending Psychiatrist, Psychiatry, NYP–Payne Whitney Manhattan, New York, New York

Lauren B. Gerlach, D.O.
Geriatric Psychiatry Fellow, University of Michigan Department of Psychiatry, Ann Arbor, Michigan

Liliya Gershengoren, M.D.
Fellow in Psychosomatic Medicine, Columbia University Medical Center and New York State Psychiatric Institute, New York, New York

Juliet A. Glover, M.D.
Assistant Professor, Department of Neuropsychiatry and Behavioral Science, University of South Carolina School of Medicine, Columbia, South Carolina

Gary J. Kennedy, M.D.
Director, Division of Geriatric Psychiatry and the Leslie and Roslyn Goldstein Geriatric Psychiatry Fellowship Program, Montefiore Medical Center; Professor of Psychiatry and Behavioral Sciences, Albert Einstein College of Medicine, Bronx, New York

Daniel Knoepflmacher, M.D.
Assistant Professor of Psychiatry, Department of Psychiatry, Weill Cornell Medical College; Assistant Attending Psychiatrist, Outpatient Department, New York-Presbyterian Hospital/Weill Cornell Medical Center, New York, New York

Rushiraj Laiwala, M.D.
Geriatric Psychiatry Fellow, Department of Neuropsychiatry, University of South Carolina, Columbia, South Carolina

Maria I. Lapid, M.D.
Associate Professor of Psychiatry and Program Director, Geriatric Psychiatry Fellowship, Mayo Clinic Department of Psychiatry and Psychology, Rochester, Minnesota

Katherine Levine, M.D.
Assistant Professor, Department of Psychiatry and Behavioral Medicine, Medical College of Wisconsin, Milwaukee, Wisconsin

Susan M. Maixner, M.D.
Associate Professor of Psychiatry, Department of Psychiatry, University of Michigan, Ann Arbor, Michigan

Kristin McArthur, M.D.
Geriatric Psychiatry Fellow, Department of Psychiatry, University of Michigan, Ann Arbor, Michigan

Philip R. Muskin, M.D., M.A.
Professor of Psychiatry, Columbia University Medical Center; Chief, Consultation-Liaison Psychiatry at New York-Presbyterian Hospital/Columbia Campus; Faculty, Columbia University Center for Psychoanalytic Training and Research, New York, New York

Mark Nathanson, M.D.
Director, Geriatric Psychiatry Fellowship, Columbia University, New York, New York

Nancy Needell, M.D.
Assistant Attending Psychiatrist, New York Presbyterian Hospital; Assistant Professor of Clinical Psychiatry, Weill Cornell Medical College, Cornell University, New York, New York

Yara A. Bonet Pagan, M.D.
Adult and Geriatric Psychiatrist, Montefiore Medical Center, Wakefield Division/Albert Einstein College of Medicine, Bronx, New York

Anusha Ranganathan, M.D.
Staff Psychiatrist, Ann Arbor VA Medical Center; Clinical Instructor, University of Michigan Division of Geriatric Psychiatry, Ann Arbor, Michigan

Swapnil Rath, M.D.
Geriatric Psychiatry Fellow, University of Michigan Department of Psychiatry, Ann Arbor, Michigan

Teri Rummans, M.D.
Professor of Psychiatry, Mayo Clinic, Rochester, Minnesota

Shilpa Srinivasan, M.D., DFAPA
Associate Professor of Clinical Psychiatry and Associate Training Director, Geriatric Psychiatry Fellowship, and Director, M4 Psychiatry Clerkship, Department of Neuropsychiatry and Behavioral Science, University of South Carolina School of Medicine, Columbia, South Carolina

Daniel Varon, M.D.
Assistant Professor of Psychiatry, Western Psychiatric Institute and Clinic, University of Pittsburgh, Pittsburgh, Pennsylvania

Marcia L. Verduin, M.D.
Associate Dean for Students and Professor of Psychiatry, College of Medicine, University of Central Florida, Orlando, Florida

Monique Yohanan, M.D., M.P.H.
Senior Physician Editor and Subject Matter Expert in Behavioral Health, MCG, San Francisco, California

Disclosure of Interests

Lisa L. Boyle, M.D., M.P.H. *Consultant:* Alzheimer's and Dementia Alliance of Wisconsin. *Grants:* HRSA.

The following contributors have indicated that they have no financial interests or other affiliations that represent a competing interest with their contributions to this book:
Ali Abbas Asghar-Ali, M.D.; Jimmy N. Avari, M.D.; Arnabh Basu, M.B., B.S.; James G. Bouknight, M.D., Ph.D.; Johanna A. Cabassa, M.D.; Jack Castro, M.D.; Adam Critchfield, M.D.; Karina Davis, M.D.; Anna L. Dickerman, M.D.; Nanette M. Dowling, D.O., M.H.P.A.; Diana Feldman, M.D.; Lauren B. Gerlach, D.O.; Liliya Gershengoren, M.D.; Juliet A. Glover, M.D.; Gary J. Kennedy, M.D.; Rushiraj Laiwala, M.D.; Maria I. Lapid, M.D.; Katherine Levine, M.D.; Susan M. Maixner, M.D.; Kristin McArthur, M.D.; Philip R. Muskin, M.D., M.A.; Mark Nathanson, M.D.; Nancy Needell, M.D.; Yara A. Bonet Pagan, M.D.

Preface

This self-examination guide is a companion to, not a replacement for, reading *The American Psychiatric Publishing Textbook of Geriatric Psychiatry*, Fifth Edition. All psychiatrists will encounter patients who are elderly in their careers, and there are special biopsychosocial considerations for older patients. The textbook will prepare readers to understand the epidemiology, neurobiology, psychology, and treatment of these patients. Therefore, we have attempted to organize questions along those domains, matching each chapter in the book. As you work through this self-examination book, let it guide you to chapters in the textbook as a path to your self-education. Some questions will seem obvious or easy, and some questions will be quite difficult. We have endeavored to use the style of question writing found in certification examinations; however, this is not a board preparation book. The contributors to this book are a group of clinicians and educators with a broad range of experience and expertise who undertook the task of writing the questions. The majority of the contributors are geriatric or consultation-liaison psychiatrists, the two subspecialties who most often treat geriatric patients. The contributors have graciously donated the proceeds from this book to charitable foundations dedicated to mental health.

Page numbers in the Answer Guide refer to *The American Psychiatric Publishing Textbook of Geriatric Psychiatry*, Fifth Edition. Visit www.appi.org for more information about this textbook.

Philip R. Muskin, M.D., M.A.
Anna L. Dickerman, M.D.

Part I

Questions

CHAPTER 1

Demography and Epidemiology of Psychiatric Disorders in Late Life

Select the single best response for each question.

1.1 What will the estimated percentage of the U.S. population of persons 65 years and older be by 2050?

A. 5%.
B. 40%.
C. 20%.
D. 15%.

1.2 What will the projected population be in 2050 of the "oldest old" segment of the United States, persons 85 and older?

A. 5.5 million.
B. 19.0 million.
C. 0.5 million.
D. 10.0 million.

1.3 What is the percentage of persons ages 85 years and older who are living in long-term care facilities?

A. 53%.
B. 14%.
C. 5.5%.
D. 87%.

1.4 By the year 2050, which of these ethnic minority groups will increase most in total number in the United States?

A. Non-Hispanic black.
B. Asian.
C. Non-Hispanic white.
D. Hispanic.

1.5 Which of the following correctly describes the findings related to the lifetime prevalence of major depression in the National Comorbidity Survey Replication (NCS-R) reported by Kessler et al. (2005)?

A. The incidence of major depressive disorder was 10.6% in participants ages 60 years and older.
B. The incidence of major depressive disorder was 40% in participants ages 18–29 years.
C. The incidence of major depressive disorder was less than 10% in participants ages 30–44 years.
D. The incidence of major depressive disorder was 12% in participants ages 45–59 years.

1.6 Which of the following is the most prevalent psychiatric disorder among persons ages 65 years and older (excluding neurocognitive disorders)?

A. Hypochondriasis.
B. Anxiety disorder.
C. Schizoaffective disorder.
D. Alcohol use disorder.

1.7 Which of these is a common syndrome confounding psychiatric and medical diagnosis in the elderly?

A. Bulimia nervosa.
B. Hypochondriasis.
C. Delusional jealousy.
D. Trichotillomania.

1.8 The Collaborative Psychiatric Epidemiology Surveys (CPES) enabled a better understanding of the relationship between major depression and which of the following?

A. Immigration status and ethnicity.
B. Medical comorbidity.
C. End of life issues.
D. Alcohol and substance use disorders.

1.9 What was the prevalence of Alzheimer's disease in persons ages 85 years and older in the East Boston Established Populations for Epidemiologic Studies of the Elderly (EPESE)?

A. 3%.
B. 47%.
C. 60%.
D. 35%.

1.10 Prevalence estimates of depressive symptoms in nursing home residents, using the Minimum Data Set, is closest to which of the following?

A. 10%.
B. 90%.
C. 30%.
D. 50%.

1.11 Which of the following statements regarding suicide mortality in the U.S. geriatric population is correct?

A. Rates of suicide are equal in males and females.
B. African American men have the highest rates of completed suicide.
C. Men ages 65 years and older have twice the rate of completed suicide than men ages 15–24 years.
D. Asian men have the highest suicide rates in the United States.

1.12 Since 2000, which group has the steepest increase in completed suicides in the United States?

A. Men ages 85 years and older.
B. Men ages 75–84 years.
C. Men ages 50–59 years.
D. Men ages 65–74 years.

1.13 Which of the following is true regarding the impact of stressful life events as measured by the Holmes-Rahe Schedule of Recent Events?

A. The impact on mental health is minimal for older adults.
B. The impact is considerable, occurring even with low Holmes-Rahe scores.
C. The relative risk for mental health impairment is >2 for those with moderate scores of 150 or greater.
D. This scale has not been used to study older adults.

1.14 With what was major depression associated in the Longitudinal Aging Study Amsterdam?

A. Poorer self-perceived health.
B. Increased social network.
C. Married status.
D. External locus of control.

1.15 When compared with a younger cohort with similar psychopathology, older patients with psychiatric illness may have which of these patterns of mental health community-based treatment?

A. Older patients are more likely to receive treatment in the health care setting.
B. Older patients are less likely to be referred to mental health specialists.
C. Older patients are more likely to perceive a need for mental health care.
D. Older patients receive more specialty mental health referral than younger patients.

CHAPTER 2

Physiological and Clinical Considerations of Geriatric Patient Care

Select the single best response for each question.

2.1   Which of the following represents age-related physiological changes in vision?

   A. There are decreases in accommodation in older people, which make it difficult to focus on near objects.
   B. Older people show a decline in the ability to view objects in motion (dynamic acuity), whereas the ability to view objects at rest (static acuity) remains relatively preserved.
   C. The ability to adapt to light often is impaired in older people because of increasing lens transparency.
   D. Age-related macular degeneration is a severe, but relatively uncommon, cause of blindness in older people.

2.2   Which of the following is characteristic of age-related hearing loss?

   A. There is loss of high-frequency hearing in older adults, but low-frequency hearing generally is preserved.
   B. Thickening of the tympanic membrane and degenerative changes in the ossicles are responsible for significant impairments in hearing.
   C. Speech discrimination ability rarely is affected in older adults.
   D. Both high- and low-frequency hearing loss are common in older adults.

2.3   A 65-year-old man presents to your clinic for routine examination. He had a sedentary lifestyle for many years. Now that he has retired, he is interested in taking up a regular exercise program. He asks if there are any concerns he should have related to his heart. He has a history of type 2 diabetes and a 20 pack a year smoking history, but he quit smoking 5 years ago. He wants to know how exercise might affect his heart. Which of the following is typical of age-related changes in the cardiovascular system?

A. The increased β-adrenergic response of the heart seen with aging increases the maximal heart rate attained during exercise.
B. A narrowing of aortic pulse pressure is seen in older adults.
C. Increased β-adrenergic responsiveness seen with age results in a higher maximum heart rate with exercise.
D. There is an age-related decline in cardiac output.

2.4   A 73-year-old man is evaluated for worsening urinary symptoms at the clinic in which you are the collaborating psychiatrist. Over the past 2 years he has had a progressive increase in nocturia and now gets up three to four times each night to urinate. He has difficulty initiating a urine stream and complains of some dribbling at the end of urination. He has no urge symptoms. He describes his energy as normal and does not complain of any decrease in libido or erectile dysfunction. Three years ago he had a screening prostate-specific antigen test result of 0.2 ng/mL. His body mass index is 24 kg/m². His blood pressure is 125/75 mm Hg. His chart indicates that he has a symmetrically enlarged prostate with no nodules. Muscle strength and bulk are normal. Body hair distribution is normal, and testicular size is normal. His internist has made a presumptive diagnosis of benign prostatic hypertrophy and recommends he begin treatment. What is likely to be the most appropriate initial therapeutic strategy?

A. The patient should begin therapy with a trial of an α-adrenergic blocking agent.
B. The patient should begin therapy with a trial of finasteride.
C. Transurethral resection of the prostate and prostatectomy should be offered.
D. The patient should be offered testosterone supplementation.

2.5   Which of the following statements related to glucose management in older persons is true?

A. Older patients have a tendency toward hypoglycemia.
B. Circulating insulin levels in older patients are low.
C. Changes in body composition associated with aging increase the risk of hyperglycemia.
D. Physical activity levels do not have an impact on blood sugar.

2.6   A 97-year-old woman collapses while outside sweeping the leaves off her front steps on an afternoon in July. The event is witnessed by a neighbor who calls 911. The woman is taken to the emergency department, where she is found to be significantly dehydrated. Which of the following represents age-related changes that may have predisposed her to volume loss?

A. The kidneys are more responsive to antidiuretic hormone (ADH) with age.
B. Impaired thirst prevents drinking adequate amounts of water to correct free water losses.

C. Increased aldosterone activity and decreased natriuretic hormone activity inhibit sodium conservation and restoration of normal volume.

D. Basal ADH levels are decreased in older individuals.

2.7 A 75-year-old woman is admitted to the hospital with a diagnosis of community-acquired pneumonia. She has a past medical history that is remarkable for osteoporosis, and she is now 2 inches shorter than she was at her peak height. She lives a sedentary lifestyle and prior to this admission rarely exercised. Which of the following age-related changes in respiratory function may have predisposed her to developing a severe pulmonary infection?

A. Low carbon dioxide levels fail to provide the same stimulus to breathing as is seen in younger patients.

B. Decreased ability to generate a strong cough increases the risk of lower lung infection.

C. Decreased residual volume is common in older patients.

D. Exercise can prevent the eventual age-related decline in pulmonary function.

2.8 A 72-year-old woman presents to her primary care provider with symptoms of urinary incontinence. She describes several recent episodes of having experienced a sudden urge to urinate but not being able to make it to the bathroom in time to avoid an episode of incontinence. She denies any problems with incontinence that are triggered by coughing or sneezing. She would rather not take medication but will follow whatever advice she is given. Which of the following represents the most appropriate initial management strategy for this patient's symptoms?

A. Her symptoms are best treated with an α-adrenergic blocking agent.

B. Her symptoms are best treated by frequent voluntary voiding and bladder retraining.

C. Her symptoms are best treated with an anticholinergic medication such as tolterodine.

D. Her symptoms are best treated with oral estrogen.

2.9 An 85-year-old woman has experienced two falls in the past month. She is at your office today for her regularly scheduled psychotherapy session. She lives in her own home, and although she is independent in caring for herself, she has an adult daughter who lives nearby and checks on her frequently. She says that neither fall resulted in injury, and this assessment is confirmed by her daughter, who brought her mother in for today's appointment. The patient is a pleasant, well-groomed woman who attributes these events to slipping on a loose throw rug on one occasion and rushing to answer the phone and losing her balance on the other. She has full recollection of the events surrounding these falls. Her medical history is remarkable only for hypertension, for which she has taken enalapril 5 mg/day for many years. On examination she is in no distress. Her blood pressure is 130/80 and no orthostatic changes are noted. The rest of her examination is relatively unremarkable, but when you ask her to get out of the chair to assess mobility and balance, you notice that she braces herself on the arms of the chair, and it takes more than 30 seconds for her to rise from the chair, walk 10 feet, turn around, return, and be seated. Her daughter asks, "Are there any interventions that might be helpful in decreasing the risk of future falls?" Which of the following is most correct with regard to fall prevention for this patient?

A. Her antihypertensive medication should be discontinued immediately.
B. Physical therapy to improve balance and gait would be an appropriate management strategy.
C. The patient should be encouraged to wear hip protectors.
D. Although vitamin D supplementation may reduce the risk of falls in institutionalized older individuals, it has not been shown to have any benefit in ambulatory persons such as this woman.

2.10   A 71-year-old woman comes to an outpatient geriatric clinic to establish primary care for herself. Her history includes diabetes mellitus, hypertension, and depression; she takes metformin, enalapril, and escitalopram to manage these conditions. For the past year she has required assistance with shopping and food preparation. Her daughter assists her with these tasks, does her housekeeping, and also helps her mother get showered and dressed daily. Which one of the following aspects of the patient's care would be considered an instrumental activity of daily living (IADL)?

A. Bathing.
B. Dressing.
C. Managing finances.
D. Toileting.

2.11   An 87-year-old woman with multiple geriatric syndromes, including incontinence and frequent falls, is admitted to inpatient care with a diagnosis of syncope. Admission to a geriatric evaluation and management unit would be expected to provide which of the following benefits?

A. Geriatric evaluation and management units are associated with positive effects on functional status.
B. Geriatric evaluation and management units provide cost savings as opposed to usual care.
C. Patients cared for on geriatric evaluation and management units have decreased morbidity, including decreased likelihood of developing malnutrition or pressure ulcers during the course of inpatient admission.
D. Patients cared for on geriatric evaluation and management units have decreased mortality as compared with patients receiving usual care.

2.12   An 87-year-old woman with advanced dementia is brought to your office for evaluation. She has been living in a skilled nursing facility for 3 years and was admitted with a diagnosis of major neurocognitive disorder due to Alzheimer's disease. She has been brought to this appointment by her son, who is visiting from out of state. He is distressed that she did not recognize her grandson when they visited her over the weekend, and he wants to know what can be done to improve his mother's memory. On examination the patient appears to be a pleasant woman in no distress. Although she is clean and well dressed, you notice that her clothes appear to be loose and hang off her. You attempt to administer a Mini-Mental State Examination (MMSE), but she declines to finish, telling you after a few questions that it's "too hard." You have access to her nursing home records, and there are records of two MMSE exams in the past year, on which she scored 15 and 10, respectively. When you compare the weight that was recorded 6 months ago in the nursing home with the weight recorded in your office today, you see that she has lost 10 pounds. The records also indicate that she walked to all activities when she was first admitted to the facility, but over the past few months she has used a wheelchair almost exclusively. During this same time period she has become incontinent of bowel and bladder and wears diapers to manage this condition. The records suggest that although she is confused, she is compliant with care, and there have been no documented episodes of agitation or other outbursts. With regard to medications for the treatment of her dementia, which of the following is most correct?

A. An acetylcholinesterase inhibitor such as donepezil would significantly improve this patient's cognition.
B. On the basis of this patient's history, the addition of an atypical antipsychotic such as risperidone should be considered at this time.
C. The addition of oxybutynin to the patient's medication regimen is recommended because it would help to improve her incontinence symptoms and is associated with improvements in cognition.
D. Acetylcholinesterase inhibitors such as donepezil have shown some effectiveness in patients with mild to moderate Alzheimer's disease, but the overall effects of these drugs may be modest.

2.13 A 76-year-old man comes to his clinic appointment asking for a testosterone prescription. When you ask him what led to this request, he says that he saw an advertisement on television for treatment of "low T" and thinks it might help him with his sexual performance. He denies any loss of libido but says he has had occasional erectile dysfunction. His chart indicates that on his last physical examination he had no obvious loss of body hair and testicular size was not reduced. Which of the following is true regarding testosterone and older men?

A. Testosterone deficiency is commonly found in men with erectile dysfunction.
B. Decreases in testosterone levels are universally seen in older men.
C. Testosterone replacement provides only minimal benefits in older men but is also generally safe, with no significant associated adverse events.
D. Declining testosterone levels are thought to have less effect on sexual function than do chronic medical or psychiatric illness, vascular disease, neuropathy, or medications.

2.14 An 89-year-old female nursing home resident falls after getting up in the middle of the night to urinate. She does not report the fall, but in the morning she awakens with severe pain in her right hip. She is transferred to acute care for evaluation, and on X ray is found to have a nondisplaced fracture of the right femoral neck. Which factor may have increased her risk of fracture?

A. High peak bone density can contribute to bone loss.
B. Lack of estrogen after menopause can lead to loss of bone mass.
C. Secondary hypoparathyroidism can contribute to bone loss.
D. Engaging in daily exercise may lead to an increase risk for bone breakdown.

2.15 Which of the following is characteristic of the effects of aging on pharmacokinetics and must be taken into account when prescribing drugs to older patients?

A. There is a significant age-related effect on drug absorption related to both lower absorption due to decreases in acid secretion, gastrointestinal perfusion, and membrane transport and decreases in gastrointestinal transit time.
B. The decreases in lean body mass and total body water that occur with aging result in a smaller volume of distribution.
C. The decrease in renal mass that commonly occurs with aging is associated with an increase in the glomerular filtration rate.
D. The elimination half-life of commonly prescribed drugs such as aspirin and calcium channel blockers is decreased, so dosages must be adjusted upward.

CHAPTER 3

Genomics in Geriatric Psychiatry

Select the single best response for each question.

3.1 Which of the following is an example of change resulting in variation of chromosome structure?

A. Base pair.
B. Phenotype.
C. Penetrance.
D. Insertion.

3.2 Located on chromosome 21, a mutation in which of the following genes is most associated with early-onset Alzheimer's disease (EOAD)?

A. Presenilin 1.
B. Presenilin 2.
C. Amyloid precursor protein.
D. Apolipoprotein ε4.

3.3 Mutation in the amyloid precursor protein (APP) gene increases risk of EOAD by which of the following mechanisms?

A. Increased γ-secretase activity.
B. Notch protein.
C. Increased β-secretase activity.
D. Apolipoprotein ε4 (*APOE*E4*).

3.4 Mutations in which of the following genes account for most familial EOAD cases?

A. *APP.*
B. *PSEN1.*
C. *PSEN2.*
D. *APOE*E4.*

3.5   A 66-year-old woman seeks genetic counseling after her 87-year-old father who has Alzheimer's disease (AD) was recently enrolled in a research study. She asks about her own risk of developing dementia after genetic testing reveals she has the *APOE*E4* allele. On the basis of the pattern of inheritance, which of the following is most likely to be the impact on her level of risk of developing AD?

A. 100% chance of developing AD.
B. Three- to fourfold increase in risk of developing AD.
C. 5%–10% increase in risk of developing AD.
D. 75% chance of developing AD.

3.6   The addition of *APOE*E4* testing to a clinical dementia assessment has which impact on a diagnosis of Alzheimer's disease?

A. Decreases specificity.
B. Increases sensitivity.
C. Increases false-positive rate.
D. Increases specificity.

3.7   The risk of late-onset Alzheimer's disease (LOAD) associated with the effect of *APOE*E4* is highest in which of the following groups?

A. Hispanics.
B. African Americans.
C. Caucasians.
D. Japanese.

3.8   Mutations in which of the following genes account for most frontotemporal dementia (FTD) cases?

A. *C9orf72*.
B. *TDP-43*.
C. *FUS*.
D. *CHMP2B*.

3.9   Mutations in which of the following genes is more likely to be associated with early-onset parkinsonism?

A. *SNCA*.
B. *LRRK2*.
C. *PINK1*.
D. *VPS35*.

3.10   Autosomal dominant Parkinson's disease (PD) is strongly associated with mutations in which of the following genes?

A. *LRRK2*.
B. *PARK2*.

C. *PINK1.*

D. *DJ1/PARK7.*

3.11 Point mutations and multiplications in which of the following genes cause cognitive/psychiatric symptoms and parkinsonism with widespread α-synuclein pathology?

A. *LRRK2.*

B. *PARK2.*

C. *SNCA.*

D. *PINK1.*

3.12 Which of the following is defined as the proportion of individuals with the mutation who exhibit clinical symptoms?

A. Penetrance.

B. Allele.

C. Phenotype.

D. Genotype.

3.13 Which of the following pairs of psychiatric disorders demonstrates a high degree of shared genotypes?

A. Schizophrenia and bipolar disorders.

B. Bipolar disorders and major depressive disorder.

C. Schizophrenia and major depressive disorder.

D. Schizophrenia and autism spectrum disorder.

3.14 A 22-year-old man with velocardiofacial syndrome develops paranoid delusions and auditory hallucinations over the course of 1 year. He has no history of substance use. Genetic testing would reveal a deletion at which of the following chromosomes?

A. Chromosome 22.

B. Chromosome 1.

C. Chromosome 3.

D. Chromosome 15.

3.15 Which of the following genes has been linked to a combination of schizophrenia, autism spectrum disorders, intellectual disability, and seizure disorder?

A. *NRXN1.*

B. *VIPR2.*

C. *DISC1.*

D. *CACNA1C.*

CHAPTER 4

The Psychiatric Interview of Older Adults

Select the single best response for each question.

4.1 Accurate genetic information can best be obtained by which of the following procedures?

A. A complete medical history.
B. A careful mental status examination.
C. A review of the patient's responses to various types of medications.
D. Interviews with family members from more than one generation.
E. A Structured Clinical Interview for DSM-IV.

4.2 Which of the following intangible supports of patients may be less important to the older patient?

A. The perception of a dependable network.
B. A sense of usefulness.
C. A sense of belonging to a network.
D. Intimacy with network members.
E. Participation or interaction in a network.

4.3 In a study by Sanford, what was the behavior least tolerated by the families of older persons?

A. Incontinence of urine.
B. Sleep disturbance.
C. Falls.
D. Physically aggressive behavior.
E. Personality conflicts.

4.4 Which of the following is the most accurate test of abstract thinking?

    A. Interpretation of a well-known proverb.
    B. The ability to perform five serial subtractions of 7 from 100.
    C. Classifying objects in a common category.
    D. Naming objects from a category.
    E. Asking the patient to repeat a series of numbers.

4.5 In assessing a patient's function and change of function, what are the most important parameters to assess?

    A. The patient's family history.
    B. Past history of symptoms and episodes.
    C. Social functioning and activities of daily living.
    D. Episodes of trauma in the past.
    E. Past response to specific medications.

4.6 When taking a medication history, older persons are generally forthcoming when asked about which of the following?

    A. Their alcohol drinking habits.
    B. Their use of substances other than alcohol.
    C. Nonprescription use of prescription drugs.
    D. Potential drug-drug interactions.
    E. The negative impact of over-the-counter medications.

4.7 Which of the following is a way to distinguish anxiety from agitation?

    A. Agitated patients typically pace, whereas anxious patients do not.
    B. Agitated patients usually display psychomotor retardation, whereas anxious patients usually do not.
    C. Anxious patients are often in a stuporous state, whereas agitated patients are usually violent.
    D. Anxious patients usually experience hallucinations, whereas hallucinations are rare in agitated patients.
    E. Agitated patients usually do not complain of a sense of impending doom or dread, whereas anxious patients may have these complaints.

4.8 Which of the following techniques would show the appropriate respect for an older patient?

    A. Addressing the patient by his or her given name.
    B. Addressing the patient by his or her surname.
    C. Speaking rapidly to the patient during the initial interview.
    D. Maintaining a distance from the patient greater than an arm's length.
    E. Ensuring that there are no periods of silence during the interview.

4.9 Which assessment tool is used to evaluate the presence of tardive dyskinesia in elderly patients?

A. Older Americans Resources and Services (OARS) Multidimensional Functional Assessment Questionnaire.
B. World Health Organization Disability Assessment Schedule 2.0 (WHODAS 2.0).
C. Geriatric Mental State Schedule.
D. Abnormal Involuntary Movement Scale (AIMS).
E. Diagnostic Interview Schedule for DSM-IV (DIS-IV).

4.10 What name is given to a patient's experiences of disvalued changes in states of being and social function?

A. Diseases.
B. Illnesses.
C. Diagnoses.
D. Symptoms.
E. Syndromes.

4.11 Which of the following statements is true regarding disturbances in thought content?

A. Older depressed patients are more likely to have delusions than are middle-aged adults.
B. After recovery from a depression, elderly persons rarely have a recurrence of delusional thoughts.
C. Older persons appear more likely to experience delusional remorse.
D. Older persons appear more likely to experience delusional guilt.
E. Older persons appear more likely to experience delusional persecution.

4.12 Older adults with a neurocognitive disorder may exhibit circumstantiality. Which of the following is the best definition of circumstantiality?

A. The intrusion of thoughts from previous conversations into a current conversation.
B. The lack of logical connections between thoughts.
C. The introduction of many apparently irrelevant details to cover a lack of clarity and memory problems.
D. False sensory perceptions not associated with real or external stimuli.
E. The irresistible intrusion of thoughts into the conscious mind.

4.13 Which of the following statements regarding suicide in the elderly is true?

A. Thoughts of death are common in late life, but spontaneous revelations of suicidal thoughts are rare.
B. Spontaneous revelations of suicidal thoughts are common in late life.

C. The clinician should never ask if there are implements for a suicide attempt because such a question may provoke suicidal thoughts.

D. It is never wise to inquire about the way in which a patient might attempt suicide.

E. Suicidal ideation in an older adult is not usually a cause for concern.

4.14 Immediate recall can be tested by which of the following methods?

A. Asking the patient to name the day, month, date, and year.

B. Asking the patient to subtract 7 from 100 and to repeat this operation on the succession of remainders.

C. Asking the patient to interpret a well-known proverb.

D. Requesting that the patient spell a word backward.

E. Asking the patient to classify objects in a common category.

4.15 Which of the following is the most frequently used structured interview instrument in the United States?

A. Diagnostic Interview Schedule for DSM-IV (DIS-IV).

B. Older Americans Resources and Services (OARS) Multidimensional Functional Assessment Questionnaire.

C. Structured Clinical Interview for DSM-IV (SCID-IV).

D. Geriatric Mental State Schedule.

E. Mini-Mental State Examination.

CHAPTER 5

Use of the Laboratory in the Diagnostic Workup of Older Adults

Select the single best response for each question.

5.1   What hematologic change is associated with lithium treatment?

   A. Leukocytosis.
   B. Leukopenia.
   C. Thrombocytopenia.
   D. Agranulocytosis.

5.2   When treating elderly depressed patients with selective serotonin reuptake inhibitors, which electrolyte disturbance can result in neurological dysfunction secondary to cerebral edema?

   A. Potassium.
   B. Calcium.
   C. Sodium.
   D. Magnesium.

5.3   The 2004 American Diabetes Association guidelines for screening and monitoring of patients taking second-generation antipsychotics recommends fasting lipid profile at baseline and at what frequency thereafter?

   A. At 12 weeks and annually.
   B. At 12 weeks and every 5 years.
   C. Every 4 weeks for 12 weeks, then quarterly.
   D. Annually.

5.4   A 65-year-old male with cognitive impairment screens positive for syphilis with the Venereal Disease Research Laboratory test. In order to distinguish true-positive results from false-positive results, what laboratory test should be performed?

A. Cerebrospinal fluid (CSF) reagin test.
B. Microhemagglutination assay for *Treponema pallidum.*
C. Rapid plasmin reagin test.
D. Blood reagin test.

5.5   What is the most frequently used screening test for thyroid disease in the elderly?

A. Thyroid-stimulating hormone (TSH).
B. Thyroxine (T_4).
C. Triiodothyronine (T_3).
D. TSH, T_3, and T_4.

5.6   A patient is found to have a high TSH level. On follow-up exam, his free T_4 and T_3 are normal. What diagnosis is suggested by these findings?

A. Euthyroid state.
B. Primary hypothyroidism.
C. Hyperthyroidism.
D. Subclinical hypothyroidism.

5.7   A 78-year-old woman is sent to the emergency department to be evaluated for a urinary tract infection (UTI). She is told that her urine sample is likely contaminated and she will need to provide the staff with a repeat sample. A urine sample containing which of the following is suggestive of contamination?

A. Red blood cells.
B. Epithelial cells.
C. White blood cells.
D. Bacteria.

5.8   Which of the following is a cerebrospinal fluid biomarker that is reduced in patients with Alzheimer's disease (AD) and mild cognitive impairment (MCI) due to AD?

A. Phosphorylated tau (p-tau).
B. Total tau (t-tau).
C. β-Amyloid peptide 1–42.
D. Progranulin (PGRN).

5.9   Which illness is highly specific for elevated plasma levels of TDP-43?

A. Creutzfeldt-Jakob disease (CJD).
B. Parkinson-plus syndromes.
C. Alzheimer's disease (AD).
D. Frontotemporal lobar degeneration (FTLD).

5.10 Testing for which biomarker is recommended by the American Academy of Neurology for confirming or rejecting the diagnosis of Creutzfeldt-Jakob disease (CJD) in clinically appropriate circumstances?

A. TDP-43 assay.
B. Progranulin (PGRN).
C. 14-3-3 protein assay.
D. β-Amyloid peptide 1–42.

5.11 Tricyclic antidepressant use in the elderly has the potential to cause which of these cardiovascular effects?

A. Shortened PR and QRS intervals.
B. Atrioventricular block.
C. Decreased QT intervals.
D. Sinoatrial block.

5.12 Which neuroimaging method can differentiate between acute and chronic infarcts?

A. Diffusion-weighted imaging (DWI).
B. Computed tomography (CT).
C. Magnetic resonance imaging (MRI).
D. Plain film radiograph.

5.13 When the clinical diagnosis is unclear, which imaging technique can be useful to distinguish Alzheimer's disease (AD) from frontotemporal dementia (FTD)?

A. MRI.
B. ^{18}Fluorodeoxyglucose positron emission tomography (FDG-PET).
C. Diffusion-weighted imaging (DWI).
D. Computed tomography (CT).

5.14 A 56-year-old man presents with a rapidly progressive dementia, leading to memory loss and hallucinations. The treatment team suspects Creutzfeldt-Jakob disease (CJD), and an electroencephalogram (EEG) is requested. What EEG pattern would you expect if CJD is the correct diagnosis?

A. Periodic sharp-wave complexes.
B. Slowing of the normal background activity.
C. Slowing of the posterior dominant rhythm.
D. Increased generalized slow-wave activity.

5.15 Which omics technology examines proteins, including posttranslational modifications such as phosphorylation, ubiquination, and glycosylation?

A. Epigenomics.
B. Metabolomics.

C. Transcriptomics.
D. Proteomics.

CHAPTER 6

Neuropsychological Assessment of Late-Life Cognitive Disorders

Select the single best response for each question.

6.1   Which of the following is true regarding neuropsychological testing?

   A. It is useful only in detecting moderate to severe cognitive impairment.
   B. It does not help differentiate among cognitive disorders.
   C. It is sensitive but not reliable in diagnosing cognitive disorders.
   D. It can be useful in establishing baseline cognitive function and monitoring treatment response.

6.2   Which of the following is a neuropsychological test commonly used to assess orientation and global mental status?

   A. Wechsler Adult Intelligence Scale, 4th Edition (WAIS-IV).
   B. Mini-Mental State Examination.
   C. Trail Making Test.
   D. Boston Naming Test.

6.3   The Wisconsin Card Sorting Test examines which cognitive domain?

   A. Executive function.
   B. Attention/concentration.
   C. Memory.
   D. Visuoperception.

6.4   Which neuropsychological test is used to assess visuoperception?

   A. Grooved Pegboard.
   B. Judgment of Line Orientation Test.

C. Minnesota Multiphasic Personality Inventory—2.

D. Color Trail Making Test.

6.5   Which of the following cognitive changes is typical of normal aging?

A. Deficits in cued recall.

B. Deficits in delayed recognition.

C. Decreased speed and efficiency of information processing.

D. Significant impairment in visuospatial skills.

6.6   Marked impairment of recent memory with rapid forgetting after a brief delay is characteristic of which neurocognitive disorder?

A. Alzheimer's disease (AD).

B. Huntington's disease.

C. Frontotemporal neurocognitive disorder.

D. Geriatric depression.

6.7   Which of the following cognitive deficit patterns is characteristic of major vascular neurocognitive disorder?

A. Marked impairment in recent memory with rapid forgetting after brief delays.

B. Fluctuations in alertness and acute confusional state.

C. Prominent personality or behavior change.

D. Multifocal "patchy" impairments.

6.8   Which neurocognitive disorder is often characterized by behavioral disinhibition or apathy with early loss of insight?

A. Alzheimer's disease (AD).

B. Major vascular neurocognitive disorder.

C. Frontotemporal lobar degeneration (FTLD).

D. Major neurocognitive disorder with Lewy bodies.

6.9   Frontotemporal lobar degeneration (FTLD) is marked by pronounced impairment in which cognitive domain?

A. Attention.

B. Visuoperception.

C. Executive function.

D. Memory.

6.10 Which neurocognitive disorder is characterized by extrapyramidal motor symptoms, visual hallucinations, and fluctuations in cognition and attention?

A. Major neurocognitive disorder with Lewy bodies.

B. Major neurocognitive disorder due to Parkinson's disease.

C. Huntington's disease.

D. Creutzfeldt-Jakob disease (CJD).

6.11 Which of the following best differentiates neurocognitive disorder due to Parkinson's disease and neurocognitive disorder with Lewy bodies?

A. Neuropsychological test results alone.

B. Clinical history and examination.

C. Neuroimaging alone.

D. Cerebrospinal fluid studies.

6.12 Which of the following neurocognitive disorders is characterized by deficits in attention, memory retrieval difficulties that improve with cues, and poor effort on tasks?

A. Alzheimer's disease (AD).

B. Major vascular neurocognitive disorder.

C. Neurocognitive disorder with Lewy bodies.

D. Neurocognitive disorder associated with geriatric depression.

6.13 What percentage of adults ages 65 years and over experience symptoms of depression?

A. 1%–5%.

B. 20%–30%.

C. 50%–60%.

D. More than 80%.

6.14 Cognitive impairment associated with geriatric depression is due to dysfunction in which brain area?

A. Temporal lobe.

B. Parietal lobe.

C. Occipital lobe.

D. Frontal lobe.

6.15 Which of the following neuropsychological testing profiles distinguishes the memory impairment of Alzheimer's disease (AD) from that associated with geriatric depression?

A. Impaired free recall but better preserved recognition memory in depression.

B. Impaired recognition memory in depression.

C. Impaired acquisition in AD.

D. Poor effort on testing in AD.

CHAPTER 7

Delirium

Select the single best response for each question.

7.1   It has been noted that differentiating dementia from delirium can be particularly difficult. Which of the following is a key diagnostic feature that aids in differentiating these two conditions?

  A. An acute and rapid onset.
  B. Laboratory tests that are pathognomonic for delirium.
  C. No alterations in attention.
  D. There is no need to differentiate the two conditions.

7.2   What is the recommended use of neuroimaging in evaluating a patient with delirium?

  A. All patients presenting with delirium should get a head computed tomography (CT) or magnetic resonance imaging (MRI) scan.
  B. Neuroimaging is recommended for the evaluation of chronic focal neurological symptoms.
  C. Neuroimaging is recommended if there is suspected or evident trauma or injury.
  D. Neuroimaging is recommended for the routine evaluation of fever.

7.3   What is the most frequently considered pathophysiological mechanism of delirium?

  A. Cholinergic dysfunction.
  B. Release of tumor necrosis factor (TNF-α).
  C. Genetic factors such as toll-like receptor 4.
  D. Hypercapnia.

7.4   Which medication or drug class poses the greatest risk for causing or precipitating delirium in older adults?

  A. Sedative-hypnotic drugs.
  B. Narcotics.

C. Anticholinergic drugs.

D. St. John's wort.

7.5 In a general medicine service, which predisposing factor poses the greatest relative risk for delirium?

A. Alcohol abuse.

B. Dementia.

C. Vision impairment.

D. Older age.

7.6 What were the clinical highlights of using haloperidol versus placebo in a randomized controlled trial of 457 noncardiac surgery patients by Wang et al. (2012)?

A. Decreased length of hospital stay.

B. Decreased incidence of delirium.

C. Fewer postoperative complications.

D. Decreased mortality.

7.7 According to the Beers Criteria, which of the following drugs should be avoided in the treatment of delirium?

A. Rivastigmine.

B. Olanzapine.

C. Haloperidol.

D. Sedative-hypnotics.

7.8 Which of the following is the most effective for alleviating symptoms associated with delirium?

A. Rivastigmine.

B. Olanzapine.

C. Primary prevention.

D. Haloperidol.

7.9 What is the first-line treatment of delirium?

A. Nonpharmacological approaches.

B. Physical restraints.

C. Normalization of sleep-wake cycle.

D. Pharmacological management.

7.10 What is the most common cause of delirium?

A. Underlying dementia.

B. Multifactorial causes.

C. Anticholinergic medications.

D. Antihistamines.

7.11 In an intensive care unit, which of the following precipitating factors poses the greatest relative risk for delirium?

A. Elevated serum urea.

B. Metabolic acidosis.

C. Infection.

D. Use of sedative-hypnotics.

7.12 In noncardiac surgical patients, which of the following predisposing factors poses the greatest relative risk for delirium?

A. Older age (≥75 years).

B. History of delirium.

C. Hearing impairment.

D. Dementia.

7.13 What is the clinical setting with the highest incidence of delirium?

A. Geriatric unit.

B. Palliative care setting.

C. Nursing home/postacute care.

D. Intensive care unit (ICU).

7.14 As a clinician, which approach would be most helpful in avoiding the common mistake of not recognizing delirium?

A. Performing a comprehensive psychiatric evaluation and supporting the findings with a Confusion Assessment Method (CAM).

B. Performing a thorough medical evaluation and running a Delirium Observation Screening Scale.

C. Combining insightful clinical judgment with a thorough medical evaluation.

D. Performing a thorough medical and psychiatric evaluation and measuring symptoms with the Delirium Rating Scale.

CHAPTER 8

Dementia and Mild Neurocognitive Disorders

Select the single best response for each question.

8.1 Which of the following is the most common neuropsychiatric symptom in a patient presenting with a diagnosis of Parkinson's disease (PD)?

A. Depression.
B. Sleep fragmentation.
C. Visual hallucinations.
D. Rapid eye movement sleep behavior disorders.

8.2 Which of the following laboratory studies is recommended by the American Academy of Neurology and the National Institute for Health and Care Excellence for the basic workup of a patient with dementia?

A. Electrocardiogram
B. Toxicology.
C. Thyroid function tests.
D. Urinalysis.

8.3 A stepwise progression with variable rates of decline is a hallmark feature in which of the following causes of dementia?

A. Lewy body disorders.
B. Cerebrovascular disease.
C. Alzheimer's disease (AD).
D. Frontotemporal lobar degeneration.

8.4 A 68-year-old man presents with early dementia, fluctuating level of consciousness, parkinsonism, and visual hallucinations. Which of the following is the most likely diagnosis?

A. Dementia due to Alzheimer's disease (AD).

B. Dementia with Lewy bodies (DLB).

C. Dementia due to frontotemporal lobar degeneration.

D. Parkinson disease dementia (PDD).

8.5   Which of the following medications has been approved by the U.S. Food and Drug Administration for the treatment of cognitive symptoms in all stages of Alzheimer's disease (AD)?

A. Memantine.

B. Donepezil.

C. Galantamine.

D. Tacrine.

8.6   Which of the following is an effective treatment modality for Alzheimer's disease (AD)?

A. Antihypertensive medications.

B. Folate.

C. *Ginkgo biloba.*

D. Anti-inflammatory agents.

8.7   Which of the following medications, used for the treatment of cognitive symptoms of Alzheimer's dementia, is the least likely to cause bradycardia as a side effect?

A. Donepezil.

B. Galantamine.

C. Rivastigmine.

D. Memantine.

8.8   Rivastigmine has been approved by the U.S. Food and Drug Administration (FDA) for the treatment of cognitive symptoms of Alzheimer's dementia. In what other condition causing dementia has the FDA approved the use of rivastigmine?

A. Vascular dementia.

B. Frontotemporal lobar degeneration

C. Parkinson's disease dementia (PDD).

D. Dementia with Lewy bodies (DLB).

8.9   What antipsychotic medication is least likely to cause extrapyramidal side effects in a patient with dementia with Lewy bodies (DLB)?

A. Risperidone.

B. Clozapine.

C. Haloperidol.

D. Olanzapine.

8.10   Which of the following behaviors in a patient with dementia is most likely to benefit from the use of antipsychotic medications?

A. Agitation in the context of hallucinations.
B. Nighttime wakefulness and wandering.
C. Refusal of care.
D. Urinating in the trash.

8.11   What agent has shown the best evidence for improving dementia-related apathy?

A. Antidepressants.
B. Antiepileptics.
C. Stimulants.
D. Cholinesterase inhibitors.

CHAPTER 9

Depressive Disorders

Select the single best response for each question.

9.1 Which of the following medications is considered first line of treatment for mild to moderate forms of depression?

A. Bupropion.
B. Trazodone.
C. Citalopram.
D. Nortriptyline.

9.2 Which of the following is the best modality of treatment for an older adult with psychotic depression?

A. Low dose of a stimulant.
B. Electroconvulsive therapy (ECT).
C. Antidepressant only.
D. St. John's wort.

9.3 Which of the following has proven to be the most robust predictor of late-life depression?

A. Religious involvement.
B. Perceived social support.
C. Personality pathology.
D. Cognitive distortions.

9.4 Which one of the following stressors was more related to severe depressive symptoms in older adults in a community survey?

A. Death of a spouse.
B. Physical illness.
C. Divorce.
D. Difficulty with the law.

9.5   Which of the following is a risk factor for the emergence of Alzheimer's disease in a depressed patient?

   A. Frailty.
   B. Poor social support.
   C. Functional limitation.
   D. Mild cognitive impairment.

9.6   Which of the following medications is most associated with agitation in older adults?

   A. Trazodone.
   B. Doxepin.
   C. Bupropion.
   D. Fluoxetine.

9.7   Which of the following is the most common type of delusion in an older adult with a psychotic depression?

   A. Nihilistic delusion.
   B. Delusion of having an incurable disease.
   C. Delusion of grandiosity.
   D. Delusion of guilt.

9.8   Which of the following adverse effects with electroconvulsive therapy is a risk for an older woman with osteoporosis?

   A. Confusion.
   B. Compression fractures.
   C. Hypotension.
   D. Amnesia.

9.9   Which of the following predictors of recovery is considered to predict faster recovery from depression for a community-dwelling patient?

   A. Religious involvement.
   B. Absence of substance abuse.
   C. Current or recent employment.
   D. Absence of major life events and serious medical illness.

9.10   Which of the following tests is not indicated in the workup of a depressed older adult?

   A. Thyroid-stimulating hormone.
   B. Magnetic resonance imaging (MRI).
   C. Vitamin B_{12}.
   D. Biological markers.

CHAPTER 10

Bipolar and Related Disorders

Select the single best response for each question.

10.1 Which of the following episodes must a patient experience to be diagnosed with bipolar I disorder?

A. Both depressed and manic episodes.
B. Depressed episode.
C. Hypomanic episode.
D. Manic episode.

10.2 How does the community prevalence of bipolar disorder in late life compare with the prevalence among younger cohorts?

A. The community prevalence of bipolar disorder in older cohorts is higher than that in younger cohorts.
B. The community prevalence of bipolar disorder in older cohorts is lower than that in younger cohorts.
C. The community prevalence of bipolar disorder in older cohorts is the same as that in younger cohorts.
D. The community prevalence of bipolar disorder in older cohorts has not been studied.

10.3 Which of the following comorbid conditions has been identified as a risk factor for late-life mania?

A. Anxiety disorder.
B. Eating disorder.
C. Neurological illness.
D. Substance abuse.

10.4 Which of the following psychiatric conditions is associated with the highest rate of type II diabetes?

A. Bipolar disorder in older psychiatric inpatients.
B. Bipolar disorder in mixed-age psychiatric inpatients.
C. Schizophrenia in older psychiatric inpatients.
D. Unipolar depression in older psychiatric inpatients.

10.5 When comparing older and younger patients with bipolar disorder, which of the following is more common in younger patients?

A. Dementia.
B. Diabetes.
C. Medical comorbidity.
D. Substance abuse.

10.6 How does the mortality rate for elderly patients with bipolar disorder compare with the mortality rate for elderly patients with unipolar depression?

A. The mortality rate for bipolar disorder is approximately a quarter of the mortality rate for unipolar depression.
B. The mortality rate for bipolar disorder is approximately half of the mortality rate for unipolar depression.
C. The mortality rate for bipolar disorder is approximately the same as the mortality rate for unipolar depression.
D. The mortality rate for bipolar disorder is approximately twice the mortality rate for unipolar depression.

10.7 Which course for bipolar disorder is more frequently experienced in older adults compared with younger adults?

A. Depressive episode followed by a long latency period of 10–20 years before onset of mania.
B. Depressive episode followed by a short latency period of 1–2 years before onset of mania.
C. Manic episode followed by a long latency period of 10–20 years before onset of depression.
D. Manic episode followed by a short latency period of 1–2 years before onset of depression.

10.8 Which cognitive functions are *least* affected by bipolar disorder?

A. Executive function.
B. Language.
C. Processing speed.
D. Verbal memory.

10.9   Which of the following neuroimaging findings has been most consistently associ-
        ated with older patients with bipolar disorder?

        A. Cortical atrophy on head computed tomography.
        B. Hyperintensities on T_2-weighted magnetic resonance imaging (MRI).
        C. Left-sided temporal lobe lesions on neuroimaging.
        D. Smaller cortical sulcal widening on MRI.

10.10   For older patients presenting with new onset of mania, which of the following
        evaluations would be *least* likely to help inform etiology?

        A. Family history.
        B. Laboratory studies.
        C. Medical and neurological examinations.
        D. Review of medications.

10.11   In a trial comparing lithium and valproate for treating late-life mania, how did
        lithium and valproate perform?

        A. Lithium was not well tolerated.
        B. Lithium led to greater reduction in mania scores.
        C. Valproate was not well tolerated.
        D. Valproate led to greater reduction in mania scores.

10.12   An older patient with bipolar disorder who has been maintained on lithium for
        many years presents to the emergency department with symptoms of lithium tox-
        icity and a lithium level of 1.3. Which of the following is the most likely cause of
        the elevated lithium level?

        A. The patient's lisinopril was discontinued.
        B. The patient's naproxen was increased.
        C. The patient's renal clearance increased with age.
        D. The patient's theophylline was increased.

10.13   Which of the following symptoms is associated with commonly reported adverse
        effects of lithium in the elderly?

        A. Cognitive impairment.
        B. New onset of psoriasis.
        C. Urinary retention.
        D. Weight loss.

10.14   Which medication is the most prescribed medication treatment for elderly per-
        sons with bipolar disorder?

        A. Carbamazepine.
        B. Lamotrigine.

C. Lithium.

D. Valproate.

10.15 An older patient will be starting valproate to treat mania. The patient is also on warfarin for atrial fibrillation and lamotrigine for seizure disorder. What should be considered for management of this patient when starting valproate?

A. As patients age, the free fraction of plasma valproate decreases.

B. The lamotrigine dose should be increased.

C. The warfarin dose should be increased.

D. Coagulation parameters should be monitored.

10.16 An elderly Hispanic woman with bipolar disorder has previously tried lithium and valproate with suboptimal response and tolerability. You are considering a trial of carbamazepine. Which laboratory test would not be a crucial part of the workup prior to starting carbamazepine in an older Hispanic woman?

A. Complete blood cell count.

B. Electrolytes.

C. Genetic blood test.

D. Liver enzymes.

10.17 Which of the following anticonvulsants may be associated with fewer cognitive side effects in older bipolar patients?

A. Carbamazepine.

B. Lamotrigine.

C. Topiramate.

D. Valproate.

10.18 When compared with lithium, lamotrigine has been demonstrated to significantly delay the time to intervention for any mood episode. In which type of mood recurrences specifically is lamotrigine most effective?

A. Depressive recurrences.

B. Manic recurrences.

C. Depressive recurrences in patients with depression associated with low cardiometabolic risk factors.

D. Depressive recurrences in patients with high level of manic symptoms.

10.19 Which of the following antidepressants is more likely to induce mania in late life?

A. Amitriptyline.

B. Bupropion.

C. Citalopram.

D. Trazodone.

10.20 Which of the following atypical antipsychotic agents has the most data to support its use in acute bipolar mania in late life?

A. Aripiprazole.
B. Clozapine.
C. Olanzapine.
D. Ziprasidone.

CHAPTER 11

Schizophrenia Spectrum and Other Psychotic Disorders

Select the single best response for each question.

11.1 When Alzheimer's disease (AD) patients with psychosis are compared with those without psychosis, which of the following is most likely to be found?

A. More rapid cognitive decline in those with psychosis.
B. Lower rates of agitation in those with psychosis.
C. A family history of dementia in those with psychosis.
D. A family history of prior psychiatric illness in those with psychosis.

11.2 Which of the following neurocognitive disorders is least likely to be associated with psychotic symptoms?

A. Lewy body dementia.
B. Parkinson's disease.
C. Vascular dementia.
D. Normal pressure hydrocephalus.

11.3 Recommended adjunctive psychosocial treatment for elderly individuals with schizophrenia includes which of the following?

A. Sensory enhancement.
B. Daily structured activities.
C. Cognitive-behavioral social skills training.
D. Social contact.

11.4 Which of the following is a distinguishing factor for late-onset schizophrenia as compared with early-onset illness?

A. Increased likelihood of first-degree relatives with a psychotic spectrum disorder.
B. Greater portion of women affected as compared to men.

C. Higher average antipsychotic dose requirement.

D. Increased severity of positive symptoms including hallucinations and delu-sions.

11.5　In choosing a medication to treat hallucinations due to neurocognitive disorders, why might a provider choose olanzapine over haloperidol?

A. Olanzapine has a U.S. Food and Drug Administration (FDA) indication for psychosis caused by Alzheimer's disease.

B. Olanzapine has a lower risk of extrapyramidal side effects compared with hal-operidol.

C. Olanzapine has a lower risk of mortality compared with treatment with halo-peridol.

D. There is no increased risk of stroke with use of olanzapine.

11.6　Compared with patients with early- or late-onset schizophrenia, patients with very-late-onset schizophrenia-like psychosis (VLOSLP) are characterized by which of the following factors?

A. Increased predominance of negative symptoms.

B. Onset after 50 years of age.

C. Decreased risk of tardive dyskinesia.

D. Decreased early childhood maladjustment.

11.7　A 65-year-old woman with no prior psychiatric history and intact cognitive func-tion develops a delusion that neighbors are poisoning her garden. Which of the following is true about older patients with delusional disorder?

A. There is higher prevalence of illness among men than among women.

B. Average age of onset is between ages 30 and 40 years.

C. Social functioning is typically preserved.

D. There is an increased risk with family history of schizoid personality disorder.

11.8　Current treatment guidelines recommend what treatment as a first-line approach for an 85-year-old woman with major neurocognitive disorder whose family com-plains she is hallucinating and seeing little children in the room?

A. Atypical antipsychotic.

B. Typical antipsychotic.

C. Behavioral intervention.

D. Selective serotonin reuptake inhibitor.

11.9　Which of the following is associated with poorer functional capacity in older pa-tients with schizophrenia?

A. High education level.

B. Positive symptoms.

C. Negative symptoms.

D. Good performance on neuropsychological testing.

11.10 What is the prevalence of schizophrenia among elderly individuals?

A. 0.1%–0.5%.

B. 2.5%.

C. 5.5%.

D. 10.1%.

11.11 The FDA issued a black box warning for elderly patients with dementia treated with antipsychotics because of an increased risk of what compared with those treated with placebo?

A. Death.

B. Metabolic syndrome.

C. Fractures.

D. Aggression.

11.12 Studies have found poorer self-assessed quality of life in persons with schizophrenia to be associated with all but which of the following?

A. Poor social skills.

B. Depression.

C. Lack of negative symptoms.

D. Financial instability.

11.13 Compared with younger adults, how does pharmacotherapy of older adults with chronic psychotic disorders differ?

A. There are no randomized controlled trials conducted in older adults.

B. Maintenance pharmacotherapy should be avoided.

C. Recommended starting and maintenance doses are lower than doses in younger adults.

D. The risk of side effects with antipsychotics is equal in both younger and older adults.

11.14 What makes the use of typical antipsychotics problematic in older adults?

A. There is a higher incidence of tardive dyskinesia in older patients compared with younger patients.

B. Higher dose of medication should be used for treatment.

C. There is a higher incidence of metabolic side effects compared with atypical antipsychotics.

D. They are less efficacious than atypical antipsychotics.

11.15 Which antipsychotic does not have evidence supporting the reduction of tardive dyskinesia in patients with preexisting tardive dyskinesia?

A. Clozapine.
B. Risperidone.
C. Olanzapine.
D. Quetiapine.

CHAPTER 1 2

Anxiety, Obsessive-Compulsive, and Trauma-Related Disorders

Select the single best response for each question.

12.1 Which of the following is a new diagnosis in DSM-5?

A. Posttraumatic stress disorder (PTSD).
B. Hoarding disorder.
C. Obsessive-compulsive disorder (OCD).
D. Panic disorder with agoraphobia.

12.2 What is the prevalence of anxiety disorders in the elderly?

A. The prevalence of late-life anxiety is currently unknown.
B. All of the anxiety disorders are less common in older adults.
C. If present, anxiety disorders are typically comorbid conditions stemming from depression and/or cognitive decline.
D. Anxiety disorders are the most prevalent disorders in older adults.

12.3 Aging may be protective from anxiety, and some reports have noted a decline in the propensity for negative affect from adulthood to "early" elderly years. What is one of the likely explanations for the protective effect of aging?

A. Older adults may be more resilient to stressors because of increased ability to regulate their emotions.
B. Aging may reduce the propensity for anxiety because of degeneration in the hippocampus.
C. The onset of anxiety disorders is in childhood or early adulthood, and symptoms of anxiety disorders rarely persist beyond three to five decades.
D. Many prescription medications used in the elderly reduce anxiety.

12.4 Which anxiety diagnosis is easiest to detect in an older adult?

A. Panic disorder.
B. Specific phobia (e.g., fear of falling).
C. Agoraphobia.
D. Generalized anxiety disorder (GAD).

12.5 Which symptom in older adults is common to all of the most common anxiety disorders and related conditions: specific phobias (including social phobia), panic disorder, obsessive-compulsive disorder (OCD), hoarding disorder, generalized anxiety disorder (GAD), and posttraumatic stress disorder (PTSD)?

A. Situational fear.
B. Situational avoidance.
C. Anticipatory worry.
D. Autonomic arousal.

12.6 A 75-year-old woman goes to her internist for a regular appointment to follow up on management of hypertension and diabetes. She appears preoccupied and keyed up and responds to her doctor's questions about the nature of her preoccupations as worries about her husband, who was just hospitalized for treatment of angina. The woman reveals that she has been having more worries as she has gotten older. Her worrying may occur as often as every day, when there are precipitants such as her family members being ill or her own health problems. She usually tries to occupy herself with either home chores or going out for a walk. Generally, this strategy works well for her. She denies any problems with her functioning and continues to be socially engaged with her friends. She also continues to enjoy her family and hobbies, such as reading and crossword puzzles. What is the most likely condition with which this woman struggles?

A. Panic disorder.
B. Generalized anxiety disorder (GAD).
C. Normal aging.
D. Specific phobia.

12.7 What is the least helpful factor to consider when making a diagnosis of generalized anxiety disorder (GAD) in older adults?

A. The amount of worry.
B. The difficulty the individual has in stopping the worry.
C. The degree of distress or functional impairment related to worrying.
D. The degree to which the worry is realistic versus excessive.

12.8 Which characteristic of the fear of falling has prevented incorporation of this condition into DSM-5?

A. Many older patients lack the insight into the excessiveness of the fear.
B. The individuals affected by the fear of falling do not avoid activities or going out of their home.

C. Fear of falling is uncommon.

D. Fear of falling is not sufficiently impairing.

12.9 The comorbidity of anxiety disorders and related conditions with late-life depression can be described by which of the following characteristics?

A. About a quarter of elderly patients with major depressive disorder (MDD) also have an anxiety disorder or significant anxiety symptoms.

B. Depressive symptoms are more stable than those of anxiety, lasting longer and precipitating anxiety conditions.

C. There is an overlap of symptoms of anxiety disorders and MDD.

D. Elderly patients with depression and anxiety experience greater suicidal ideation but not greater risk of suicide.

12.10 An 86-year-old woman has a 6-year history of generalized anxiety disorder (GAD) as well as a fear of falling. She recently had an increase in intensity of her anxiety symptoms, along with the onset of mild cognitive impairment. What is the most likely explanation of her symptoms?

A. The patient has a separate anxiety disorder that is now co-occurring with either stable mild cognitive impairment or early dementia.

B. The patient likely had a prodromal anxiety disorder (diagnosed as GAD) that manifested before symptoms of dementia were recognized, and anxiety is now exacerbated by the presence of cognitive impairment.

C. All of the patient's anxiety symptoms are a direct result of the patient's age.

D. The patient's mild cognitive impairment is a direct result of years of experiencing anxiety symptoms.

12.11 What is the best approach to treatment of generalized anxiety disorder (GAD) in older adults?

A. An antidepressant, particularly a selective serotonin reuptake inhibitor (SSRI).

B. Psychotherapy, especially cognitive-behavioral therapy (CBT).

C. Combination of benzodiazepine and CBT.

D. Combination of SSRI and CBT.

CHAPTER 13

Somatic Symptom and Related Disorders

Select the single best response for each question.

13.1   Which of the following disorders is no longer classified under somatic symptom and related disorders in DSM-5?

A. Illness anxiety disorder.
B. Factitious disorder.
C. Conversion disorder.
D. Body dysmorphic disorder.

13.2   Which of the following symptoms is unlikely to be associated with somatic symptom and related disorders in older adults?

A. Depression.
B. Delusional thinking.
C. Anxiety.
D. Substance abuse.

13.3   Which of the following features is commonly seen across somatic symptom and related disorders?

A. Reduced pain sensitivity.
B. Absence of functional disability.
C. Excessive fears about health status.
D. Attenuated sensitivity to somatic sensations.

13.4   Which of the following DSM-5 disorders is a more common somatic symptom and related disorder in the elderly?

A. Body dysmorphic disorder.
B. Conversion disorder.

C. Factitious disorder.

D. Unspecified somatic symptom and related disorder.

13.5 A 68-year-old woman with hypertension, type 2 diabetes mellitus, and hyperlip-idemia presents for psychiatric evaluation on referral from the emergency depart-ment, where she has presented six times in the last year because of her concern that she has pancreatic cancer. She reports generalized abdominal discomfort that "comes and goes." A thorough medical workup, including imaging and evalua-tion by a gastroenterologist, is negative. She is anxious and complains of poor sleep due to her concerns about her health. She has no other psychiatric symp-toms or prior history. Which of the following somatic symptom and related dis-orders is the most likely diagnosis?

A. Malingering.

B. Illness anxiety disorder, care-seeking type.

C. Conversion disorder.

D. Delusional disorder.

13.6 Which of the following symptoms is most common in elderly persons with so-matic symptom disorder?

A. Depression.

B. Substance abuse.

C. Insomnia.

D. Pain.

13.7 Which of the following symptoms is more common in younger versus older per-sons with conversion disorder?

A. Pseudoseizures.

B. Paralysis.

C. Swallowing difficulty.

D. Weakness.

13.8 The prevalence of which of the following somatic symptom and related disorders is associated with increased age?

A. Somatic symptom disorder.

B. Illness anxiety disorder.

C. Alexithymia.

D. Dissociative amnesia.

CHAPTER 14

Sexuality and Aging

Select the single best response for each question.

14.1   According to major studies and recent surveys of sexual activity, which of the following accurately describes sexual behaviors in individuals ages 65 years and older?

A. A majority of older men and women continue to be sexually active.
B. The quality of the relationship is the most influential factor for both men and women.
C. Previous level of sexual activity has little influence on late-life sexual activity.
D. Older gay and lesbian individuals report low levels of satisfaction with their sex lives.

14.2   Which of the following accurately describes normal age-related changes in sexual function?

A. In older men, the resolution or refractory stage decreases.
B. Compared with women, sexual changes in aging men occur more gradually and are less predictable.
C. The effects of physiological changes in sexual function are rarely influenced by psychosocial factors.
D. Erections take longer to achieve but are easier to sustain.

14.3   Which of the following best describes the more common sexual dysfunctions seen in late life?

A. Oral erectogenic agents are ineffective in men with psychogenic erectile dysfunction.
B. The physiological cause of female sexual interest/arousal disorder in older women is primarily due to reduced levels of free testosterone.
C. In older women, female orgasmic disorder is often permanent and unresponsive to treatment.
D. Premature (early) ejaculation is most common in younger men and almost always resolves with normal aging.

14.4 Which of the following medications is *least likely* to cause sexual dysfunction in late life?

A. Antidepressants (tricyclic antidepressants, selective serotonin reuptake inhibitors, monoamine oxidase inhibitors).
B. Antiandrogens (e.g., leuprolide, ketoconazole).
C. Mood stabilizers (e.g., lithium, valproic acid, carbamazepine)
D. Phosphodiesterase type 5 inhibitors (e.g., sildenafil, tadalafil)

14.5 A geriatric psychiatry fellow is preparing to provide nursing home staff with education about how dementia affects sexuality. Which of the following is most consistent with current knowledge?

A. Sexual desire in individuals with dementia may remain strong and even increase.
B. The percentage of individuals with dementia who demonstrate sexual aggression or inappropriate sexual behaviors is high.
C. Sexual disinhibition and innocuous behaviors are easy for staff and caregivers to differentiate.
D. In nursing home settings, health care professionals are not required to inquire about ethical issues associated with sexuality and dementia.

14.6 Which of the following is most accurate concerning sexually transmitted diseases (STDs) in people 65 years and older since 2008?

A. Rates of STDs (chlamydia, gonorrhea, syphilis) have significantly increased.
B. Extensive data on STDs have been collected in published surveys about late-life sexuality.
C. With respect to HIV and AIDS, the rates of individuals living with HIV infection have not changed appreciably.
D. Older individuals remain at risk for STDs but may neglect safe sex practices.

14.7 Which of the following is most accurate with regard to sexuality in long-term-care settings?

A. Many residents report the desire for sexual relationships is extinguished.
B. Common barriers to sexual activity in facilities include negative attitudes of staff.
C. Obtaining a sexual history during long-term-care facility intake is often irrelevant.
D. Couples wishing to be intimate must arrange for visits outside the care facility.

14.8   A couple in their early 70s recently started dating. They come for a consultation regarding issues with fear of intimacy. Which of the following best describes current sex therapy treatment models in older adults?

A. Sex therapy is best done conjointly with sexual partners.
B. A psychodynamic model is often more successful than cognitive-behavioral techniques.
C. Sensate focus exercises should be avoided in older, anxious couples.
D. Cognitive distortions toward sexual activity in older adults are often fixed and treatment resistant.

14.9   Which of the following antidepressants is associated with lower rates of sexual dysfunction?

A. Tricyclic antidepressants (TCAs).
B. Venlafaxine.
C. Bupropion.
D. Serotonin selective reuptake inhibitors (SSRIs).

14.10   Which of the following options most accurately describes antipsychotic medications and sexual function in older adults?

A. Higher rates of dysfunction occur with prolactin-sparing agents.
B. All antipsychotics can cause sexual dysfunction, usually in proportion to the dose.
C. Less potent agents with higher anticholinergic effects may cause less dysfunction.
D. Atypical antipsychotics are used to enhance libido and sexual arousal.

C H A P T E R 1 5

Bereavement

Select the single best response for each question.

15.1 Which of the following events that can cause bereavement is the most common and traumatic in late life?

A. Death of spouse.
B. Death of an adult child.
C. Deterioration of one's health.
D. Divorce.

15.2 How does the mortality rate compare for men and women in the first year after a spouse's death?

A. The rate is 2 times less for men than for women.
B. The rate is the same for men as for women.
C. The rate is 2 times greater for men than for women.
D. The rate is 12 times greater for men than for women.

15.3 Which of the following is a significant differentiating factor between grieving and major depression?

A. Problems with sleep.
B. Poor appetite.
C. Feelings of global dejection or complete anhedonia.
D. Attention and concentration problems.

15.4 Which of the following approaches to a loss is found in those individuals having the best psychological outcome from bereavement?

A. Focusing on the individual who died and his or her contributions.
B. Accepting the loss as a part of life.
C. Constructing a meaning in life from the loss.
D. Focusing on finding a balance between loss-oriented stressors and restoration-oriented stressors.

15.5 Which of the following coping strategies is more likely to be used by resilient individuals?

A. Supportive counseling.
B. Religious or faith-based coping.
C. Physical exercise.
D. Medications to maximize sleep.

15.6 Which of the following statements best characterizes chronic or abnormal grief?

A. Individuals with chronic grief display both intrusive symptoms and signs of avoidance and failure to adapt more than a year after the loss.
B. Individuals with chronic grief display episodic symptoms of distress for up to a year after the loss.
C. Individuals with chronic grief display signs of avoidance and failure to adapt for only the first month after the loss.
D. Individuals with chronic grief display both intrusive symptoms and signs of avoidance and failure to adapt within the first 6 months after the loss.

15.7 Cultural differences exist among bereaved individuals in different parts of the world. What pattern best describes Chinese bereavement?

A. Emotional experiences.
B. Spiritual rituals.
C. Cognitive practices.
D. Behavioral rituals.

15.8 Which of the following is true regarding gender differences in bereavement?

A. Widowers are at relatively higher risk of death than widows.
B. Bereavement has a greater impact on depression scores in women than in men.
C. Following the loss of a spouse, men experience more personal growth than women.
D. In the "dual process" model, men are more focused on psychological aspects of coping with the loss, whereas women are more focused on restoring their life pattern without the loved one.

15.9 Of the risk factors for complicated bereavement, which of the following is associated with poor coping with loss 2 years later?

A. Clinically significant depression within the first 2 weeks postloss.
B. Intense negative emotions at 2 months postloss, such as a desire to die and frequent crying.
C. Self-reported depression in the mild range.
D. Spouse died of violent causes.

15.10 Which of the following psychological treatments for complicated grief has been found to be more effective than other form of therapies?

A. Cognitive-behavioral therapy.
B. Supportive therapy.
C. Interpersonal therapy.
D. Waitlist control conditions.

15.11 Which of the following reflects the use of pharmacological interventions in bereavement?

A. Antidepressants should be prescribed to reduce symptoms of grief whether or not the person has symptoms of depression.
B. The empirical literature is equivocal with regard to effectiveness of medication use in uncomplicated grief.
C. Antidepressants, including tricyclic antidepressants (TCAs) and selective serotonin reuptake inhibitors (SSRIs), have not been found to be effective in reducing symptoms of grief that are also present in depression.
D. World Health Organization (WHO) guidelines in management of stress and trauma-related disorders recommend the use of benzodiazepines in the management of bereavement.

15.12 Which of the following is one of the eight developmental levels in the Assimilation of Problematic Experiences Sequence model?

A. Full immersion in the painful situation.
B. Development of heightened awareness of the painful situation.
C. Reduction of understanding/insight.
D. Integration/mastery.

CHAPTER 16

Sleep and Circadian Rhythm Disorders

Select the single best response for each question.

16.1 Which of the following correctly states the prevalence of sleep problems in geriatric patients?

A. Sleep complaints are rarely reported by seniors with Parkinson's disease.
B. More than half of all seniors who live at home report sleep difficulties.
C. Restless legs syndrome (RLS) is reported by less than 10% of patients older than 65 years.
D. Nocturia is reported by less than 50% of seniors as a cause of sleep difficulties.

16.2 Which of the following is true regarding the changes in sleep with aging?

A. Decreased total sleep time, reduced sleep efficiency, and increased awakenings.
B. Increased total sleep time, increased sleep efficiency, and increased awakenings.
C. Decreased total sleep time, increased sleep efficiency, and reduced awakenings.
D. Increased total sleep time, reduced sleep efficiency, and reduced awakenings.

16.3 An 85-year-old man comes to your office with concerns that his family has noticed changes in his sleep pattern. His grandson complains that he goes to bed too early, and his daytime napping worries his daughter. The patient admits that he is more tired than he used to be and he goes to bed and wakes up earlier than in the past. Which statement most adequately addresses the concerns of this patient?

A. The increased likelihood of napping is associated with aging, but the tendency to fall asleep and wake earlier is not.
B. The tendency to fall asleep and wake earlier is associated with aging, but an increased likelihood of napping is not.
C. Aging is not associated with the increased likelihood of napping or the tendency to fall asleep and wake earlier.
D. Aging is associated with an increased likelihood of napping and a tendency to fall asleep and wake up earlier.

16.4   A divorced 78-year-old man comes to your office for an evaluation. He has a medical history significant for obesity, hypertension, coronary artery disease, and diabetes mellitus. The patient complains of excessive daytime sleepiness and foggy thinking. He falls asleep between 10 and 11 P.M. and wakes up between 6 and 7 A.M. What is the most appropriate next step?

A. Obtain a subjective sleep log.
B. Order a brain magnetic resonance imaging (MRI) scan.
C. Start actigraphy.
D. Get a polysomnogram.

16.5   A 68-year-old woman comes to your office reporting sleep difficulties. She notes that when she is falling asleep her legs become very uncomfortable and she has to kick her legs back and forth to relieve the sensation. What is the best next step?

A. Start ropinerole or pramipexole.
B. Check glucose, complete blood count (CBC), and ferritin.
C. Start clonazepam or gabapentin.
D. Get a polysomnogram.

16.6   An 86-year-old patient with moderate Alzheimer's disease (AD) is brought to your office by his family. Concerns are voiced around the patient's going to bed at 7 P.M. and waking up around 2 A.M. The patient needs a significant amount of attention, and the family is having difficulties being up in the middle of the night. The family hopes to keep their loved one at home as long as possible. What would you recommend for managing the patient's sleep?

A. Begin evening bright light therapy.
B. Give evening melatonin.
C. Start a cholinesterase inhibitor.
D. Place the patient in a nursing facility.

16.7   What would you advise to a family practice colleague who has questions about managing the sleep complaints of depressed patients?

A. Treating depressed patients' insomnia will not affect their mood.
B. Improving their sleep will decrease their suicide risk.
C. You can expect an antidepressant to fix patients' insomnia.
D. If the depression has resolved, there is no need to treat insomnia.

16.8   A middle-aged man presents with his wife for consultation. He reports sleeping well, but his wife reports that he "fights" in his sleep and has accidentally injured her in the past. Which condition is he most likely to develop in the next 5 years?

A. Alzheimer's disease.
B. Frontotemporal dementia.
C. Vascular dementia.
D. Parkinson's disease.

16.9   A 52-year-old man presents complaining of sleep difficulties. He notes that he wakes "countless" times a night to urinate and feels that he can never sleep more than an hour or two at a time. His home medications include hydrochlorothiazide, simvastatin, and finasteride. Which of the following recommendations is most appropriate at this time for this patient?

A. Restrict evening fluids.
B. Take diuretics in the afternoon.
C. Restrict alcohol intake to moderate evening consumption.
D. Lower finasteride dose.

16.10 A middle-aged woman with no significant medical conditions reports ongoing sleep difficulties since menopause. She notes that she used to wake in the middle of the night with hot flashes and now continues to wake regularly, but she doesn't know why. She would like a long-term solution to this issue. What would you recommend?

A. Hormone replacement therapy.
B. Low-dose venlafaxine.
C. Cognitive-behavioral therapy.
D. Zolpidem before bedtime.

16.11 A middle-aged woman with a history of degenerative joint disease and diabetes mellitus presents with sleep difficulties that started during perimenopause. She reports that when she gets hot flashes and night sweats, she awakens and cannot get back to sleep. She sleeps well when she is not experiencing vasomotor symptoms. What treatment would you recommend for her sleep complaints?

A. Hormone replacement therapy.
B. Low-dose venlafaxine.
C. Cognitive-behavioral therapy.
D. Zolpidem before bedtime.

16.12 A 71-year-old man comes to your office complaining of difficulties falling asleep, noting that he goes to bed at 10 P.M. but cannot fall asleep until 2 or 3 A.M. He often does not wake up until noon. What is the best step in evaluating this patient?

A. Order a polysomnogram.
B. Order a thorough urologic evaluation.
C. Monitor symptoms with a sleep log and actigraphy.
D. Administer the Multiple Sleep Latency Test.

16.13 An 83-year-old man with hypertension, presbycusis, degenerative joint disease, diabetes mellitus, and cataracts reports difficulty sleeping at night. What is the most likely cause of his insomnia?

A. Unplanned daytime napping.
B. Untreated major depression.

C. Unrecognized sleep apnea.

D. Undiagnosed midbrain lesion.

16.14   Which of the following describes stimulus control to treat insomnia?

A. Using the bed only for sleeping, not napping, and having a routine schedule.

B. Using a sleep log to determine how much time to spend in bed at night.

C. Using relaxation therapies that decrease sleep latency and manage night awakenings.

D. Addressing dysfunctional beliefs and encouraging increased daytime activity.

16.15   Which agent has been found to improve sleep maintenance and decrease early morning awakenings for older adults?

A. Ramelteon.

B. Mirtazapine.

C. Doxepin.

D. Trazodone.

CHAPTER 1 7

Substance-Related and Addictive Disorders

Select the single best response for each question.

17.1   What effect do the physiological changes associated with aging have on the pharmacokinetics of alcohol?

   A. Decreased serum concentration and absorption and increased distribution.
   B. Increased serum concentration and absorption and decreased distribution.
   C. Increased serum concentration, absorption, and distribution.
   D. Decreased serum concentration, absorption, and distribution.

17.2   According to national guidelines, which of the following represents the upper limit of recommended alcohol consumption for adults older than age 65 years?

   A. 1 standard drink per day or 7 standard drinks per week.
   B. 2 standard drinks per day or 14 standard drinks per week.
   C. No more than 3 standard drinks per drinking occasion.
   D. At least 1 standard drink per day for health benefits unless there is a medical comorbidity or past history of alcohol use disorder.

17.3   An elderly individual who consumes 10 standard drinks per week and has no substance-related health, social, or emotional problems would be classified as which of the following?

   A. Low-risk drinker.
   B. Moderate drinker.
   C. Social drinker.
   D. At-risk drinker.

17.4 Which of the following symptoms of substance use disorder is valid for young to middle-aged adults but may be of questionable validity in diagnosing the disorder in later life?

A. Unsuccessful attempts to cut down on use.
B. Cravings or a strong desire to use the substance.
C. Presence of withdrawal.
D. Failure to fulfill major role obligations at work or home.

17.5 Which of the following substances is more likely to be misused by older women than older men?

A. Alcohol.
B. Marijuana.
C. Cocaine.
D. Psychoactive medications.

17.6 Older adults who are moderate drinkers are at increased risk of developing which of the following?

A. Type 2 diabetes mellitus.
B. Hemorrhagic stroke.
C. Cardiovascular disease.
D. Physical limitations.

17.7 Which of the following techniques is considered the gold standard for assessing the frequency and quantity of alcohol use by patients?

A. Prospective diary method.
B. Timeline followback (TLFB) method.
C. Assessing average drinking practices.
D. CAGE questionnaire.

17.8 Among individuals who participated in age-integrated residential treatment, older adults were as likely as middle-aged adults to do which of the following?

A. Contact a sponsor.
B. Self-identify as being a 12-step group member.
C. Engage in 12-step programs.
D. Call a fellow group member for help.

17.9 Which of the following medications has the most evidence to support its use in reducing heavy drinking and craving in older adults with alcohol use disorders?

A. Disulfiram.
B. Naltrexone.
C. Acamprosate.
D. Lorazepam.

17.10 Which of the following symptoms, when present with other withdrawal symptoms, is an indicator of severe alcohol withdrawal?

A. Autonomic hyperactivity.
B. Tremor.
C. Nausea.
D. Hallucinations.

17.11 Which of the following changes in sleep patterns is associated with alcohol use?

A. Decrease in stage 4 sleep.
B. Increase in rapid eye movements (REM).
C. Increased sleep latency.
D. Decrease in stage 3 sleep.

17.12 In the modified version of the CAGE questionnaire, problem drinking in older adults is indicated by a minimum of how many positive responses?

A. One.
B. Two.
C. Three.
D. Four.

17.13 In older adults, what is the minimum score on the Alcohol Use Disorders Identification Test (AUDIT-C) that indicates a positive screen and the need for further evaluation?

A. 1.
B. 3.
C. 5.
D. 10.

17.14 The majority of drugs of abuse will remain detectable in a urine drug screen for a minimum of how many days?

A. 4.
B. 7.
C. 10.
D. 14.

17.15 What is the rate of heavy and binge drinking among adults older than 65 years?

A. 3%.
B. 10%.
C. 15%.
D. 25%.

CHAPTER 18

Personality Disorders

Select the single best response for each question.

18.1 Which of the following is true about personality disorders in the geriatric population?

A. Personality disorders are unlikely to have an effect on comorbid depressive disorders in elderly persons.

B. Because of the high prevalence of chronic medical disorders in this population, functional impairment leads to an increase in the prevalence of personality disorders.

C. Problems related to personality disorders are less frequently a focus in the patients of geriatric psychiatrists than their general psychiatrist colleagues.

D. The prevalence of cluster B personality disorders is higher in the elderly than in the young.

18.2 Which of the following correctly identifies the relationship between the specified personality disorder and aspects of aging?

A. Elderly paranoid patients may improve from forced intimate contact associated with hospital stays and nursing facilities.

B. Narcissistic patients are particularly susceptible to losses associated with retirement and bereavement, which aggravate regulation of self-esteem.

C. Borderline patients continue to have problems with impulsivity and self-harm at high rates as they age, whereas their sense of self becomes more stable over time.

D. Antisocial personality disorder is as prevalent in the elderly as in younger adults.

18.3 Using the five-factor model of personality, nonclinical samples of older persons are more likely to display which of the following traits in comparison with younger persons?

A. Extraversion.

B. Neuroticism.

C. Openness.

D. Conscientiousness.

18.4 An older patient with a personality disorder is likely to display fewer of which of the following diagnostic criteria?

A. Feelings of emptiness.

B. Impaired affect regulation.

C. Intense anger.

D. Breaking the law.

18.5 Which of the following best represents Erikson's stage theory of late development?

A. Older adults develop more mature defense mechanisms than do younger adults.

B. The development of mature defenses has been found to be independent of education and social privilege.

C. Cluster B personality disorders become less severe as people age.

D. The major goal of adjustment to old age is to look back across the lifespan in order to find meaning.

18.6 A well-adjusted elderly person might be expected to make frequent use of which one of these defense mechanisms?

A. Anticipation.

B. Projection.

C. Splitting.

D. Problem-focused coping.

18.7 Patients with frontal lobe syndromes are more likely to show preservation in which of the following domains?

A. Executive function, including planning.

B. Obeying rules of interpersonal social behavior.

C. Memory.

D. Verbal reasoning.

18.8 Which symptom if it appears independently should raise suspicion for organic brain pathology when onset is late in life?

A. Obsessive-compulsive traits.

B. Irritability.

C. Fatigue.

D. Suicidal ideation.

18.9   Which of the following is a core feature of any successful psychotherapy for geriatric patients?

A. Global revision of maladaptive aspects of personality.
B. Empathic and respectful listening.
C. Cognitive restructuring.
D. Behavioral analysis.

18.10   Which of the following is a component of a good pharmacological treatment plan to target symptoms of personality disorder?

A. Use of repeatable self-report assessments.
B. Use of selective serotonin reuptake inhibitors (SSRIs) as first-line treatment.
C. Development of a plan for continued long-term use of the medication.
D. Use of antipsychotics as first-line treatment.

CHAPTER 19

Agitation in Older Adults

Select the single best response for each question.

19.1 You are asked to see a 75-year-old man with a known diagnosis of Alzheimer's disease. The patient has lived in a nursing facility for many years, and staff note that the patient is agitated, intermittently confused, and combative over the course of the night. Nursing notes indicate that this is new behavior for the patient, and staff have never known him to be violent in the past. Which of the following is the most likely underlying diagnosis?

A. Delirium due to a general medical etiology.
B. Change in the patient's routine.
C. Gradual progression of Alzheimer's disease.
D. Change in staffing and in patient's caregiver.

19.2 What is the preferred approach to management of agitation in neurocognitive disorders?

A. Pharmacological approach.
B. Nonpharmacological approach.
C. Relocating the patient to a new, unfamiliar setting.
D. Ignoring agitation because it usually occurs without a distinct reason.

19.3 Which of the following strategies to reduce agitation in older adults should be considered as a first-line approach?

A. Immediately calling social services to investigate the home or nursing facility.
B. Prescribing a high-dose antipsychotic.
C. Assessing patient preferences.
D. Increasing the patient's physical activity throughout the day.

19.4 What is the best approach when trying to communicate with an agitated person with dementia?

A. Do not repeat yourself because it will further agitate the person.
B. Speak loudly if the person is hard of hearing.

C. Make eye contact.

D. Do not ask any questions if you are unsure of the person's meaning because that may agitate him or her further.

19.5 Which of the following is a true statement regarding agitation in frail elderly patients?

A. Agitation occurs only in the context of delirium.

B. Agitation most commonly occurs in the context of delirium superimposed on dementia.

C. Agitation often occurs without a cause.

D. Agitation is never a feature of depression.

19.6 When are benzodiazepines the appropriate treatment for agitation in older adults?

A. Only in the context of suspected delirium.

B. When agitation is the result of hypoxia in patients with chronic obstructive pulmonary disease.

C. In late-life depression.

D. In cases of alcohol withdrawal.

19.7 Management of agitation in the context of delirium should be focused on which of the following interventions?

A. Administration of anticholinergic medications.

B. Ensuring proper use of physical restraints.

C. Identification and treatment of the underlying causes.

D. Administration of psychoactive medication.

19.8 You are called to see a 75-year-old man with Alzheimer's disease who has been verbally abusive and physically violent with hospital staff over the course of the day. He is refusing to take medication orally. The team plans to give the patient intravenous (IV) haloperidol. Which of the following is true regarding IV haloperidol?

A. IV haloperidol is known to cause hypotension.

B. IV haloperidol is associated with significant sedation.

C. IV haloperidol is best used in patients with parkinsonism.

D. IV haloperidol is associated with prolongation of the QT interval.

19.9 You are asked to evaluate a 75-year-old man with cirrhosis who has been confused and agitated with staff in his nursing facility over the course of the night. Medical workup is significant for electrocardiogram with QTc interval of 515 ms and an elevated ammonia level. What treatment should you consider in this case?

A. IV haloperidol.

B. IV lorazepam.

C. Lactulose.

D. Oral clonazepam.

19.10 When evaluating a patient with Alzheimer's disease with acute onset of agitation, what is the first step in the evaluation?

A. Identifying potential precipitants associated with acute onset of agitation.
B. Prescribing opiates because the patient is likely in pain.
C. Prescribing antipsychotics to manage agitation.
D. Prescribing benzodiazepines to ensure sedation.

19.11 Older adults who are receiving carbamazepine for management of agitation should be monitored for which of the following abnormalities?

A. Hypernatremia.
B. Leukocytosis.
C. Hyponatremia.
D. Eosinophilia.

19.12 A 70-year-old woman with Alzheimer's disease living in a nursing home has been intermittently agitated, yelling and cursing at staff over the course of the week. The patient has also been noted to be tearful, lamenting over the infrequency of her family's visits. The consulting psychiatrist's differential diagnosis includes late-life depression. Which of the following medications has been shown to be effective for treating agitation in depressed patients with dementia?

A. Carbamazepine.
B. Citalopram.
C. Trazodone.
D. Valproic acid.

19.13 A family brings their 65-year-old grandmother to the emergency department for evaluation of ongoing agitation in the context of pronounced visual hallucinations over the course of the past 6 months. The family has also noted memory difficulties during this time, and most recently, the patient has been walking very slowly with a slight resting tremor involving her arms. Medical workup is unrevealing, and the consulting psychiatrist suspects a neurocognitive disorder. Which of the following medications can the physician consider for management of agitation in this patient?

A. Rivastigmine.
B. Haloperidol.
C. Quetiapine.
D. Lorazepam.

19.14 Which of the following classes of medications used to treat agitation in older adults has a black box warning regarding increased mortality rates issued by the U.S. Food and Drug Administration (FDA) in 2008?

A. Antidepressants.
B. Mood stabilizers.

C. Benzodiazepines.

D. Antipsychotics.

19.15 A family brings their 70-year-old grandmother with no prior psychiatric history to the emergency department for evaluation of approximately 1 year of verbal agitation that has worsened over the past 2 months. After a thorough medical and psychiatric evaluation, the evaluating physician determines that the patient likely has Alzheimer's dementia and is considering treatment for agitation. Which of the following is important for the physician to consider when deciding on treatment?

A. Pharmacological approaches are always preferred for treatment of agitation in older adults.

B. Antipsychotics are the safest treatments available for agitation.

C. Antipsychotics should be prescribed in high doses when used in agitation in older adults.

D. Antipsychotics should be used at the lowest possible dosages for the shortest possible duration.

CHAPTER 20

Psychopharmacology

Select the single best response for each question.

20.1 Which of the following describes the efficacy data regarding treatment of depression in the elderly?

A. Antidepressants have not demonstrated efficacy for any disorder in this population.
B. No class of antidepressants is considered first-line treatment.
C. Antidepressants have not demonstrated efficacy in the treatment of depression in elderly patients with dementia.
D. Antidepressants work for depressive disorders but not for anxiety disorders.

20.2 Which physiological change in the elderly results in an increase in the elimination half-life of lipid-soluble drugs?

A. Decreases in concentration of plasma albumin.
B. Decreases in hepatic blood flow.
C. Decreases in intestinal blood flow.
D. Decreases in lean body mass.

20.3 Which of the following antidepressants has linear plasma concentrations across the entire dosing range?

A. Sertraline.
B. Fluoxetine.
C. Paroxetine.
D. Fluvoxamine.

20.4 Which of the following medications has the highest potential to cause clinically significant drug-drug interactions secondary to the pharmacokinetic effects on hepatic metabolism?

A. Sertraline.
B. Fluoxetine.

C. Escitalopram.

D. Venlafaxine.

20.5 Which of the following considerations limits the use of medications such as desipramine and nortriptyline in elderly patients?

A. High propensity to cause orthostasis and falls.

B. Effects on cardiac conduction.

C. Inability to use serum levels to monitor dosing.

D. Untreatable impact of bowel function.

20.6 In which of the following conditions should discontinuation of antipsychotics be considered for elderly patients?

A. Schizophrenia.

B. Major depressive disorder with psychosis.

C. Bipolar disorder.

D. Dementia with psychosis.

20.7 Which of the following is correct regarding the use of antipsychotics in the treatment of behavioral and psychological symptoms of dementia?

A. Second-generation antipsychotics have been shown to be significantly more likely to cause mortality compared with first-generation antipsychotics.

B. There is a tenfold increase in the rate of death in older patients treated with atypical antipsychotics compared with placebo.

C. Antipsychotics should be prescribed only to patients who have failed to respond to nonpharmacological interventions or alternative medications.

D. There is a substantially higher rate of falls in patients receiving second-generation antipsychotics compared with first-generation antipsychotics.

20.8 Which of the following antipsychotic medications is considered to be the first-line treatment for agitation in elderly patients with dementia and distressing psychosis or agitation?

A. Olanzapine.

B. Quetiapine.

C. Risperidone.

D. Paliperidone.

20.9 Which of the following issues in an elderly patient would limit the use of paliperidone?

A. There are no data on its use in the elderly.

B. The patient has reduced hepatic function.

C. The patient is receiving a potent CYP2D6 inhibitor.

D. The patient has end-stage renal disease.

20.10 Which of the following antipsychotic medications is often used as a first-line treatment in older patients with Parkinson's disease because of its low propensity to cause extrapyramidal symptoms?

A. Haloperidol.
B. Risperidone.
C. Quetiapine.
D. Olanzapine.

20.11 Aripiprazole treatment for older individuals with dementia is limited by which of the following concerns?

A. Orthostatic hypotension.
B. Lack of efficacy.
C. Akathisia.
D. Anticholinergic effects.

20.12 Which of the following is a limitation to the use of lithium in older patients with bipolar disorder?

A. Lack of efficacy in suicidality.
B. Definitive evidence of adverse renal effects.
C. Changes in pharmacokinetics.
D. Need to reach very high serum lithium levels in order to achieve therapeutic effects.

20.13 Which of the following is a true statement regarding the use of bupropion for treatment of geriatric depression?

A. There is no evidence base to support the safety or efficacy of bupropion in geriatric depression.
B. Expert consensus favors the use of bupropion as a first-line agent in older depressed patients.
C. Bupropion has been reported to be safe and effective in older patients who were partial responders to SSRIs or venlafaxine.
D. Bupropion can be helpful for patients who complain of nausea, diarrhea, unbearable fatigue, or sexual dysfunction during SSRI treatment.

20.14 Which of the following was a finding in the Sequenced Treatment Alternatives to Relieve Depression (STAR*D) study regarding geriatric depression?

A. STAR*D established the safety of combination treatment with mirtazapine and venlafaxine XR in older patients with geriatric depression.
B. The STAR*D trial found that a combination of mirtazapine and venlafaxine XR was less effective than the monoamine oxidase inhibitor (MAOI) tranylcypromine for treatment-resistant depression.
C. Only a few STAR*D participants were elderly.

D. Data from the STAR*D trial suggest that a combination of mirtazapine and venlafaxine is safe but ineffective for treatment-resistant depression.

20.15 Which of the following is a true statement regarding the use of trazodone in geriatric patients?

A. Trazodone has no role in the treatment of agitation or aggression in patients with dementia.
B. Trazodone is more efficacious than placebo in the treatment of sleep disturbances of patients with Alzheimer's disease.
C. Adverse effects of trazodone are not dose-dependent.
D. At doses typically used to treat insomnia, trazodone may cause dry mouth, orthostatic hypotension, and QT prolongation.

20.16 Which of the following is the most evidence-based indication for use of psychostimulants in geriatric patients?

A. Treatment of depression in medically burdened elders.
B. Adjunctive treatment for negative symptoms of schizophrenia.
C. Treatment of apathy and fatigue in patients taking SSRIs.
D. Treatment augmentation for depressed patients taking SSRIs.

20.17 Which of the following statements correctly reflects drug-drug interactions among the mood stabilizers?

A. Valproate decreases lamotrigine concentration.
B. Carbamazepine doubles lamotrigine concentrations.
C. Oxcarbazepine is more likely to be involved in drug interactions than carbamazepine.
D. Carbamazepine can lower its own concentration.

CHAPTER 21

Electroconvulsive Therapy and Other Forms of Brain Stimulation

Select the single best response for each question.

21.1 Which of the following is a true statement regarding the effectiveness of electroconvulsive therapy (ECT) in the treatment of psychiatric disorders?

A. ECT is effective in the treatment of melancholic depression, nonmelancholic depression, and unipolar depression but is *not* effective in the treatment of bipolar depression.
B. In the treatment of acute mania, lithium is superior to ECT.
C. There is an abundance of evidence showing that ECT effectively treats rapid-cycling bipolar disorder.
D. Case series suggest that patients with schizoaffective disorder have a more robust response to ECT treatment than do those with schizophrenia.

21.2 You recommend ECT for a 73-year-old woman with treatment-refractory depression. She has concerns about this modality because of stories she heard about "shock treatment" in the past. Which of the following would be an accurate statement about ECT treatment for someone in her age group?

A. ECT is more effective in young individuals than in elderly individuals.
B. ECT is at least as effective in elderly individuals as it is in middle-aged individuals.
C. ECT prevents recurrence of neuropsychiatric disorders.
D. ECT has a higher mortality rate than treatment with tricyclic antidepressants.

21.3 Which of the following is a factor at the time of treatment that can worsen the cognitive side effects of ECT?

A. Using bifrontal instead of bitemporal electrode placement.
B. Stopping lithium while undergoing treatment.

C. The presence of basal ganglia disease.

D. The presence of pseudodementia.

21.4 What is the only absolute contraindication to the use of ECT?

A. Unstable angina.

B. Unstable bone fractures.

C. Hyperkalemia.

D. There are no absolute contraindications.

21.5 Why is an anticholinergic medication, such as glycopyrrolate or atropine, administered before anesthesia during ECT treatment?

A. To prevent seizure-related tachycardia and hypertension.

B. To counteract the increased sympathetic effects of agents such as dexmedetomidine.

C. To counter the anticonvulsant properties of certain anesthetics.

D. To minimize the risk of stimulus-related asystole.

21.6 What must an anesthesiologist consider when administering medications and monitoring an older adult during ECT treatment?

A. Because of altered metabolism or tolerance, older adults often need higher doses of medications than younger patients.

B. Time to effect may be longer in elderly patients.

C. Individuals with osteoporosis should be given less succinylcholine.

D. Haloperidol should be avoided in the treatment of postictal delirium or agitation.

21.7 Which type of stimulus electrode placement during ECT is associated with the least number of cognitive side effects?

A. Unilateral nondominant.

B. Bitemporal.

C. Bifrontal.

D. Cognitive side effects have been found to be equivalent among the three major types of stimulus electrode placement.

21.8 Which of the following statements is true regarding seizures induced during ECT?

A. It is easier to determine the quality of a seizure in geriatric patients.

B. ECT-induced seizures are identical to complex partial seizures in terms of electroencephalogram (EEG) findings.

C. The higher seizure threshold in older adults increases the risk of their being unable to receive a stimulus of sufficient intensity during ECT.

D. In unilateral ECT, there is no difference in therapeutic effect between a barely suprathreshold seizure and a moderately suprathreshold of the same duration.

21.9 What is the most commonly recommended frequency and duration of ECT treatments in the United States?

A. Two times per week, between 4 and 8 treatments.
B. Two times per week, between 8 and 16 treatments.
C. Three times per week, between 3 and 9 treatments.
D. Three times per week, between 6 and 12 treatments.

21.10 Which of the following is a true statement regarding pharmacotherapy after an initial treatment of ECT?

A. Studies of maintenance pharmacotherapy after ECT treatment for major depression suggest that antidepressants should be augmented with a mood stabilizer.
B. A randomized trial showed that maintenance ECT is superior to maintenance pharmacological treatment with nortriptyline and lithium.
C. Initial ECT treatment typically eliminates preexisting resistance to antidepressants used prior to the initiation of ECT treatment.
D. Several studies of maintenance pharmacotherapy after ECT treatment for mania or schizophrenia suggest avoiding aggressive treatment with medications from different classes.

21.11 Which of the following is a true statement regarding the use of repetitive transcranial magnetic stimulation (rTMS) in geriatric patients?

A. Elderly patients have shown a higher incidence of cognitive side effects.
B. The difficult side effects of rTMS cause more than a third of patients to discontinue treatment before completion.
C. Cortical atrophy in geriatric patients limits magnetic stimulation of deep brain structures.
D. rTMS is not associated with increased potential for seizure induction.

21.12 Which of the following is a reason why transcranial direct current stimulation (tDCS) may be a promising treatment for the geriatric population?

A. Multiple tDCS studies in the geriatric population have shown efficacy in the treatment of major depression.
B. Like rTMS, tDCS has shown specific benefits in the treatment of depression with psychosis and severe suicidal ideation.
C. tDCS provides a noninvasive method of stimulating neuronal excitation in cortical tissue, which is relatively well tolerated by patients.
D. tDCS is not associated with any adverse effects related to its administration.

21.13 Direct stimulation of which of the following targets has been approved by the FDA as an invasive treatment for refractory major depression?

A. Vagus nerve.
B. Nucleus accumbens.

C. Ventral striatum.

D. Brodmann area 25.

21.14 Which of the following is an accurate statement regarding deep brain stimulation (DBS) in the treatment of chronic refractory depression?

A. DBS has not been shown to increase the risk of seizures.

B. DBS has not been shown to negatively affect cognitive functioning.

C. DBS targets various deep brain structures but does not target cortical areas.

D. DBS has not been effective for treating depression in patients with Parkinson's disease.

CHAPTER 2 2

Nutrition and Physical Activity

Select the single best response for each question.

22.1 An 84-year-old woman with diabetes is brought in by her family for concerns of weight loss, weakness, and confusion. Which of the following dietary factors is least likely contributing to her current symptoms?

A. Negative energy balance from chronic inadequate food intake.
B. Decreased fluid intake due to the diminished thirst response.
C. A 20-year history of drinking 3 ounces of red wine nightly with dinner.
D. Poor glycemic control due to noncompliance with diabetic dietary restrictions.

22.2 Which of the following aspects of the diet is associated with a reduced risk of cognitive decline, stroke, and depression?

A. High intake of monounsaturated fats.
B. High intake of saturated fats.
C. Low intake of polyunsaturated fats.
D. Consumption of a Western-style diet.

22.3 Which of the following is true regarding nutritional status and cognitive function?

A. Reduced dietary folate intake is not associated with the development of dementia.
B. Excessive vitamin B_{12} intake has been associated with dementia.
C. Vitamin D plays a role in cognitive function.
D. High plasma antioxidant levels are associated with cognitive impairment.

22.4 Which of the following outcomes is *not* associated with adherence to a Mediterranean diet?

A. Lower rates of vascular diseases.
B. Increased risk of depression.

C. Decreased risk of stroke.

D. Decreased risk of cognitive impairment.

22.5   What is the mechanism by which moderate alcohol intake helps in the preservation of cognitive function?

A. It increases generation of thromboxane A_2.

B. It increases white matter lesions.

C. It increases prostacyclin concentrations.

D. It increases platelet function.

22.6   Which of the following is true regarding physical activity and cognition?

A. Physical activity has been associated with decreased white matter integrity.

B. Physical activity has been associated with higher Mini-Mental State Examination scores.

C. Aerobic exercise has been associated with improved cognitive speed but not auditory and visual attention.

D. Physical activity does not affect brain volume.

22.7   Which statement is accurate regarding physical activity in healthy older adults?

A. Low to moderate physical activity is associated with a reduced risk of cognitive decline in older adults compared with sedentary individuals.

B. Vigorous, but not moderate, activity is associated prospectively with fewer depressive symptoms.

C. Living in a less walkable neighborhood is not associated with depressive symptoms.

D. Physical activity does not influence quality of life.

22.8   Which of the following is accurate regarding nutritional screening methods?

A. The Subjective Global Assessment (SGA) detects nutritional deficiencies in patients who are overweight at baseline.

B. The patient's body weight is the most important clinical measure of undernutrition.

C. The Mini Nutritional Assessment (MNA) is superior to other instruments in detecting nutritional deficiencies in patients who are overweight at baseline.

D. Serum albumin should be checked frequently in protein repletion.

22.9   What is the recommendation regarding physical activity for older adults?

A. At least 150 minutes per week of moderate-intensity aerobic exercise is recommended.

B. When older adults are physically unable to complete 150 minutes of moderate-intensity physical activity, they should not be physically active.

C. To promote and maintain health, older adults should be physically active once a week.

D. Vigorous-intensity physical activity is not recommended for older adults.

22.10 Which of the following is a true statement regarding the nutritional status of older adults?

A. Serum albumin increases slightly with age.

B. Dietary intake is affected when older adults eat in social settings versus eating alone.

C. Risk of compromised nutritional status is reduced by residing in an assisted living facility.

D. Serum albumin is recommended as the sole marker of nutritional status.

22.11 Which of the following is a true statement regarding weight and nutritional status in older adults?

A. Unintentional weight loss is associated with increased mortality.

B. Vitamin D deficiency is not common in older adults.

C. Weight loss of 5% of usual body weight in 180 days should trigger activating protocols for clinical assessment.

D. Nutritional status should not affect ability to taste or smell.

22.12 Which of the following is a true statement regarding the use of psychotropic medications in older adults?

A. Considering a patient's nutritional status is not necessary prior to starting the psychotropic.

B. Use of multiple medications is infrequent in elderly individuals.

C. The potential for drug-food interactions should be assessed.

D. Alcohol consumption does not have a bearing on the medication used.

22.13 Which of the following is true regarding vitamins?

A. Pyridoxine (B_6) deficiency causes depression.

B. Prolonged cobalamin (B_{12}) deficiency causes reversible neurological damage.

C. L-Methylfolate has been used as an adjunctive therapy for selective serotonin reuptake inhibitor (SSRI) resistant depression.

D. Vitamin D does not help reduce risk of fractures.

22.14 Which of the following nutrients is known to promote vascular disease?

A. Monounsaturated fat.

B. Polyunsaturated fats.

C. Trans-unsaturated fat.

D. Moderate alcohol intake.

22.15 Which of the following statements is true regarding depression in the elderly?

A. Corticotrophin-releasing factor (CRF) is known to be elevated in depressed individuals.
B. The antidepressant effect of aerobic exercise is less than that of antidepressant medications.
C. Corticotrophin-releasing factor can be used as an appetite stimulant for depressed patients.
D. Tricyclic antidepressants are often associated with weight loss.

22.16 Which of the following is true regarding the dietary intake of nutrients for older adults?

A. Total daily energy expenditures increase with age.
B. Older adults need less dietary protein than younger adults.
C. The recommended daily water intake for healthy older adults is 1.5 L (six glasses) of water a day.
D. The recommended dietary fiber intake for older adults is 15 grams, the same as younger adults.

CHAPTER 23

Individual and Group Psychotherapy

Select the single best response for each question.

23.1 Cognitive-behavioral therapy (CBT) for people with moderate to severe cognitive impairment focuses on which of the following?

A. Challenging assumptions of being a burden to family.
B. Helping to generate realistic assessment of the risk of falls.
C. Incorporating caregivers into the therapeutic process.
D. Adapting to the environment.

23.2 Which of the following is true about problem-solving therapy (PST)?

A. It comprises 4–10 sessions.
B. The therapist "assigns" problems to the patient to solve.
C. The dropout rate from PST is higher than from other interventions.
D. Sessions must be conducted in person.

23.3 Which of the following is true regarding psychotherapy with older adults?

A. Psychotherapy can be beneficial for people who cannot tolerate the side effects of medication.
B. Older patients are more likely than their younger counterparts to go to a therapist's office rather than see a therapist in a primary care setting.
C. Older adults are more concerned about stigma than are younger adults.
D. Older adults are less particular about the race, ethnicity, and culture of their therapists than are their younger counterparts.

23.4 Which of the following is the most studied psychotherapy modality for depression in older adults?

A. Psychodynamic psychotherapy.
B. Interpersonal therapy.

C. Cognitive-behavioral therapy (CBT).

D. Problem-solving therapy.

23.5 Which of the following is true regarding substance abuse in older adults?

A. Rates of illicit drug use have not changed since 2002.

B. Prescription medications and alcohol are the most commonly abused substances.

C. Well-established treatment protocols exist for treating substance abuse in late life.

D. Older adults should always be treated alongside younger people in addiction programs.

23.6 Cognitive reappraisal is the ability to reflect on and revise previously held beliefs. Which of the following is true regarding cognitive reappraisal?

A. Cognitive reappraisal is unrelated to executive functioning.

B. Cognitive reappraisal is not a part of CBT.

C. People with even minimal diminution in cognitive reappraisal are not appropriate candidates for psychotherapy.

D. Cognitive reappraisal requires patients to attend to their thoughts, hold them in working memory, generate alternative thoughts, and then implement these alternative thoughts.

23.7 What is the most commonly diagnosed anxiety disorder in older adults?

A. Substance/medication-induced anxiety disorder.

B. Agoraphobia.

C. Generalized anxiety disorder.

D. Panic disorder.

23.8 Which of the following is true regarding relaxation training in older adults?

A. Relaxation training should be taught in the patient's home, where he or she is most relaxed.

B. Relaxation training can be helpful for treating mild anxiety.

C. Relaxation training takes months to show efficacy.

D. Efficacy is achieved relatively rapidly, but gains are not maintained.

23.9 Which of the following is true regarding comorbid personality disorders and depressive disorders in older persons?

A. Rates of personality disorders are lower in older adults with depression than in the general population of older adults.

B. Older adults with depression and personality disorders are less likely to have depressive symptoms recur than are those with depression alone.

C. Studies have shown that selective serotonin reuptake inhibitors (SSRIs) alone are the best treatment for older adults with personality disorders and depression.

D. Modified dialectical-behavioral therapy (DBT) has been shown to be effective in treating comorbid personality disorders and depressive disorders in older adults.

23.10 Which of the following is *not* a common psychological problem addressed through interpersonal therapy (IPT) for depression?

A. Loss and grief.
B. Interpersonal disputes and conflicts.
C. Role transitions.
D. Insomnia and hypersomnia.

23.11 What percentage of older adults who might benefit from psychotherapy actually receives treatment?

A. 1%.
B. 10%.
C. 25%.
D. 50%.

23.12 Which of the following is true about reminiscence psychotherapy?

A. It takes place between one patient and one therapist.
B. There is no evidence that it has any therapeutic efficacy.
C. It is less effective than CBT.
D. It draws on a patient's personal memories and life experiences with the goal of improving self-esteem and developing a sense of social cohesiveness.

23.13 Which of the following is true regarding cognitive-behavioral therapy (CBT) for anxiety disorders in older persons?

A. It does not help patients who cannot distinguish between medical and psychiatric symptoms.
B. It includes repeated exposure to feared stimuli.
C. It has been proven ineffective.
D. It is less effective than medication management.

23.14 Which of the following is true regarding acceptance and commitment therapy (ACT)?

A. It aims to increase a patient's acceptance of unwanted thoughts or experiences.
B. It aims to teach patients to commit to a strategy of avoiding unwanted thoughts and experiences.
C. It consistently has higher dropout rates than more traditional therapies.
D. It targets the frequency and intensity of anxiety symptoms.

23.15 What is the prevalence rate of personality disorders in the overall population of older adults?

    A. Less than 5%.
    B. Between 5% and 10%.
    C. Between 10% and 20%.
    D. Between 25% and 30%.

C H A P T E R   2 4

Working With Families of Older Adults

Select the single best response for each question.

24.1   What percentage of older adults with moderate to severe dementia live alone, using extensive supervision and assistance from local and long-distance family caregivers?

    A. 10%.
    B. 30%.
    C. 5%.
    D. 50%.

24.2   Psychiatrists working collaboratively with social workers or nurses can help provide timely or sustained assistance for families. Which of the following specific interventions has been shown to delay nursing home placement by more than a year?

    A. Treating substance-related or anxiety disorders in caregivers.
    B. Closely monitoring for abuse, exploitation, or neglect of patients.
    C. Providing individual and family counseling for spouse caregivers.
    D. Providing care management and monitoring the family's capacity and tolerance.

24.3   Which of the following strategies may be helpful in adequately assessing, counseling, and treating dementia patients and their families in the office setting?

    A. Patients with dementia should not be interviewed without a family member present.
    B. Family caregivers should be allowed to talk privately with the psychiatrist to avoid having to confront the older adult about his or her symptoms and declining condition.

C. Only one family member should accompany the patient to the visit because having too many family members during the evaluation may be confusing to the patient.

D. To avoid confronting doubt or denial initially, the clinician might suggest to caregivers that they not worry about Alzheimer's disease until a diagnosis has been confirmed.

24.4 When providing information and education for older spouses who are caregivers, which of the following principles should be kept in mind?

A. Older spouses in first marriages are generally more comfortable facing threatening health information together rather than apart.

B. They do not appreciate the psychiatrist asking about what else is going on in their lives because they may see this as unrelated to the care of their loved one.

C. Subtle or vague suggestions that they need to take care of themselves can help families who are overwhelmed by caregiving responsibilities.

D. When dealing with a combative patient, asking the family about guns in the house early on may be interpreted as an invasion of privacy.

24.5 Which of the following is true in assessing family caregivers of older adults with dementia?

A. Family caregivers who report being frustrated, overwhelmed, edgy, or exhausted will acknowledge having depression and anxiety.

B. Older husband caregivers may be particularly at risk of increased alcohol use in response to care demands.

C. Poor nutrition should prompt a suggestion to have all meals at home in order to adequately meet the patient's nutritional needs.

D. If the family belongs to an ethnic minority group, the psychiatrist should monitor for legal protections or fully sanctioned empowerment to make care decisions.

24.6 Which intervention is most effective for families of older adults?

A. Unimodal strategies concentrating resources on family counseling.

B. Didactic educational approaches.

C. Participation in support groups.

D. Problem-solving and/or active participatory skill-building strategies.

24.7 Which of the following is the most common symptom reported by caregivers of patients with Alzheimer's disease?

A. Fatigue.

B. Irritability.

C. Anxiety.

D. Insomnia.

24.8   When considering educational strategies for families, what should be done during the initial evaluation?

A. Offer as much information regarding diagnosis and treatment as possible.
B. Talk about potential problems in the future, such as psychosis.
C. Provide the family with a complete list of suggestions and referrals.
D. Avoid overwhelming families with too many treatment suggestions or too much information.

24.9   When working with dementia patients and their families, which of the following general principles is not accurate?

A. Denial is a common defense of family caregivers.
B. Overutilization of services and overreporting of burden occur frequently.
C. Successful family caregivers are flexible in adjusting expectations of themselves, the older adult, and other family members.
D. A primary caregiver at home is generally preferred.

24.10 Which one of the following is not a correct key message for family caregivers?

A. Be willing to listen to the older adult and know that it will get easier.
B. It is tempting for distant relatives to second-guess or criticize.
C. The older adult is not unhappy or upset because of what you have done.
D. Considering what is best for your family involves compromise among competing needs, loyalties, and commitments.

CHAPTER 25

Clinical Psychiatry in the Nursing Home

Select the single best response for each question.

25.1 Which of the following is true regarding nursing home admission in patients with dementia?

A. Performance of activities of daily living (ADLs) does not have an impact on nursing home admission.
B. Disturbances of behavior are among the most common reasons for nursing home admission.
C. Dementia with Lewy bodies is highly prevalent among nursing home populations.
D. Depression is the most common psychiatric diagnosis among nursing home residents.

25.2 Which of the following has *not* been shown to be associated with depression among nursing home residents?

A. Diabetes.
B. Increase in pain complaints.
C. Risk of delirium.
D. Unchanged nutritional status.

25.3 Which of the following has been associated with poor antidepressant treatment response in nursing home residents?

A. Absence of cognitive impairment.
B. Depressive symptoms associated with vascular risk factors and executive dysfunction.
C. Preserved self-care abilities.
D. High serum levels of albumin.

25.4 Which of the following nonpharmacological interventions emphasizes a multi-component psychosocial approach?

A. Snoezelen rooms.
B. Namaste Care.
C. VA Community Living Centers program.
D. Standardized nonpharmacological interventions.

25.5 Which of the following is an institutional and systemic factor associated with physical restraint use?

A. Insufficient staffing.
B. Agitation and behavior problems.
C. Presence of monitoring or treatment devices.
D. Need to promote body alignment.

25.6 Which of the following best describes the purpose of a second-stage assessment at the time of admission to a nursing home?

A. To evaluate the patient for dementia.
B. To provide acute psychiatric treatment after admission to a nursing home rather than a psychiatric facility.
C. To make a specific psychiatric diagnosis.
D. To allow for appropriate admission to nursing homes of patients who have a severe psychiatric disorder.

25.7 Which of the following is true regarding the surveyor guidelines based on the Centers of Medicare and Medicaid Services regulations related to quality of care?

A. The guidelines address psychotropic medication use only.
B. The guidelines have not been updated since original publication.
C. The guidelines do not address the provision of care for residents with mental health problems.
D. The guidelines address upper limits for daily dosages and acceptable indications for medications.

25.8 Which of the following is true regarding the Nursing Home Quality Initiative?

A. The information is available only to health care providers.
B. It includes only long-stay quality measures.
C. Antipsychotic medication administration is not addressed.
D. Information is posted on the Medicare.gov Web site.

25.9 Which of the following is true regarding short-stay residents at nursing homes?

A. Addressing their depression and anxiety is not a primary objective of mental health care during their stay.

B. They are more likely than long-term-care patients to have a primary diagnosis of stroke.

C. They are more likely than long-term-care patients to have ambulatory dysfunction.

D. They are less likely than long-term-care patients to be admitted directly from an acute care hospital.

25.10 Which of the following is a component of the intrinsic system of mental health care in nursing homes?

A. Optimizing the ways staff and residents interact.

B. Evaluating the interactions between medical and mental health problems.

C. Establishing psychiatric diagnoses.

D. Administering specific treatments for mental disorders.

Part II

Answer Guide

C H A P T E R   1

Demography and Epidemiology of Psychiatric Disorders in Late Life

1.1   What will the estimated percentage of the U.S. population of persons 65 years and older be by 2050?

A. 5%.
B. 40%.
C. 20%.
D. 15%.

The correct response is option C: 20%.

With the aging of the baby boomer cohort (those born between 1946 and 1964), the size of the elderly population is projected to continue to increase over the next several decades and to reach 72.1 million by the year 2030 and 88.5 million by 2050, accounting for an estimated 20.2% of the population (Federal Interagency Forum on Aging-Related Statistics 2012) (option C; options A, B, and D are incorrect). **(p. 3)**

1.2   What will the projected population be in 2050 of the "oldest old" segment of the United States, persons 85 and older?

A. 5.5 million.
B. 19.0 million.
C. 0.5 million.
D. 10.0 million.

The correct response is option B: 19.0 million.

The number of oldest old, or persons ages 85 years and older, was 5.5 million in 2010 (option A) and is projected to reach 19.0 million by 2050 (option B; options C and D are incorrect) (Federal Interagency Forum on Aging-Related Statistics 2012). **(p. 3)**

1.3   What is the percentage of persons ages 85 years and older who are living in long-term care facilities?

A. 53%.
B. 14%.
C. 5.5%.
D. 87%.

The correct response is option B: 14%.

Among individuals ages 85 years and older, 14% resided in long-term care facilities (Federal Interagency Forum on Aging-Related Statistics 2012) (option B; options A, C, and D are incorrect). Many of these residents are placed in residential care because of psychiatric disorders, especially the behavior problems that result from Alzheimer's disease. **(p. 4)**

1.4   By the year 2050, which of these ethnic minority groups will increase most in total number in the United States?

A. Non-Hispanic black.
B. Asian.
C. Non-Hispanic white.
D. Hispanic.

The correct response is option D: Hispanic.

By 2050, the proportion of non-Hispanic blacks is projected to be 12% (option A), Asians 9% (option B), and Hispanics of any race 20% (option D), whereas the proportion of non-Hispanic whites is expected to decrease to 58% (option C) (Federal Interagency Forum on Aging-Related Statistics 2012). **(p. 4)**

1.5   Which of the following correctly describes the findings related to the lifetime prevalence of major depression in the National Comorbidity Survey Replication (NCS-R) reported by Kessler et al. (2005)?

A. The incidence of major depressive disorder was 10.6% in participants ages 60 years and older.
B. The incidence of major depressive disorder was 40% in participants ages 18–29 years.
C. The incidence of major depressive disorder was less than 10% in participants ages 30–44 years.
D. The incidence of major depressive disorder was 12% in participants ages 45–59 years.

The correct response is option A: The incidence of major depressive disorder was 10.6% in participants ages 60 years and older.

The World Mental Health Survey version of the Composite International Diagnostic Interview was used in the NCS-R, which reported that the lifetime prevalence of major depressive disorder was 10.6% among participants ages 60 years and older compared with 15.4% among those ages 18–29 years, 19.8% among those ages 30–44 years, and 18.8% among those ages 45–59 years (Kessler et al. 2005) (option A; options B, C, and D are incorrect). **(p. 6)**

1.6   Which of the following is the most prevalent psychiatric disorder among persons ages 65 years and older (excluding neurocognitive disorders)?

A. Hypochondriasis.
B. Anxiety disorder.
C. Schizoaffective disorder.
D. Alcohol use disorder.

The correct response is option B: Anxiety disorder.

The National Institute of Mental Health (NIMH) established the ECA program to determine the prevalence of specific psychiatric disorders in both community and institutional populations (Regier et al. 1984). Of persons ages 65 and older, 12.3% (13.6% of the women and 10.5% of the men) met criteria for one or more psychiatric disorders in the month prior to the interview. The two most prevalent disorders in this age group were any anxiety disorder (5.5%) (option B) and severe cognitive impairment (4.9%) (Regier et al. 1988). Hypochondriasis (option A), schizoaffective disorder (option C), and alcohol use disorder (option D) are not as prevalent as the group of anxiety disorders. **(pp. 8, 11, 15; Table 1–5, "Prevalence of selected psychiatric symptoms and disorders among older adults in selected treatment settings," p. 19)**

1.7   Which of these is a common syndrome confounding psychiatric and medical diagnosis in the elderly?

A. Bulimia nervosa.
B. Hypochondriasis.
C. Delusional jealousy.
D. Trichotillomania.

The correct response is option B: Hypochondriasis.

Psychiatric syndromes—rather than discrete disorders—are more realistic as diagnostic entities in geriatric psychiatry. The most common of these syndromes are memory loss, confusion, depression, anxiety, suspiciousness and agitation, sleep disturbance, and hypochondriasis (Blazer 2000) (option B). Bulimia nervosa, delusional jealousy, and trichotillomania are not common syndromes that may confound a psychiatric diagnosis in geriatrics (options A, C, and D). **(p. 7)**

1.8　The Collaborative Psychiatric Epidemiology Surveys (CPES) enabled a better under-standing of the relationship between major depression and which of the following?

A. Immigration status and ethnicity.
B. Medical comorbidity.
C. End of life issues.
D. Alcohol and substance use disorders.

The correct response is option A: Immigration status and ethnicity.

The CPES initiative sponsored by NIMH combined three nationally representative studies that used the same research methods: the National Comorbidity Survey Replication (NCS-R), the National Survey of American Life, and the National Latino and Asian American Study, all conducted in the United States between 2001 and 2003. The CPES provided the opportunity to examine the prevalence of major depression by racial/ethnic group and immigration status (option A) (Heeringa et al. 2004). Medical comorbidity (option B), end of life issues (option C), and alcohol and substance use disorders (option D) were not the focus of CPES. **(p. 9)**

1.9　What was the prevalence of Alzheimer's disease in persons ages 85 years and old-er in the East Boston Established Populations for Epidemiologic Studies of the El-derly (EPESE)?

A. 3%.
B. 47%.
C. 60%.
D. 35%.

The correct response is option B: 47%.

In EPESE, the prevalence of probable Alzheimer's disease increased with age. Specifically, the prevalence was 3.0% in those ages 65–74 years, 18.7% in those ages 75–84 years, and 47.2% in those ages 85 years and older (option B; options A, C, and D are incorrect) (Evans et al. 1989). **(p. 11)**

1.10　Prevalence estimates of depressive symptoms in nursing home residents, using the Minimum Data Set, is closest to which of the following?

A. 10%.
B. 90%.
C. 30%.
D. 50%.

The correct response is option D: 50%.

Data collected using the Minimum Data Set showed the prevalence of mental health conditions in older nursing home residents to be high: depression 49.6% (option D), anxiety disorders 16.1%, bipolar disorder 2.8%, and schizophrenia

3.6% (Eden et al. 2012). The prevalence of major depression in nursing homes or long-term-care facilities is estimated to be 6.0% to over 14.0% (option A), and the prevalence of minor depression is estimated to be as high as 30.5% (option C). No mental health conditions were found with the prevalence of 90% (option B). **(p. 18)**

1.11   Which of the following statements regarding suicide mortality in the U.S. geriatric population is correct?

A. Rates of suicide are equal in males and females.
B. African American men have the highest rates of completed suicide.
C. Men ages 65 years and older have twice the rate of completed suicide than men ages 15–24 years.
D. Asian men have the highest suicide rates in the United States.

The correct response is option C: Men ages 65 years and older have twice the rate of completed suicide than men ages 15–24 years.

Suicide mortality is positively correlated with age. Suicide mortality in the United States in 2010 was almost twice as high for men ages 65 years and older (29.0 per 100,000 men) than for men ages 15–24 years (16.9 per 100,000 men) (option C). Among women, suicide mortality has long been lower than among men (option A). In 2010, the suicide rate was 3.9 per 100,000 women ages 15–24 years versus 4.2 per 100,000 women ages 65 years and older (National Center for Health Statistics 2012). In 2010 in the United States, suicide rates among men ages 65 years and older varied by race and ethnicity: the suicide rate for non-Hispanic white men was 32.7 per 100,000, compared with 8.3 for non-Hispanic black men (option B), 14.9 for Asian men (option D), and 15.7 for Hispanic men. Rates for women ages 65 years and older were 4.7 for non-Hispanic white women, 4.3 for Asian women, and 2.2 for Hispanic women (National Center for Health Statistics 2012). **(p. 20)**

1.12   Since 2000, which group has the steepest increase in completed suicides in the United States?

A. Men ages 85 years and older.
B. Men ages 75–84 years.
C. Men ages 50–59 years.
D. Men ages 65–74 years.

The correct response is option C: Men ages 50–59 years.

Among men, the greatest increases in completed suicide rates were observed among those ages 50–54 years (49.4%, from 20.6 to 30.7) and those ages 55–59 years (47.8%, from 20.3 to 30.0) (option C). Among women, the greatest increase was among those ages 60–64 years (59.7%, from 4.4 to 7.0) (Centers for Disease Control and Prevention (CDC) 2013). The suicide rate among U.S. adults ages 65 years and older was 30.0 per 100,000 in 1950 but decreased to 14.9 per 100,000 in 2010 (options A, B, and D). **(p. 20)**

1.13 Which of the following is true regarding the impact of stressful life events as measured by the Holmes-Rahe Schedule of Recent Events?

A. The impact on mental health is minimal for older adults.
B. The impact is considerable, occurring even with low Holmes-Rahe scores.
C. The relative risk for mental health impairment is >2 for those with moderate scores of 150 or greater.
D. This scale has not been used to study older adults.

The correct response is option C: The relative risk for mental health impairment is >2 for those with moderate scores of 150 or greater.

By far the most frequently investigated environmental factors associated with psychiatric disorders are social factors. Many investigators believe that the changing roles and circumstances of older adults can cause stress and thereby contribute to the onset of psychiatric disorders and cognitive difficulties. In a study of 986 community-dwelling older adults, Blazer (1980) found the crude estimate of relative risk for mental health impairment to be 2.14, given a life event score of 150 or greater on the Schedule of Recent Events (Holmes and Rahe 1967) (option C; options A, B, and D are incorrect). A relative risk of 1.73 ($P<0.01$) was estimated when a binary regression procedure was used, controlling for physical health, economic status, social support, and age. **(p. 22)**

1.14 With what was major depression associated in the Longitudinal Aging Study Amsterdam?

A. Poorer self-perceived health.
B. Increased social network.
C. Married status.
D. External locus of control.

The correct response is option A: Poorer self-perceived health.

In the Longitudinal Aging Study Amsterdam, major depression was associated with unmarried status (option C), functional limitation, perceived loneliness (option B), internal locus of control (option D), poorer self-perceived health (option A), and lack of instrumental social support (Beekman et al. 1995). **(p. 23)**

1.15 When compared with a younger cohort with similar psychopathology, older patients with psychiatric illness may have which of these patterns of mental health community-based treatment?

A. Older patients are more likely to receive treatment in the health care setting.
B. Older patients are less likely to be referred to mental health specialists.
C. Older patients are more likely to perceive a need for mental health care.
D. Older patients receive more specialty mental health referral than younger patients.

The correct response is option B: Older patients are less likely to be referred to mental health specialists.

Klap et al. (2003) reported that older adults who met criteria for a psychiatric disorder were less likely than younger adults to perceive a need for mental health care (option C), to receive specialty mental health care or counseling (option D), and to receive referrals from primary care to mental health specialty care (option B). In the NCS-R, participants ages 60 years and older were less likely than those in younger age groups to receive any mental health treatment in the previous 12 months. Among individuals who received treatment, those ages 60 years and older were less likely to receive treatment in the health care setting (option A), and those older adults who did receive treatment in the health care setting were less likely to receive treatment in a mental health specialty (Wang et al. 2005). **(p. 24)**

References

Beekman ATF, Deeg DJH, van Tilburg T, et al: Major and minor depression in later life: a study of prevalence and risk factors. J Affect Disord 36(1-2):65–75, 1995 8988267

Blazer D: Life events, mental health functioning and the use of health care services by the elderly. Am J Public Health 70(11):1174–1179, 1980 7425190

Blazer DG: Psychiatry and the oldest old. Am J Psychiatry 157(12):1915–1924, 2000 11097951

Centers for Disease Control and Prevention (CDC): Suicide among adults aged 35-64 years—United States, 1999-2010. MMWR Morb Mortal Wkly Rep 62(17):321–325, 2013 23636024

Eden J, Le M, Maslow K, et al: The Mental Health and Substance Use Workforce for Older Adults: In Whose Hands? Washington, DC, National Academies Press, 2012

Evans DA, Funkenstein HH, Albert MS, et al: Prevalence of Alzheimer's disease in a community population of older persons. Higher than previously reported. JAMA 262(18):2551–2556, 1989 2810583

Federal Interagency Forum on Aging-Related Statistics: Older Americans 2012: Key Indicators of Well-Being. Washington, DC, US Government Printing Office, 2012

Heeringa SG, Wagner J, Torres M, et al: Sample designs and sampling methods for the Collaborative Psychiatric Epidemiology Studies (CPES). Int J Methods Psychiatr Res 13(4):221–240, 2004 15719530

Holmes TH, Rahe RH: The social readjustment rating scale. J Psychosom Res 11(2):213–218, 1967

Kessler RC, Berglund P, Demler O, et al: Lifetime prevalence and age-of-onset distributions of DSM-IV disorders in the National Comorbidity Survey Replication. Arch Gen Psychiatry 62(6):593–602, 2005 15939837

Klap R, Unroe KT, Unützer J: Caring for mental illness in the United States: a focus on older adults. Am J Geriatr Psychiatry 11(5):517–524, 2003 14506085

National Center for Health Statistics: Health, United States, 2012: With Special Feature on Emergency Care. Hyattsville, MD, U.S. Government Printing Office, 2012

Regier DA, Myers JK, Kramer M, et al: The NIMH Epidemiologic Catchment Area program. Historical context, major objectives, and study population characteristics. Arch Gen Psychiatry 41(10):934–941, 1984 6089692

Regier DA, Boyd JH, Burke JD Jr, et al: One-month prevalence of mental disorders in the United States. Based on five Epidemiologic Catchment Area sites. Arch Gen Psychiatry 45(11):977–986, 1988 3263101

Wang PS, Lane M, Olfson M, et al: Twelve-month use of mental health services in the United States: results from the National Comorbidity Survey Replication. Arch Gen Psychiatry 62(6):629–640, 2005 15939840

CHAPTER 2

Physiological and Clinical Considerations of Geriatric Patient Care

2.1 Which of the following represents age-related physiological changes in vision?

A. There are decreases in accommodation in older people, which make it difficult to focus on near objects.
B. Older people show a decline in the ability to view objects in motion (dynamic acuity), whereas the ability to view objects at rest (static acuity) remains relatively preserved.
C. The ability to adapt to light often is impaired in older people because of increasing lens transparency.
D. Age-related macular degeneration is a severe, but relatively uncommon, cause of blindness in older people.

The correct response is option A: There are decreases in accommodation in older people, which make it difficult to focus on near objects.

The weakening of the ciliary muscle, combined with decreased curvature of the lens, results in a loss of accommodation; therefore, it becomes difficult for an individual to focus on near objects, and bifocals may be needed (option A). Elderly people show a decline in their ability to view objects at rest (static acuity) and in motion (dynamic acuity) (option B). It is difficult for elderly people to adapt to light because of rigidity of the pupil and increasing size and opacity of the lens (option C). Age-related macular degeneration is the most common cause of blindness in elderly people in the United States (Harvey 2003; Hubschman et al. 2009) (option D). **(p. 35)**

2.2 Which of the following is characteristic of age-related hearing loss?

A. There is loss of high-frequency hearing in older adults, but low-frequency hearing generally is preserved.

B. Thickening of the tympanic membrane and degenerative changes in the ossicles are responsible for significant impairments in hearing.
C. Speech discrimination ability rarely is affected in older adults.
D. Both high- and low-frequency hearing loss are common in older adults.

The correct response is option D: Both high- and low-frequency hearing loss are common in older adults.

Older adults can expect alterations in the ear, which may lead to hearing loss in both high and low frequencies (option D). In the inner ear, cochlear neurons are lost, and changes in the organ of Corti, basilar membrane, stria vascularis, and spiral ligament also affect hearing. The degeneration of the organ of Corti is associated with high-frequency sensorineural hearing loss, whereas atrophy of the stria vascularis may cause hearing loss across all frequencies (option A). In the middle ear, thickening of the tympanic membrane and degenerative changes in the ossicles occur, but these changes have an insignificant effect on function (option B). The stiffening of the basilar membrane and atrophy of the spiral ligament both can result in loss of speech discrimination (Huang and Tang 2010) (option C). **(p. 35)**

2.3   A 65-year-old man presents to your clinic for routine examination. He had a sedentary lifestyle for many years. Now that he has retired, he is interested in taking up a regular exercise program. He asks if there are any concerns he should have related to his heart. He has a history of type 2 diabetes and a 20 pack a year smoking history, but he quit smoking 5 years ago. He wants to know how exercise might affect his heart. Which of the following is typical of age-related changes in the cardiovascular system?

A. The increased β-adrenergic response of the heart seen with aging increases the maximal heart rate attained during exercise.
B. A narrowing of aortic pulse pressure is seen in older adults.
C. Increased β-adrenergic responsiveness seen with age results in a higher maximum heart rate with exercise.
D. There is an age-related decline in cardiac output.

The correct response is option D: There is an age-related decline in cardiac output.

In elderly patients, the β-adrenergic response of the heart during exercise is attenuated; a lower maximum heart rate and decreased force of contraction are the result (option A). With age, human blood vessels stiffen. The vessels are thicker and less distensible. The physiological results are a greater pulse wave velocity, early reflected pulse waves, and higher systolic blood pressures and aortic pulse pressures in older individuals (option B). The β-adrenergic response of the heart during exercise is attenuated with age; a lower maximum heart rate and decreased force of contraction are the result (option C). The older heart dilates during exercise to increase end-diastolic volume and maintain stroke volume, but cardiac output nonetheless declines with age. Because the heart stiffens, it empties less completely. The decline in cardiac output adversely affects oxygen use in older adults (Lakatta 1999) (option D). **(pp. 35–36)**

2.4   A 73-year-old man is evaluated for worsening urinary symptoms at the clinic in which you are the collaborating psychiatrist. Over the past 2 years he has had a progressive increase in nocturia and now gets up three to four times each night to urinate. He has difficulty initiating a urine stream and complains of some dribbling at the end of urination. He has no urge symptoms. He describes his energy as normal and does not complain of any decrease in libido or erectile dysfunction. Three years ago he had a screening prostate-specific antigen test result of 0.2 ng/mL. His body mass index is 24 kg/m^2. His blood pressure is 125/75 mm Hg. His chart indicates that he has a symmetrically enlarged prostate with no nodules. Muscle strength and bulk are normal. Body hair distribution is normal, and testicular size is normal. His internist has made a presumptive diagnosis of benign prostatic hypertrophy and recommends he begin treatment. What is likely to be the most appropriate initial therapeutic strategy?

A. The patient should begin therapy with a trial of an α-adrenergic blocking agent.
B. The patient should begin therapy with a trial of finasteride.
C. Transurethral resection of the prostate and prostatectomy should be offered.
D. The patient should be offered testosterone supplementation.

The correct response is option A: He should begin therapy with a trial of an α-adrenergic blocking agent.

In clinical trials, α-adrenergic blocking agents have been proven most effective for benign prostatic hypertrophy (option A). Finasteride may be useful as a second-line treatment for benign prostatic hypertrophy (option B). Transurethral resection of the prostate and prostatectomy are the available options for cases that fail to respond to medical therapy (option C). The patient's history and examination are not suggestive of androgen deficiency. Testosterone supplementation is not a general recommendation at this time and, in any case, would not be a first-line approach to management (option D). **(pp. 49–50)**

2.5   Which of the following statements related to glucose management in older persons is true?

A. Older patients have a tendency toward hypoglycemia.
B. Circulating insulin levels in older patients are low.
C. Changes in body composition associated with aging increase the risk of hyperglycemia.
D. Physical activity levels do not have an impact on blood sugar.

The correct response is option C: Changes in body composition associated with aging increase the risk of hyperglycemia.

Elderly patients have a tendency toward hyperglycemia (option A). Circulating insulin levels may rise with age but are less efficiently utilized (option B). Although insulin secretion by the pancreatic β cells is preserved with age, insulin clearance declines and insulin levels increase. Elderly individuals have decreased muscle mass and a higher percentage of fat and therefore an increased number of adipocytes. Peripheral uptake of insulin is affected by insulin resistance in peripheral tissues; some of these tissues, particularly adipocytes, have fewer receptors, thereby decreasing their sensitivity to insulin (option C). Reduction in physical activity is one of the factors associated with high rates of type II diabetes in adults ages 65–79 years (option D). **(p. 41)**

2.6 A 97-year-old woman collapses while outside sweeping the leaves off her front steps on an afternoon in July. The event is witnessed by a neighbor who calls 911. The woman is taken to the emergency department, where she is found to be significantly dehydrated. Which of the following represents age-related changes that may have predisposed her to volume loss?

A. The kidneys are more responsive to antidiuretic hormone (ADH) with age.
B. Impaired thirst prevents drinking adequate amounts of water to correct free water losses.
C. Increased aldosterone activity and decreased natriuretic hormone activity inhibit sodium conservation and restoration of normal volume.
D. Basal ADH levels are decreased in older individuals.

The correct response is option B: Impaired thirst prevents drinking adequate amounts of water to correct free water losses.

The kidneys are less responsive to ADH with age (option A), which impairs the kidney's efforts to make more concentrated urine. The impaired thirst mechanism in elderly individuals prevents them from drinking adequate amounts of fluid to correct free water losses (option B), thereby contributing further to dehydration (Gruenewald and Matsumoto 2003; Oskvig 1999; Perry 1999). Aldosterone activity decreases and natriuretic hormone activity increases, both of which inhibit renal conservation of sodium and restoration of normal volume (option C). Basal ADH levels are normal to increased in older individuals; because renal free water clearance decreases with age, hyponatremia can more easily occur. However, when volume loss takes place, with subsequent hypotension, less ADH is released in older individuals (option D). **(p. 38)**

2.7 A 75-year-old woman is admitted to the hospital with a diagnosis of community-acquired pneumonia. She has a past medical history that is remarkable for osteoporosis, and she is now 2 inches shorter than she was at her peak height. She lives a sedentary lifestyle and prior to this admission rarely exercised. Which of the following age-related changes in respiratory function may have predisposed her to developing a severe pulmonary infection?

A. Low carbon dioxide levels fail to provide the same stimulus to breathing as is seen in younger patients.
B. Decreased ability to generate a strong cough increases the risk of lower lung infection.

C. Decreased residual volume is common in older patients.

D. Exercise can prevent the eventual age-related decline in pulmonary function.

The correct response is option B: Decreased ability to generate a strong cough increases the risk of lower lung infection.

Low oxygen tension and high carbon dioxide levels fail to provide the same physiological stimulus to breathe, but the decreased response to hypercapnia is not consistent in all studies (option A). With age, the person's ability to generate a sufficiently strong cough declines. The development of higher closing volumes further complicates defense against infection by making it harder to expel secretions from the lower areas of the lungs (option B). Higher closing volumes make full expansion of the airways more difficult, especially in the dependent areas of the lung (option C). Although exercise is helpful, it cannot prevent the eventual decline in pulmonary function (Schwartz and Kohrt 2003) (option D). **(pp. 36–37)**

2.8   A 72-year-old woman presents to her primary care provider with symptoms of urinary incontinence. She describes several recent episodes of having experienced a sudden urge to urinate but not being able to make it to the bathroom in time to avoid an episode of incontinence. She denies any problems with incontinence that are triggered by coughing or sneezing. She would rather not take medication but will follow whatever advice she is given. Which of the following represents the most appropriate initial management strategy for this patient's symptoms?

A. Her symptoms are best treated with an α-adrenergic blocking agent.

B. Her symptoms are best treated by frequent voluntary voiding and bladder retraining.

C. Her symptoms are best treated with an anticholinergic medication such as tolterodine.

D. Her symptoms are best treated with oral estrogen.

The correct response is option B: Her symptoms are best treated by frequent voluntary voiding and bladder retraining.

Overflow incontinence in men may be addressed with an α-adrenergic blocking agent to treat benign prostatic hypertrophy. This patient is female, and her symptoms are consistent with urge, rather than overflow, incontinence (option A). Urge incontinence is best treated by frequent voluntary voiding and bladder retraining (option B). Patients are placed on a voiding schedule that corresponds to their usual minimal interval of urination. They are taught how to voluntarily inhibit the urge to void. The goal of therapy is to increase gradually the interval between urination. Although medications such as oxybutynin, tolterodine, solifenacin, or imipramine may be helpful, they are best reserved for patients in whom behavioral methods have been unsuccessful (option C). Patients who are given these medications to treat incontinence symptoms should be monitored carefully for anticholinergic side effects. Although oral or topical estrogen therapy may be beneficial in the treatment of stress urinary incontinence, this patient's symptoms are most consistent with urge incontinence (option D). **(p. 49)**

2.9   An 85-year-old woman has experienced two falls in the past month. She is at your office today for her regularly scheduled psychotherapy session. She lives in her own home, and although she is independent in caring for herself, she has an adult daughter who lives nearby and checks on her frequently. She says that neither fall resulted in injury, and this assessment is confirmed by her daughter, who brought her mother in for today's appointment. The patient is a pleasant, well-groomed woman who attributes these events to slipping on a loose throw rug on one occasion and rushing to answer the phone and losing her balance on the other. She has full recollection of the events surrounding these falls. Her medical history is remarkable only for hypertension, for which she has taken enalapril 5 mg/day for many years. On examination she is in no distress. Her blood pressure is 130/80 and no orthostatic changes are noted. The rest of her examination is relatively unremarkable, but when you ask her to get out of the chair to assess mobility and balance, you notice that she braces herself on the arms of the chair, and it takes more than 30 seconds for her to rise from the chair, walk 10 feet, turn around, return, and be seated. Her daughter asks, "Are there any interventions that might be helpful in decreasing the risk of future falls?" Which of the following is most correct with regard to fall prevention for this patient?

A. Her antihypertensive medication should be discontinued immediately.
B. Physical therapy to improve balance and gait would be an appropriate management strategy.
C. The patient should be encouraged to wear hip protectors.
D. Although vitamin D supplementation may reduce the risk of falls in institutionalized older individuals, it has not been shown to have any benefit in ambulatory persons such as this woman.

The correct response is option B: Physical therapy to improve balance and gait would be an appropriate management strategy.

Although some medications predispose patients to falls, this patient has been treated for many years with a stable dose of a blood pressure medication. Given that her blood pressure is well controlled and there are no signs or symptoms of orthostasis on examination, discontinuing her antihypertensive medication would not be the best initial strategy in preventing falls in this patient (option A). Physical therapy to improve balance and gait (option B) would be an appropriate management strategy. This patient took more than 30 seconds to complete the "get up and go" test; a time greater than 20 seconds is abnormal and suggests that more extensive evaluation is needed. Although hip protectors are a protective factor, their primary benefit is in decreasing the risk of hip or pelvic fractures rather than the risk of falls themselves (option C). A meta-analysis of five randomized clinical trials suggested that vitamin D supplementation may reduce the risk of falls in ambulatory or institutionalized older individuals by more than 20% (Bischoff-Ferrari et al. 2004) (option D). **(pp. 47–48, 52)**

2.10 A 71-year-old woman comes to an outpatient geriatric clinic to establish primary care for herself. Her history includes diabetes mellitus, hypertension, and depression; she takes metformin, enalapril, and escitalopram to manage these conditions. For the past year she has required assistance with shopping and food preparation. Her daughter assists her with these tasks, does her housekeeping, and also helps her mother get showered and dressed daily. Which one of the following aspects of the patient's care would be considered an instrumental activity of daily living (IADL)?

A. Bathing.
B. Dressing.
C. Managing finances.
D. Toileting.

The correct response is option C: Managing finances.

Bathing (option A), dressing (option B), and toileting (option D) are each considered an activity of daily living (ADL). Managing finances (option C) is an IADL. Other examples of IADLs include driving, shopping, cooking, housekeeping, and using the telephone. **(p. 52)**

2.11 An 87-year-old woman with multiple geriatric syndromes, including incontinence and frequent falls, is admitted to inpatient care with a diagnosis of syncope. Admission to a geriatric evaluation and management unit would be expected to provide which of the following benefits?

A. Geriatric evaluation and management units are associated with positive effects on functional status.
B. Geriatric evaluation and management units provide cost savings as opposed to usual care.
C. Patients cared for on geriatric evaluation and management units have decreased morbidity, including decreased likelihood of developing malnutrition or pressure ulcers during the course of inpatient admission.
D. Patients cared for on geriatric evaluation and management units have decreased mortality as compared with patients receiving usual care.

The correct response is option A: Geriatric evaluation and management units are associated with positive effects on functional status.

A multi-institutional randomized controlled trial of geriatric evaluation and management units in the Veterans Affairs Health Care System showed a positive effect on functional status (Cohen et al. 2002) (option A). In this trial, overall costs were equivalent to those for usual care (option B), and there was no effect on morbidity (option C) or mortality (option D) (Cohen et al. 2002). **(pp. 52–53)**

2.12 An 87-year-old woman with advanced dementia is brought to your office for evaluation. She has been living in a skilled nursing facility for 3 years and was admitted with a diagnosis of major neurocognitive disorder due to Alzheimer's disease. She has been brought to this appointment by her son, who is visiting from out of state. He is distressed that she did not recognize her grandson when they visited her over the weekend, and he wants to know what can be done to improve his mother's memory. On examination the patient appears to be a pleasant woman in no distress. Although she is clean and well dressed, you notice that her clothes appear to be loose and hang off her. You attempt to administer a Mini-Mental State Examination (MMSE), but she declines to finish, telling you after a few questions that it's "too hard." You have access to her nursing home records, and there are records of two MMSE exams in the past year, on which she scored 15 and 10, respectively. When you compare the weight that was recorded 6 months ago in the nursing home with the weight recorded in your office today, you see that she has lost 10 pounds. The records also indicate that she walked to all activities when she was first admitted to the facility, but over the past few months she has used a wheelchair almost exclusively. During this same time period she has become incontinent of bowel and bladder and wears diapers to manage this condition. The records suggest that although she is confused, she is compliant with care, and there have been no documented episodes of agitation or other outbursts. With regard to medications for the treatment of her dementia, which of the following is most correct?

A. An acetylcholinesterase inhibitor such as donepezil would significantly improve this patient's cognition.
B. On the basis of this patient's history, the addition of an atypical antipsychotic such as risperidone should be considered at this time.
C. The addition of oxybutynin to the patient's medication regimen is recommended because it would help to improve her incontinence symptoms and is associated with improvements in cognition.
D. Acetylcholinesterase inhibitors such as donepezil have shown some effectiveness in patients with mild to moderate Alzheimer's disease, but the overall effects of these drugs may be modest.

The correct response is option D: Acetylcholinesterase inhibitors such as donepezil have shown some effectiveness in patients with mild to moderate Alzheimer's disease, but the overall effects of these drugs may be modest.

Although acetylcholinesterase inhibitors, such as donepezil, galantamine, and rivastigmine, have been shown to have some effectiveness in patients with mild to moderate Alzheimer's disease, their overall effects may be modest (Raina et al. 2008). This patient's history suggests a more advanced stage of disease, for which these drugs would not likely lead to significant improvement in cognition (option A). Because agitation may be a prevalent symptom for patients with dementia, particularly in patients with late disease, this symptom also may require treatment; atypical antipsychotic agents such as risperidone may be helpful in this context (Defilippi and Crismon 2000; Tune 2001). However, the U.S. Food and Drug Administration has issued black box warnings regarding the use of antipsychotics in treating patients with dementia-related psychosis (U.S. Food and Drug Administration 2008). Both conventional and atypical antipsychotics carry increased mortality risk in dementia. Although this patient's history is consistent with advanced dementia, there is no suggestion of agitation, and the addition of an antipsychotic to her regimen would not be appropriate (option B). Although oxybutynin may be used to help treat urge incontinence symptoms, it is an anticholinergic medication and would be more likely to worsen, rather than improve, cognitive dysfunction (option C). Acetylcholinesterase inhibitors, including donepezil, galantamine, and rivastigmine, have shown some effectiveness in clinical trials of patients with mild to moderate Alzheimer's disease, with documented improvements in the Alzheimer's Disease Assessment Scale Cognitive Subscale score (Birks and Cochrane Dementia and Cognitive Improvement Group 2006), but the overall effects of these drugs may be modest (Raina et al. 2008) (option D). **(pp. 47, 49, 225–226)**

2.13 A 76-year-old man comes to his clinic appointment asking for a testosterone prescription. When you ask him what led to this request, he says that he saw an advertisement on television for treatment of "low T" and thinks it might help him with his sexual performance. He denies any loss of libido but says he has had occasional erectile dysfunction. His chart indicates that on his last physical examination he had no obvious loss of body hair and testicular size was not reduced. Which of the following is true regarding testosterone and older men?

A. Testosterone deficiency is commonly found in men with erectile dysfunction.
B. Decreases in testosterone levels are universally seen in older men.
C. Testosterone replacement provides only minimal benefits in older men but is also generally safe, with no significant associated adverse events.
D. Declining testosterone levels are thought to have less effect on sexual function than do chronic medical or psychiatric illness, vascular disease, neuropathy, or medications.

The correct response is option D: Declining testosterone levels are thought to have less effect on sexual function than do chronic medical or psychiatric illness, vascular disease, neuropathy, or medications.

Only 2% of men with erectile dysfunction have an endocrine disorder (Sadovsky et al. 2007) (option A). Changes in testosterone secretion are common but not universal, and some men have normal serum testosterone levels as they age (Gruenewald and Matsumoto 2003; Perry 1999) (option B). Testosterone replacement is associated with a greater risk of all-cause mortality, myocardial infarction, and ischemic stroke 3 years after angiography (Vigen et al. 2013) (option C). Declining testosterone levels are thought to have less effect on sexual function than chronic medical or psychiatric illness, vascular disease, neuropathy, or medications (option D). Testing for testosterone deficiency is generally recommended only for those patients with clinical symptoms of hypogonadism, including both specific symptoms—decreased libido, erectile dysfunction, loss of body hair, small testes, loss of height, and reduced muscle size and strength—and nonspecific symptoms—decreased energy, depression, anemia, and decline in physical performance (Bhasin et al. 2010; Sadovsky et al. 2007). **(p. 40)**

2.14 An 89-year-old female nursing home resident falls after getting up in the middle of the night to urinate. She does not report the fall, but in the morning she awakens with severe pain in her right hip. She is transferred to acute care for evaluation, and on X ray is found to have a nondisplaced fracture of the right femoral neck. Which factor may have increased her risk of fracture?

A. High peak bone density can contribute to bone loss.
B. Lack of estrogen after menopause can lead to loss of bone mass.
C. Secondary hypoparathyroidism can contribute to bone loss.
D. Engaging in daily exercise may lead to an increase risk for bone breakdown.

The correct response is option B: Lack of estrogen after menopause can lead to loss of bone mass.

Low peak bone density (option A), poor calcium intake, secondary hyperparathyroidism (option C), and insufficient exercise (option D) can contribute to bone loss (option A) (Prestwood and Duque 2003). Without estrogen replacement, women can lose significant bone mass after menopause (option B). **(pp. 41–42)**

2.15 Which of the following is characteristic of the effects of aging on pharmacokinetics and must be taken into account when prescribing drugs to older patients?

A. There is a significant age-related effect on drug absorption related to both lower absorption due to decreases in acid secretion, gastrointestinal perfusion, and membrane transport and decreases in gastrointestinal transit time.
B. The decreases in lean body mass and total body water that occur with aging result in a smaller volume of distribution.
C. The decrease in renal mass that commonly occurs with aging is associated with an increase in the glomerular filtration rate.
D. The elimination half-life of commonly prescribed drugs such as aspirin and calcium channel blockers is decreased, so dosages must be adjusted upward.

The correct response is option B: The decreases in lean body mass and total body water that occur with aging result in a smaller volume of distribution.

Age has no significant effect on drug absorption. Although acid secretion, gastrointestinal perfusion, and membrane transport all may decrease and thereby lower absorption, gastrointestinal transit time is prolonged and increases absorption, and thus no net change occurs (option A). The decreases in lean body mass and total body water that occur with aging result in a smaller volume of distribution. This is particularly relevant when choosing proper dosages for drugs, such as antibiotics or lithium, that are primarily distributed in water (option B). With age, renal mass and renal blood flow are decreased, resulting in a decline in glomerular filtration rate (option C). The elimination half-life—the time required for the drug concentration to decrease by half—of certain drugs increases in older adults. This may require adjustment of the drug dosing interval. For example, aspirin, certain antibiotics (e.g., vancomycin), digoxin, and the calcium channel blockers (diltiazem, felodipine, and nifedipine) all have higher elimination half-lives, and the dosages must be adjusted downward (option D). **(pp. 44–45)**

References

Bhasin S, Cunningham GR, Hayes FJ, et al; Task Force, Endocrine Society: Testosterone therapy in men with androgen deficiency syndromes: an Endocrine Society clinical practice guideline. J Clin Endocrinol Metab 95(6):2536–2559, 2010 20525905

Birks J, Cochrane Dementia and Cognitive Improvement Group: Cholinesterase inhibitors for Alzheimer's disease. The Cochrane Library 2006. Available at: http://onlinelibrary.wiley.com/doi/10.1002/14651858.CD005593/abstract;jsessionid=4FA2F34374EC93993955F67AD324F922.f03t02. Accessed April 8, 2014.

Bischoff-Ferrari HA, Dawson-Hughes B, Willett WC, et al: Effect of vitamin D on falls: a meta-analysis. JAMA 291(16):1999–2006, 2004 15113819

Cohen HJ, Feussner JR, Weinberger M, et al: A controlled trial of inpatient and outpatient geriatric evaluation and management. N Engl J Med 346(12):905–912, 2002 11907291

Defilippi JL, Crismon ML: Antipsychotic agents in patients with dementia. Pharmacotherapy 20(1):23–33, 2000 10641973

Gruenewald DA, Matsumoto AM: Aging of the endocrine system, in Principles of Geriatric Medicine and Gerontology, 5th Edition. Edited by Hazzard WR, Blass JP, Halter JB, et al. New York, McGraw-Hill, 2003, pp 819–836

Harvey PT: Common eye diseases of elderly people: identifying and treating causes of vision loss. Gerontology 49(1):1–11, 2003 12457044

Huang Q, Tang J: Age-related hearing loss or presbycusis. Eur Arch Otorhinolaryngol 267(8):1179–1191, 2010 20464410

Hubschman JP, Reddy S, Schwartz SD: Age-related macular degeneration: current treatments. Clin Ophthalmol 3:155–166, 2009 19668560

Lakatta EG: Cardiovascular aging research: the next horizons. J Am Geriatr Soc 47(5):613–625, 1999 10323658

Oskvig RM: Special problems in the elderly. Chest 115(5)(suppl):158S–164S, 1999 10331350

Perry HM III: The endocrinology of aging. Clin Chem 45(8 Pt 2):1369–1376, 1999 10430820

Prestwood K, Duque G: Osteoporosis, in Principles of Geriatric Medicine and Gerontology, 5th Edition. Edited by Hazzard WR, Blass JP, Halter JB, et al. New York, McGraw-Hill, 2003, pp 973–985

Raina P, Santaguida P, Ismaila A, et al: Effectiveness of cholinesterase inhibitors and memantine for treating dementia: evidence review for a clinical practice guideline. Ann Intern Med 148(5):379–397, 2008 18316756

Sadovsky R, Dhindsa S, Margo K: Testosterone deficiency: which patients should you screen and treat? J Fam Pract 56 (5 suppl Testosterone):S1–S20, 2007

Schwartz RS, Kohrt WM: Exercise in elderly people: physiological and functional effects, in Principles of Geriatric Medicine and Gerontology, 5th Edition. Edited by Hazzard WR, Blass JP, Halter JB, et al. New York, McGraw-Hill, 2003, pp 931–946

Tune LE: Risperidone for the treatment of behavioral and psychological symptoms of dementia. J Clin Psychiatry 62(Suppl 21):29–32, 2001 11584986

U.S. Food and Drug Administration: FDA Drug Safety and Availability: Information for Healthcare Professionals: Conventional Antipsychotics, 2008. Available at: http://www.fda.gov/Drugs/DrugSafety/ucm124830.htm. Accessed March 1, 2013.

Vigen R, O'Donnell CI, Barón AE, et al: Association of testosterone therapy with mortality, myocardial infarction, and stroke in men with low testosterone levels. JAMA 310(17):1829–1836, 2013 24193080

C H A P T E R   3

Genomics in Geriatric Psychiatry

3.1 Which of the following is an example of change resulting in variation of chromosome structure?

A. Base pair.
B. Phenotype.
C. Penetrance.
D. Insertion.

The correct response is option D: Insertion.

Structural variation is variation in the structure of an organism's chromosome, usually involving changes such as deletions, duplications (copy-number variants), insertions (option D), and translocations. Base pair refers to the building blocks of the DNA double helix, each containing two complementary nucleotides (option A). Penetrance is the proportion of individuals carrying a particular genotype that also expresses an associated phenotype. In medical genetics, penetrance is defined as the proportion of individuals with the mutation who exhibit clinical symptoms (option C). Phenotype is the observable composite of an organism's genetic characteristics and traits (option B). **(Table 3–1, "Definitions of importance," pp. 63–64)**

3.2 Located on chromosome 21, a mutation in which of the following genes is most associated with early-onset Alzheimer's disease (EOAD)?

A. Presenilin 1.
B. Presenilin 2.
C. Amyloid precursor protein.
D. Apolipoprotein ε4.

The correct response is option C: Amyloid precursor protein.

Rare nonsynonymous mutations at three genetic loci associated with EOAD have been identified. The first was the amyloid precursor protein gene *APP* located on chromosome 21 (Goate et al. 1991) (option C). A second Alzheimer's disease (AD) locus was found on chromosome 14 (Schellenberg et al. 1992; St George-Hyslop et al. 1992) and is now called presenilin 1 (*PSEN1*) (Sherrington et al. 1995) (option A). A third EOAD gene has been localized to chromosome 1 and is known as presenilin 2 (*PSEN2*) (Levy-Lahad et al. 1995a, 1995b) (option B). Apolipoprotein ε4 (*APOE*E4*) is most associated with late-onset Alzheimer's disease (LOAD) (option D). **(pp. 68, 70)**

3.3   Mutation in the amyloid precursor protein (APP) gene increases risk of EOAD by which of the following mechanisms?

A. Increased γ-secretase activity.
B. Notch protein.
C. Increased β-secretase activity.
D. Apolipoprotein ε4 (*APOE*E4*).

The correct response is option C: Increased β-secretase activity.

The identification of a mutation in *APP* that selectively enhances metabolism of APP protein by β-secretase (known as the Swedish mutation) (option C) provided the assay necessary for the successful identification of β-secretase (Vassar et al. 1999). The identification of AD-causing mutations in proteins PSEN1 and PSEN2 led to a search for their function and ultimately converged on their identification as constituents of the proteolytic site in γ-secretase (option A) (Hardy et al. 2006; Selkoe et al. 2004). Efforts to identify γ-secretase inhibitors for the treatment of AD are also under way (Eder et al. 2007), although these are not as far advanced as the development of β-secretase inhibitors due to the potential toxicity associated with inhibiting the actions of γ-secretase on proteins other than APP, such as Notch protein (option B). *APOE* is clearly associated with LOAD, with increased risk of AD found in individuals carrying *APOE*E4* (option D) in both familial and sporadic cases (Brousseau et al. 1994; Mayeux et al. 1993; Rebeck et al. 1993; Saunders et al. 1993; Schmechel et al. 1993). **(pp. 69–70)**

3.4   Mutations in which of the following genes account for most familial EOAD cases?

A. *APP.*
B. *PSEN1.*
C. *PSEN2.*
D. *APOE*E4.*

The correct response is option B: *PSEN1.*

Some reports have suggested that *PSEN1* mutations (option B) account for most familial EOAD cases (Campion et al. 1995, 1999; Hutton et al. 1996), whereas others have reported that a more realistic estimate is 20% or fewer of such cases, with *PSEN2* (option C) and *APP* (option A) accounting for 1% and 5%, respectively

(Cruts et al. 1998). *APOE*E4* (option D) accounts for up to 50% of the genetic contribution to late-onset AD, in contrast to early-onset AD (Pericak-Vance and Haines 1995). **(pp. 69, 71)**

3.5   A 66-year-old woman seeks genetic counseling after her 87-year-old father who has Alzheimer's disease (AD) was recently enrolled in a research study. She asks about her own risk of developing dementia after genetic testing reveals she has the *APOE*E4* allele. On the basis of the pattern of inheritance, which of the following is most likely to be the impact on her level of risk of developing AD?

A. 100% chance of developing AD.
B. Three- to fourfold increase in risk of developing AD.
C. 5%–10% increase in risk of developing AD.
D. 75% chance of developing AD.

The correct response is option B: Three- to fourfold increase in risk of developing AD.

The effect of a specific genetic variation on disease risk may be extremely large (e.g., with complete penetrance, 100% of individuals with the genetic lesion who live to the age of risk develop the disease) (option A) or very small (e.g., the 5%–10% increase in disease risk often seen for common variants detected in genome-wide association studies of complex diseases) (option C). However, the risk is moderate (e.g., a three- to fourfold increase in risk) for AD because of an allele that produces *APOE*E4*) (option B). Approximately 50%–70% of people with AD carry at least one ε4 allele, and *APOE*E4* accounts for 50% of the genetic contribution to late-onset AD (Pericak-Vance and Haines 1995). It has been estimated that of the *APOE*E4* homozygotes who are disease-free at age 65, at most 50% will develop AD within their lifetime (option D). **(pp. 66, 71)**

3.6   The addition of *APOE*E4* testing to a clinical dementia assessment has which impact on a diagnosis of Alzheimer's disease?

A. Decreases specificity.
B. Increases sensitivity.
C. Increases false-positive rate.
D. Increases specificity.

The correct response is option D: Increases specificity.

In general, the addition of *APOE*E4* testing to a clinical dementia assessment lowers the sensitivity (option B) and enhances the specificity (option D; option A is incorrect) of an AD diagnosis (Ertekin-Taner 2007), ultimately reducing the false-positive rate (option C). **(p. 71)**

3.7 The risk of late-onset Alzheimer's disease (LOAD) associated with the effect of *APOE*E4* is highest in which of the following groups?

A. Hispanics.
B. African Americans.
C. Caucasians.
D. Japanese.

The correct response is option D: Japanese.

Although the effect of *APOE*E4* on increased risk for LOAD was evident in both sexes and in all age and ethnic groups, the magnitude of the risk varied by age and ethnicity. The risk appeared to be attenuated in older individuals and in African Americans (option B) and Hispanics (option A) (relative to Caucasians) (option C), whereas the risk conferred by *APOE*E4* was increased in individuals of Japanese ethnicity (option D) (Farrer et al. 1997). **(pp. 70–71)**

3.8 Mutations in which of the following genes account for most frontotemporal dementia (FTD) cases?

A. *C9orf72.*
B. *TDP-43.*
C. *FUS.*
D. *CHMP2B.*

The correct response is A: *C9orf72.*

Major causes of FTD include mutations in the following genes: *MAPT*, *PGRN* or *GRN*, and *C9orf72* (Wang et al. 2013). A significant discovery identified mutation in *C9orf72* (DeJesus-Hernandez et al. 2011) as perhaps the most common genetic abnormality in both familial behavioral variant FTD (11.7% of cases) and motor neuron disease (23.5%) (option A). A minority of cases are caused by mutations in the following genes: *TDP-43* (option B), *VCP*, *CHMP2B* (option D), and *FUS* (option C). **(p. 73)**

3.9 Mutations in which of the following genes is more likely to be associated with early-onset parkinsonism?

A. *SNCA.*
B. *LRRK2.*
C. *PINK1.*
D. *VPS35.*

The correct response is option C: *PINK1.*

Autosomal dominant Parkinson's disease (PD) is robustly associated with mutations in the following genes: *SNCA* (option A), *LRRK2* (option B), *EIF4G1*, and *VPS35* (option D). *LRRK2* mutations may lead to a clinical phenotype closely resembling idiopathic PD, with a variety of neuropathology. Mutations in *PARK2*, *PINK1* (option C), and *DJ1/PARK7*, on the other hand, may cause early-onset parkinsonism with limited risk for cognitive decline. **(p. 74)**

3.10   Autosomal dominant Parkinson's disease (PD) is strongly associated with mutations in which of the following genes?

A. *LRRK2*.
B. *PARK2*.
C. *PINK1*.
D. *DJ1/PARK7*.

The correct response is option A: *LRRK2*.

Autosomal dominant PD is robustly associated with mutations in the following genes: *SNCA*, *LRRK2* (option A), *EIF4G1*, and *VPS35*. Recessive PD is associated with mutations in *PARK2* (option B), *PINK1* (option C), and *DJ1/PARK7* (option D) (Puschmann 2013). However, many cases of PD are thought to arise sporadically. The mutations account for a small number of affected families and are primarily associated with earlier lifetime onset. **(p. 74)**

3.11   Point mutations and multiplications in which of the following genes cause cognitive/psychiatric symptoms and parkinsonism with widespread α-synuclein pathology?

A. *LRRK2*.
B. *PARK2*.
C. *SNCA*.
D. *PINK1*.

The correct response is option C: *SNCA*.

Point mutations and multiplications in *SNCA*, the gene encoding α-synuclein protein, cause cognitive or psychiatric symptoms and parkinsonism, with widespread α-synuclein pathology in the central and peripheral nervous system (Puschmann 2013) (option C). *LRRK2* mutations (option A) may lead to a clinical phenotype closely resembling idiopathic PD, with a variety of neuropathology. Mutations in *PARK2* (option B), *PINK1* (option D), and *DJ1/PARK7*, on the other hand, may cause early-onset parkinsonism with limited risk for cognitive decline. **(p. 74)**

3.12   Which of the following is defined as the proportion of individuals with the mutation who exhibit clinical symptoms?

A. Penetrance.
B. Allele.
C. Phenotype.
D. Genotype.

The correct response is option A: Penetrance.

In medical genetics, penetrance is defined as the proportion of individuals with the mutation who exhibit clinical symptoms (option A). Phenotype is defined as the observable composite of an organism's genetic characteristics and traits (option C). Genotype is defined as the genetic makeup of an organism (option D). Allele is defined as one of a number of different forms of the same gene. Alleles may or may not result in different observable phenotypic traits (option B). **(Table 3–1, "Definitions of importance," pp. 63–64)**

3.13 Which of the following pairs of psychiatric disorders demonstrates a high degree of shared genotypes?

A. Schizophrenia and bipolar disorders.
B. Bipolar disorders and major depressive disorder.
C. Schizophrenia and major depressive disorder.
D. Schizophrenia and autism spectrum disorder.

The correct response is option A: Schizophrenia and bipolar disorders.

Evidence demonstrated a high degree of shared genotypes between schizophrenia and bipolar disorders (option A), a moderate degree between bipolar disorders and major depressive disorder (option B), and a moderate degree between schizophrenia and major depressive disorder (option C). In addition, a moderate degree of genetic correlation existed between major depressive disorder and attention-deficit/hyperactivity disorder, and a small degree was present between schizophrenia and autism spectrum disorder (option D). **(pp. 75–76)**

3.14 A 22-year-old man with velocardiofacial syndrome develops paranoid delusions and auditory hallucinations over the course of 1 year. He has no history of substance use. Genetic testing would reveal a deletion at which of the following chromosomes?

A. Chromosome 22.
B. Chromosome 1.
C. Chromosome 3.
D. Chromosome 15.

The correct response is option A: Chromosome 22.

There is an increased risk for schizophrenia in individuals with a large deletion at chromosome (chr) 22q11.2 (option A), which is associated with the developmental disorder velocardiofacial syndrome, in which about 25% of individuals develop schizophrenia. Deletions at chr1q21.1 (option B), chr3q29 (option C), and chr15q13.3 (option D) have been associated with increased risk of schizophrenia but not with velocardiofacial syndrome. **(p. 77)**

3.15   Which of the following genes has been linked to a combination of schizophrenia, autism spectrum disorders, intellectual disability, and seizure disorder?

A. *NRXN1.*
B. *VIPR2.*
C. *DISC1.*
D. *CACNA1C.*

The correct response is option A: *NRXN1.*

All of the genes mentioned here are associated with schizophrenia; however, only deletions and duplications affecting the gene *NRXN1* (option A) have been found to be associated with autism spectrum disorder, intellectual disability, and seizure disorder (Doherty et al. 2012). A duplication affecting the vasoactive intestinal peptide receptor 2 gene (*VIPR2*) (option B) has been associated with schizophrenia and autism spectrum disorders but not with intellectual disability and seizure disorder. Studies have provided supportive but not unequivocal evidence for an association of *DISC1* (option C) with schizophrenia, depressive disorders, and autism spectrum disorders but not intellectual disability (Thomson et al. 2013). A significant association of genes involved in calcium signaling, including the calcium channel, voltage-dependent, L type, alpha 1C subunit gene (*CACNA1C*) (option D) and the calcium channel, voltage-dependent, beta 2 subunit gene (*CACNB2*), has been shown with schizophrenia but not autism spectrum disorders, intellectual disability, or seizure disorder. **(pp. 77–78)**

References

Brousseau T, Legrain S, Berr C, et al: Confirmation of the epsilon 4 allele of the apolipoprotein E gene as a risk factor for late-onset Alzheimer's disease. Neurology 44(2):342–344, 1994 8309588

Campion D, Flaman JM, Brice A, et al: Mutations of the presenilin I gene in families with early-onset Alzheimer's disease. Hum Mol Genet 4(12):2373–2377, 1995 8634712

Campion D, Dumanchin C, Hannequin D, et al: Early-onset autosomal dominant Alzheimer disease: prevalence, genetic heterogeneity, and mutation spectrum. Am J Hum Genet 65(3):664–670, 1999 10441572

Cruts M, van Duijn CM, Backhovens H, et al: Estimation of the genetic contribution of presenilin-1 and -2 mutations in a population-based study of presenile Alzheimer disease. Hum Mol Genet 7(1):43–51, 1998 9384602

DeJesus-Hernandez M, Mackenzie IR, Boeve BF, et al: Expanded GGGGCC hexanucleotide repeat in noncoding region of C9ORF72 causes chromosome 9p-linked FTD and ALS. Neuron 72(2):245–256, 2011 21944778

Doherty JL, O'Donovan MC, Owen MJ: Recent genomic advances in schizophrenia. Clin Genet 81(2):103–109, 2012 21895634

Eder J, Hommel U, Cumin F, et al: Aspartic proteases in drug discovery. Curr Pharm Des 13(3):271–285, 2007 17313361

Ertekin-Taner N: Genetics of Alzheimer's disease: a centennial review. Neurol Clin 25(3):611–667, v, 2007

Farrer LA, Cupples LA, Haines JL, et al; APOE and Alzheimer Disease Meta Analysis Consortium: Effects of age, sex, and ethnicity on the association between apolipoprotein E genotype and Alzheimer disease: a meta-analysis. JAMA 278(16):1349–1356, 1997 9343467

Goate A, Chartier-Harlin MC, Mullan M, et al: Segregation of a missense mutation in the amyloid precursor protein gene with familial Alzheimer's disease. Nature 349(6311):704–706, 1991 1671712

Hardy J, Cai H, Cookson MR, et al: Genetics of Parkinson's disease and parkinsonism. Ann Neurol 60(4):389–398, 2006 17068789

Hutton M, Busfield F, Wragg M, et al: Complete analysis of the presenilin 1 gene in early onset Alzheimer's disease. Neuroreport 7(3):801–805, 1996 8733749

Levy-Lahad E, Wasco W, Poorkaj P, et al: Candidate gene for the chromosome 1 familial Alzheimer's disease locus. Science 269(5226):973–977, 1995a 7638622

Levy-Lahad E, Wijsman EM, Nemens E, et al: A familial Alzheimer's disease locus on chromosome 1. Science 269(5226):970–973, 1995b 7638621

Mayeux R, Stern Y, Ottman R, et al: The apolipoprotein epsilon 4 allele in patients with Alzheimer's disease. Ann Neurol 34(5):752–754, 1993 8239575

Pericak-Vance MA, Haines JL: Genetic susceptibility to Alzheimer disease. Trends Genet 11(12):504–508, 1995 8533168

Puschmann A: Monogenic Parkinson's disease and parkinsonism: clinical phenotypes and frequencies of known mutations. Parkinsonism Relat Disord 19(4):407–415, 2013 23462481

Rebeck GW, Reiter JS, Strickland DK, Hyman BT: Apolipoprotein E in sporadic Alzheimer's disease: allelic variation and receptor interactions. Neuron 11(4):575–580, 1993 8398148

Saunders AM, Strittmatter WJ, Schmechel D, et al: Association of apolipoprotein E allele epsilon 4 with late-onset familial and sporadic Alzheimer's disease. Neurology 43(8):1467–1472, 1993 8350998

Schellenberg GD, Bird TD, Wijsman EM, et al: Genetic linkage evidence for a familial Alzheimer's disease locus on chromosome 14. Science 258(5082):668–671, 1992 1411576

Schmechel DE, Saunders AM, Strittmatter WJ, et al: Increased amyloid beta-peptide deposition in cerebral cortex as a consequence of apolipoprotein E genotype in late-onset Alzheimer disease. Proc Natl Acad Sci USA 90(20):9649–9653, 1993 8415756

Selkoe DJ; American College of Physicians; American Physiological Society: Alzheimer disease: mechanistic understanding predicts novel therapies. Ann Intern Med 140(8):627–638, 2004 15096334

Sherrington R, Rogaev EI, Liang Y, et al: Cloning of a gene bearing missense mutations in early-onset familial Alzheimer's disease. Nature 375(6534):754–760, 1995 7596406

St George-Hyslop P, Haines J, Rogaev E, et al: Genetic evidence for a novel familial Alzheimer's disease locus on chromosome 14. Nat Genet 2(4):330–334, 1992 1303289

Thomson PA, Malavasi EL, Grünewald E, et al: DISC1 genetics, biology and psychiatric illness. Front Biol (Beijing) 8(1):1–31, 2013 23550053

Vassar R, Bennett BD, Babu-Khan S, et al: Beta-secretase cleavage of Alzheimer's amyloid precursor protein by the transmembrane aspartic protease BACE. Science 286(5440):735–741, 1999 10531052

Wang X, Shen Y, Chen W: Progress in frontotemporal dementia research. Am J Alzheimers Dis Other Demen 28(1):15–23, 2013 23221030

CHAPTER 4

The Psychiatric Interview of Older Adults

4.1 Accurate genetic information can best be obtained by which of the following procedures?

A. A complete medical history.
B. A careful mental status examination.
C. A review of the patient's responses to various types of medications.
D. Interviews with family members from more than one generation.
E. A Structured Clinical Interview for DSM-IV.

The correct response is option D: Interviews with family members from more than one generation.

Accurate genetic information can be better obtained when family members from more than one generation are interviewed (option D). Many psychiatric disorders are characterized by a variety of symptoms, so asking the patient or one family member for a history of depression is insufficient. Research on the genetic expression of psychiatric disorders in families requires the psychiatric investigator to interview directly as many family members as possible to determine accurately the distribution of disorders throughout the family. Options A, B, C, and E provide invaluable information about the geriatric patient, but they are unlikely to aid in the identification of a genetic pattern of illness. Given the high likelihood of comorbid medical problems associated with psychiatric disorders in late life, a comprehensive medical history is essential (option A). The mental status examination of the older psychiatric patient is central to the diagnostic workup (option B). It is essential to evaluate the medication history of the older adult. A careful review of current and past medications by the clinician, a nurse, or a physician's assistant is essential (option C). The most frequently used structured interview instrument in the United States is the Structured Clinical Interview for DSM-IV (SCID-IV; First et al. 1997) (now Structured Clinical Interview for DSM-5 [SCID-5; First et al. 2016]) (option E). **(pp. 92–93, 95, 101)**

4.2 Which of the following intangible supports of patients may be less important to the older patient?

A. The perception of a dependable network.
B. A sense of usefulness.
C. A sense of belonging to a network.
D. Intimacy with network members.
E. Participation or interaction in a network.

The correct response is option B: A sense of usefulness.

Regardless of the level and types of services provided by the family to the older person, if these services are to be effective, it is beneficial for the older person to perceive that he or she lives in a supportive environment. Intangible supports include the perception of a dependable network (option A), participation or interaction in the network (option E), a sense of belonging to the network (option C), intimacy with network members (option D), and a sense of usefulness to the family (option B) (Blazer and Kaplan 1983). The sense of usefulness may be of less importance to some older adults who believe they have contributed to the family for many years and therefore deserve reciprocal services in their waning years. Unfortunately, family members, frequently stressed across generations, may not recognize this reciprocal responsibility. **(pp. 94–95)**

4.3 In a study by Sanford, what was the behavior least tolerated by the families of older persons?

A. Incontinence of urine.
B. Sleep disturbance.
C. Falls.
D. Physically aggressive behavior.
E. Personality conflicts.

The correct response is option B: Sleep disturbance.

Family tolerance of specific behaviors may not correlate with overall support. Every person has a level of tolerance for specific behaviors that are especially difficult to manage. Sanford (1975) found that the following behaviors were tolerated by families of older persons with impairments (in decreasing percentages): incontinence of urine (81%) (option A), personality conflicts (54%) (option E), falls (52%) (option C), physically aggressive behavior (44%) (option D), inability to walk unaided (33%), daytime wandering (33%), and sleep disturbance (16%) (option B). These relative frequencies may appear counterintuitive, because incontinence is generally considered particularly aversive to family members; however, although the outcome of incontinence can be corrected easily enough, a few nights of no sleep can easily extend family members beyond their capabilities for serving a parent, sibling, or spouse. **(p. 95)**

4.4   Which of the following is the most accurate test of abstract thinking?

   A. Interpretation of a well-known proverb.
   B. The ability to perform five serial subtractions of 7 from 100.
   C. Classifying objects in a common category.
   D. Naming objects from a category.
   E. Asking the patient to repeat a series of numbers.

The correct response is option C: Classifying objects in a common category.

A capacity for abstract thinking is often tested by asking the patient to interpret a well-known proverb, such as "A rolling stone gathers no moss" (option A). A more accurate test of abstraction, however, is classifying objects in a common category (option C). For example, the patient is asked to state the similarity between an apple and a pear. Whereas naming objects from a category, such as fruits, is retained despite moderate and sometimes marked declines in cognition, the opposite process of classifying two different objects in a common category is not retained as well. Immediate recall can be tested by asking the older person to repeat a word, phrase, or series of numbers (option E). Tests of simple arithmetic calculation and fund of knowledge, supplemented by portions of well-known psychiatric tests, are helpful for superficial assessment of intelligence. The classic test for calculation is to ask a patient to subtract 7 from 100 and to repeat this operation on the succession of remainders. Usually, five calculations are sufficient to determine the older adult's ability to complete this task (option B). **(p. 98)**

4.5   In assessing a patient's function and change of function, what are the most important parameters to assess?

   A. The patient's family history.
   B. Past history of symptoms and episodes.
   C. Social functioning and activities of daily living.
   D. Episodes of trauma in the past.
   E. Past response to specific medications.

The correct response is option C: Social functioning and activities of daily living.

Critical to the assessment of the present illness is an assessment of function and change in function. The two parameters that are most important (and not included in usual assessments of physical and psychiatric illness) are social functioning and activities of daily living (option C). Other psychiatric and medical problems should be reviewed as well (option B), especially medical illnesses that have led to hospitalization and the use of medication (option E). Not infrequently, an older adult has experienced a major illness or trauma in childhood or as a younger adult (option D) but views this information as being of no relevance to the present episode and therefore dismisses it. Probes to elicit these data are essential. The distribution of psychiatric symptoms and illnesses in the family should be determined next (option A). **(pp. 91–92)**

4.6 When taking a medication history, older persons are generally forthcoming when asked about which of the following?

A. Their alcohol drinking habits.
B. Their use of substances other than alcohol.
C. Nonprescription use of prescription drugs.
D. Potential drug-drug interactions.
E. The negative impact of over-the-counter medications.

The correct response is option A: Their alcohol drinking habits.

Although older persons do not usually volunteer information about their substance intake (option B), they are generally forthcoming when asked about their drinking habits (option A). Older persons are less likely than younger persons to have a substance use disorder, but a careful history of alcohol and drug intake (especially nonprescription use of prescription medications) (option C) is essential to the diagnostic workup. Both prescription and over-the-counter drugs (option E), such as laxatives and vitamins, should be recorded. The clinician can then identify the medications that potentially lead to drug-drug interactions and ask about them during subsequent patient visits. Most elderly persons take a variety of medicines simultaneously, and the potential for drug-drug interaction is high (option D). Some medications prescribed for older persons—such as the β-blocker propranolol and calcium channel blockers—can exacerbate or produce depressive symptoms. Options B, C, D, and E represent important questions to ask, but either the patient is unlikely to be forthcoming or he or she frequently will not understand the importance of this information. **(p. 93)**

4.7 Which of the following is a way to distinguish anxiety from agitation?

A. Agitated patients typically pace, whereas anxious patients do not.
B. Agitated patients usually display psychomotor retardation, whereas anxious patients usually do not.
C. Anxious patients are often in a stuporous state, whereas agitated patients are usually violent.
D. Anxious patients usually experience hallucinations, whereas hallucinations are rare in agitated patients.
E. Agitated patients usually do not complain of a sense of impending doom or dread, whereas anxious patients may have these complaints.

The correct response is option E: Agitated patients usually do not complain of a sense of impending doom or dread while anxious patients may have these complaints.

Options A, B, C, and D are incorrect because they describe behaviors that do not distinguish agitation from anxiety. Pacing is often observed when the older adult is admitted to a hospital ward (option A). Psychomotor retardation or underactivity is characteristic of major depression and severe schizophreniform symptoms, as well as of some variants of primary degenerative neurocognitive disorder. Psychiatrically impaired older persons, except some who have advanced neurocognitive disorder, are more likely to exhibit hyperactivity or agitation (option B). Agitation can usually be distinguished from anxiety, for the agitated individual does not complain of a sense of impending doom or dread (option E). Occasionally, the older adult with psychomotor retardation may actually be experiencing a disturbance in consciousness and may even reach an almost stuporous state (option C). Hallucinations often take the form of false auditory perceptions, false perceptions of movement or body sensation (e.g., palpitations), and false perceptions of smell, taste, and touch. The older patient who is severely depressed may have frank auditory hallucinations that condemn or encourage self-destructive behavior (option D). **(pp. 95–96)**

4.8 Which of the following techniques would show the appropriate respect for an older patient?

A. Addressing the patient by his or her given name.
B. Addressing the patient by his or her surname.
C. Speaking rapidly to the patient during the initial interview.
D. Maintaining a distance from the patient greater than an arm's length.
E. Ensuring that there are no periods of silence during the interview.

The correct response is option B: Addressing the patient by his or her surname.

The older person should be approached with respect. The clinician should knock before entering a patient's room and should greet the patient by surname (e.g., Mr. Jones, Mrs. Smith) (option B) rather than by a given name (option A), unless the clinician also wishes to be addressed by a given name. After taking a position near the older person—near enough to reach out and touch the patient (option D)—the clinician should speak clearly and slowly and use simple sentences in case the person's hearing is impaired (option C). The interview should be paced so that the older individual has enough time to respond to questions. Most elders are not uncomfortable with silence, because it gives them an opportunity to formulate their answers to questions and elaborate certain points they wish to emphasize (option E). **(p. 103)**

4.9 Which assessment tool is used to evaluate the presence of tardive dyskinesia in elderly patients?

A. Older Americans Resources and Services (OARS) Multidimensional Functional Assessment Questionnaire.
B. World Health Organization Disability Assessment Schedule 2.0 (WHODAS 2.0).
C. Geriatric Mental State Schedule.
D. Abnormal Involuntary Movement Scale (AIMS).
E. Diagnostic Interview Schedule for DSM-IV (DIS-IV).

The correct response is option D: Abnormal Involuntary Movement Scale.

Any discussion of clinical rating scales is not complete without a discussion of the Abnormal Involuntary Movement Scale (AIMS; National Institute of Mental Health 1975) (option D). There has been an increased incidence of tardive dyskinesia among older adults, coupled with the need for better documentation of this outcome due to prolonged use of antipsychotic agents. Regular ratings of patients on the AIMS by clinicians have therefore become essential to the practice of inpatient and outpatient geriatric psychiatry. The Older Americans Resources and Services (OARS) Multidimensional Functional Assessment Questionnaire (Duke University Center for the Study of Aging and Human Development 1978) (option A), administered by a lay interviewer, produces functional impairment ratings in five dimensions: mental health, physical health, social functioning, economic functioning, and activities of daily living. DSM-5 has adopted the World Health Organization Disability Assessment Schedule 2.0 (WHODAS 2.0) (option B) to assess disability in adults age 18 years and older (World Health Organization 2010; the scale is also available in DSM-5 Section III, "Emerging Measures and Models"). The Geriatric Mental State Schedule (Copeland et al. 1976) (option C), an adaptation of the Present State Exam (Wing et al. 1974) and the Psychiatric Status Schedule (Spitzer et al. 1968), is a semistructured interviewing guide that allows the rater to inventory symptoms associated with psychiatric disorders. The Diagnostic Interview Schedule for DSM-IV (DIS-IV; Robins et al. 2000) (option E) is a highly structured, computer-scored interview that can be administered by a lay interviewer and allows psychiatric diagnoses to be made according to DSM-IV criteria and Feighner criteria (Feighner et al. 1972). **(pp. 100–102)**

4.10 What name is given to a patient's experiences of disvalued changes in states of being and social function?

A. Diseases.
B. Illnesses.
C. Diagnoses.
D. Symptoms.
E. Syndromes.

The correct response is option B: Illnesses.

Patients have illnesses—experiences of disvalued changes in states of being and in social function (option B). Disease and illness do not maintain a one-to-one relationship. Symptoms (option D) should be defined in such a way that if multiple clinicians independently obtain equivalent information, they would have minimal disagreement about the presence or absence of a symptom. The decision about whether those symptoms form a syndrome (option E) or derive from a particular etiology must be determined independently of the data collection on symptoms. Even so, the clinical interaction may be confounded by bias when a clinician communicates with an older adult about psychiatric symptoms. As many insightful clinicians, such as Eisenberg (1977), have recognized, physicians diagnose (option C) and treat diseases (option A)—that is, abnormalities in the structure and function of body organs and systems. **(p. 90)**

4.11   Which of the following statements is true regarding disturbances in thought content?

A. Older depressed patients are more likely to have delusions than are middle-aged adults.
B. After recovery from a depression, elderly persons rarely have a recurrence of delusional thoughts.
C. Older persons appear more likely to experience delusional remorse.
D. Older persons appear more likely to experience delusional guilt.
E. Older persons appear more likely to experience delusional persecution.

The correct response is option A: Older depressed patients are more likely to have delusions than are middle-aged adults.

Meyers and Greenberg (1986) found delusional depression to be more prevalent among older depressed patients than among middle-aged adults (option A). Of 161 patients with endogenous depression, 72 (45%) were found to be delusional. Delusions included beliefs such as "I've lost my mind," "My body is disintegrating," "I have an incurable illness," and "I have caused some great harm." Even after elderly persons recover from depression, they may still experience periodic recurrences of delusional thoughts, which can be most disturbing to otherwise rational older adults (option B). Older patients appear less likely to experience delusional remorse (option C), guilt (option D), or persecution (option E). **(p. 96)**

4.12   Older adults with a neurocognitive disorder may exhibit circumstantiality. Which of the following is the best definition of circumstantiality?

A. The intrusion of thoughts from previous conversations into a current conversation.
B. The lack of logical connections between thoughts.
C. The introduction of many apparently irrelevant details to cover a lack of clarity and memory problems.
D. False sensory perceptions not associated with real or external stimuli.
E. The irresistible intrusion of thoughts into the conscious mind.

The correct response is option C: The introduction of many apparently irrelevant details to cover a lack of clarity and memory problems.

Some older adults with a neurocognitive disorder exhibit circumstantiality—that is, the introduction of many apparently irrelevant details to cover a lack of clarity and memory problems (option C). Interviews with patients who have this problem can be most frustrating because they proceed at a very slow pace. The intrusion of thoughts from previous conversations into a current conversation is a prime example of the disturbance in association found in patients with major neurocognitive disorder associated with Alzheimer's disease (option A). Elderly patients may appear incoherent, with no logical connection to their thoughts, or they may produce irrelevant answers (option B). Disturbances of perception include hallucinations—that is, false sensory perceptions not associated with real or external stimuli (option D). Even if delusions are not obvious, preoccupation with a particular thought or idea is common among depressed elderly persons. Such preoccupation is closely associated with obsessional thinking or irresistible intrusion of thoughts into the conscious mind (option E). **(pp. 96–97)**

4.13 Which of the following statements regarding suicide in the elderly is true?

A. Thoughts of death are common in late life, but spontaneous revelations of suicidal thoughts are rare.
B. Spontaneous revelations of suicidal thoughts are common in late life.
C. The clinician should never ask if there are implements for a suicide attempt because such a question may provoke suicidal thoughts.
D. It is never wise to inquire about the way in which a patient might attempt suicide.
E. Suicidal ideation in an older adult is not usually a cause for concern.

The correct response is option A: Thoughts of death are common in late life, but spontaneous revelations of suicidal thoughts are rare.

Suicidal thoughts are critical to assess in the elderly patient with psychiatric impairment. Although thoughts of death are common in late life (option A), spontaneous revelations of suicidal thoughts are rare (option B). A stepwise probe is the best means of assessing the presence of suicidal ideation (Blazer 1982). First, the clinician should ask the patient if he or she has ever thought that life was not worth living. If so, has the patient considered acting on that thought? If so, how would the patient attempt to inflict such harm (option D)? If definite plans are revealed, the clinician should probe to determine whether the implements for a suicide attempt are available (option C). For example, if a patient has considered shooting himself, the clinician should ask, "Do you have a gun available and loaded at home?" Suicidal ideation in an older adult is always of concern (option E), but intervention is necessary when suicide has been considered seriously and the implements are available. **(p. 97)**

4.14 Immediate recall can be tested by which of the following methods?

A. Asking the patient to name the day, month, date, and year.
B. Asking the patient to subtract 7 from 100 and to repeat this operation on the succession of remainders.
C. Asking the patient to interpret a well-known proverb.
D. Requesting that the patient spell a word backward.
E. Asking the patient to classify objects in a common category.

The correct response is option D: Requesting the patient to spell a word backward.

Immediate recall can be tested by asking the older person to repeat a word, phrase, or series of numbers, but it can also be tested in conjunction with cognitive skills by requesting that a word be spelled backward (option D) or that elements of a story be recalled. Disturbances of recall can be tested directly in a number of ways. The most common are tests of orientation to time, place, person, and situation (option A). Tests of simple arithmetic calculation are helpful for superficial assessment of intelligence. The classic test for calculation is to ask a patient to subtract 7 from 100 and to repeat this operation on the succession of remainders (option B). A capacity for abstract thinking is often tested by asking the patient to interpret a well-known proverb, such as "A rolling stone gathers no moss" (option C). A more accurate test of abstraction, however, is classifying objects in a common category (option E). For example, the patient is asked to state the similarity between an apple and a pear. **(p. 98)**

4.15 Which of the following is the most frequently used structured interview instrument in the United States?

A. Diagnostic Interview Schedule for DSM-IV (DIS-IV).
B. Older Americans Resources and Services (OARS) Multidimensional Functional Assessment Questionnaire.
C. Structured Clinical Interview for DSM-IV (SCID-IV).
D. Geriatric Mental State Schedule.
E. Mini-Mental State Examination.

The correct response is option C: Structured Clinical Interview for DSM-IV (SCID).

The most frequently used structured interview instrument in the United States is the Structured Clinical Interview for DSM-IV (SCID-IV; First et al. 1997) (now Structured Clinical Interview for DSM-5 [SCID-5; First et al. 2016]) (option C). The Diagnostic Interview Schedule for DSM-IV (DIS-IV; Robins et al. 2000) (option A) is a highly structured, computer-scored interview that can be administered by a lay interviewer and allows psychiatric diagnoses to be made according to DSM-IV criteria and Feighner criteria (Feighner et al. 1972). The Older Americans Resources and Services (OARS) Multidimensional Functional Assessment Questionnaire (Duke University Center for the Study of Aging and Human Development 1978) (option B), administered by a lay interviewer, produces functional impairment ratings in five dimensions: mental health, physical health, social functioning, economic functioning, and activities of daily living. The Geriatric Mental State Schedule (Copeland et al. 1976) (option D), an adaptation of the Present State Exam (Wing et al. 1974) and the Psychiatric Status Schedule (Spitzer et al. 1968), is a semistructured interviewing guide that allows the rater to inventory symptoms associated with psychiatric disorders. The Mini-Mental State Examination (Folstein et al. 1975) (option E) is a 30-item screening instrument that assesses orientation, registration, attention and calculation, recall, and language. **(pp. 99–102)**

References

Blazer DG: Depression in Late Life. St Louis, MO, CV Mosby, 1982

Blazer DG, Kaplan BH: The assessment of social support in an elderly community population. Am J Soc Psychiatry 3:29–36, 1983

Copeland JRM, Kelleher MJ, Kellett JM, et al: A semi-structured clinical interview for the assessment of diagnosis and mental state in the elderly: the Geriatric Mental State Schedule, I: development and reliability. Psychol Med 6(3):439–449, 1976 996204

Duke University Center for the Study of Aging and Human Development: Multidimensional Functional Assessment: The OARS Methodology—A Manual, 2nd Edition. Durham, NC, Duke University Center for the Study of Aging and Human Development, 1978

Eisenberg L: Disease and illness: distinctions between professional and popular ideas of sickness. Cult Med Psychiatry 1(1):9–23, 1977 756356

Feighner JP, Robins E, Guze SB, et al: Diagnostic criteria for use in psychiatric research. Arch Gen Psychiatry 26(1):57–63, 1972 5009428

First MB, Spitzer RL, Gibbon M: Structured Clinical Interview for DSM-IV. Washington, DC, American Psychiatric Press, 1997

First MB, Williams JBW, Karg RS, Spitzer RL: Structured Clinical Interview for DSM-5 Disorders—Clinician Version (SCID-5-CV). Arlington, VA, American Psychiatric Association, 2016

Folstein MF, Folstein SE, McHugh PR: "Mini-mental state." A practical method for grading the cognitive state of patients for the clinician. J Psychiatr Res 12(3):189–198, 1975 1202204

Meyers BS, Greenberg R: Late-life delusional depression. J Affect Disord 11(2):133–137, 1986 2948986

National Institute of Mental Health: Development of a Dyskinetic Movement Scale (Publ No 4). Rockville, MD, National Institute of Mental Health, Psychopharmacology Research Branch, 1975

Robins LN, Cottler L, Bucholz K, et al: Diagnostic Interview Schedule for the DSM-IV (DIS-IV). St. Louis, MO, Washington University School of Medicine, 2000

Sanford JRA: Tolerance of debility in elderly dependants by supporters at home: its significance for hospital practice. BMJ 3(5981):471–473, 1975 1156826

Spitzer RL, Endicott J, Cohen GM: Psychiatric Status Schedule, 2nd Edition. New York, New York State Department of Mental Hygiene, Evaluation Unit, Biometrics Research, 1968

Wing JK, Cooper JE, Sartorius N: The Measurement and Classification of Psychiatric Symptoms. London, Cambridge University Press, 1974

World Health Organization: Measuring Health and Disability: Manual for WHO Disability Assessment Schedule (WHO-DAS 2.0). Edited by Üstün TB, Kostanjsek N, Chatterji S, Rehm J. Geneva, Switzerland, World Health Organization, 2010. Available at: http://whqlibdoc.who.int/publications/2010/9789241547598_eng.pdf. Accessed October 2014.

CHAPTER 5

Use of the Laboratory in the Diagnostic Workup of Older Adults

5.1 What hematologic change is associated with lithium treatment?

A. Leukocytosis.
B. Leukopenia.
C. Thrombocytopenia.
D. Agranulocytosis.

The correct response is option A: Leukocytosis.

A complete blood cell count (CBC) is a standard part of any evaluation. It screens for multiple problems, including infections and anemia. It also provides a platelet count, a value important to monitor in psychiatric medications associated with thrombocytopenia (option C), such as divalproex sodium or carbamazepine. This concern is particularly important in elderly patients, because the risk of drug-induced thrombocytopenia may increase with age. Lithium, in contrast, may result in mild leukocytosis (option A; option B is incorrect). Because of the risk of agranulocytosis (option D), CBC testing is required weekly or biweekly for patients taking clozapine and may be needed more frequently if the patient develops signs of infection. Mirtazapine can also lead to agranulocytosis in rare cases. **(p. 108)**

5.2 When treating elderly depressed patients with selective serotonin reuptake inhibitors, which electrolyte disturbance can result in neurological dysfunction secondary to cerebral edema?

A. Potassium.
B. Calcium.
C. Sodium.
D. Magnesium.

The correct response is option C: Sodium.

Hyponatremia—commonly defined as a serum sodium concentration (option C) less than 135 mEq/L—has been reported with selective serotonin reuptake inhibitors, particularly in the elderly. The signs and symptoms of hyponatremia result from neurological dysfunction secondary to cerebral edema. Of all the electrolyte abnormalities, potassium (option A) disorders may be the most crucial to identify. These rarely cause psychiatric symptoms but may result in severe cardiac arrhythmias. Although not always included in routine chemistry screens, calcium (option B) and magnesium (option D) levels are also important to consider, because abnormal levels may result in paranoid ideation or frank psychosis. **(pp. 108–109)**

5.3   The 2004 American Diabetes Association guidelines for screening and monitoring of patients taking second-generation antipsychotics recommends fasting lipid profile at baseline and at what frequency thereafter?

A. At 12 weeks and annually.
B. At 12 weeks and every 5 years.
C. Every 4 weeks for 12 weeks, then quarterly.
D. Annually.

The correct response is option B: At 12 weeks and every 5 years.

Fasting lipid profile should be assessed at baseline, at 12 weeks, and every 5 years (option B). Personal and family history should be taken at baseline and annually (option D). Weight should be taken at baseline, every 4 weeks for 12 weeks, then quarterly (option C). Waist circumference should be measured at baseline and annually (option D). Blood pressure and fasting plasma glucose should be taken at baseline, at 12 weeks, and annually (option A). **(Table 5–1, "Guidelines for screening and monitoring of patients taking second-generation antipsychotics," p. 109)**

5.4   A 65-year-old male with cognitive impairment screens positive for syphilis with the Venereal Disease Research Laboratory test. In order to distinguish true-positive results from false-positive results, what laboratory test should be performed?

A. Cerebrospinal fluid (CSF) reagin test.
B. Microhemagglutination assay for *Treponema pallidum*.
C. Rapid plasmin reagin test.
D. Blood reagin test.

The correct response is option B: Microhemagglutination assay for *Treponema pallidum*.

If a clinician suspects syphilis infection, the Venereal Disease Research Laboratory and the rapid plasmin reagin tests (option C) are screening tools for infection with

Treponema pallidum, the cause of syphilis. These tests are unfortunately nonspecific; false-positive results may occur in acute infections and chronic illnesses such as systemic lupus erythematosus. More specific tests, the fluorescent treponemal antibody and the microhemagglutination assay for *Treponema pallidum* (option B), may distinguish false-positive from true-positive results and may aid in diagnosing late syphilis when blood reagin (option D) and even CSF (option A) tests are negative. **(p. 110)**

5.5　What is the most frequently used screening test for thyroid disease in the elderly?

A. Thyroid-stimulating hormone (TSH).
B. Thyroxine (T_4).
C. Triiodothyronine (T_3).
D. TSH, T_3, and T_4.

The correct response is option A: Thyroid-stimulating hormone (TSH).

A serum TSH test (option A) is the most frequently used screen for thyroid disease; it is an excellent screening test because of its high negative predictive value (Klee and Hay 1997). A physical examination and measurement of T_4, T_3, and TSH (options B, C, and D) may be required for a definitive diagnosis of thyroid disease. **(pp. 110–111)**

5.6　A patient is found to have a high TSH level. On follow-up exam, his free T_4 and T_3 are normal. What diagnosis is suggested by these findings?

A. Euthyroid state.
B. Primary hypothyroidism.
C. Hyperthyroidism.
D. Subclinical hypothyroidism.

The correct response is option D: Subclinical hypothyroidism.

High TSH, normal free T_4, and normal T_3 suggest a diagnosis of subclinical hypothyroidism (option D). High TSH, low free T_4, and low or normal T_3 suggest a diagnosis of primary hypothyroidism (option B). Low TSH, high or normal free T_4, and high T_3 suggest a diagnosis of hyperthyroidism (option C). Normal results on all three tests suggest a euthyroid diagnosis (option A). **(Table 5–2, "Patterns of thyroid function tests," p. 111)**

5.7　A 78-year-old woman is sent to the emergency department to be evaluated for a urinary tract infection (UTI). She is told that her urine sample is likely contaminated and she will need to provide the staff with a repeat sample. A urine sample containing which of the following is suggestive of contamination?

A. Red blood cells.
B. Epithelial cells.

C. White blood cells.

D. Bacteria.

The correct response is option B: Epithelial cells.

A UTI is suggested when a microscopic examination shows high levels of white blood cells (option C), bacteria (option D), positive leukocyte esterase and nitrite, and possibly red blood cells (option A); high numbers of epithelial cells (option B) make the results difficult to interpret, because their presence suggests contamination. **(p. 112)**

5.8   Which of the following is a cerebrospinal fluid biomarker that is reduced in patients with Alzheimer's disease (AD) and mild cognitive impairment (MCI) due to AD?

A. Phosphorylated tau (p-tau).

B. Total tau (t-tau).

C. β-Amyloid peptide 1–42.

D. Progranulin (PGRN).

The correct response is option C: β-Amyloid peptide 1–42.

In patients with AD and MCI due to AD, CSF levels of β-amyloid peptide 1–42 are reduced (option C), whereas levels of p-tau (option A) and t-tau (option B) are increased (Blennow et al. 2010; Hansson et al. 2006). Two promising assays for frontotemporal lobar degeneration (FTLD) include the measurement of plasma levels of PGRN (option D) and transactive response DNA-binding protein of 43 kDa molecular weight (TDP-43). TDP-43 proteinopathy has also been associated with both FTLD and amyotrophic lateral sclerosis. **(pp. 112–113)**

5.9   Which illness is highly specific for elevated plasma levels of TDP-43?

A. Creutzfeldt-Jakob disease (CJD).

B. Parkinson-plus syndromes.

C. Alzheimer's disease (AD).

D. Frontotemporal lobar degeneration (FTLD).

The correct response is option D: Frontotemporal lobar degeneration (FTLD).

Two promising assays for FTLD include the measurement of plasma levels of PGRN and TDP-43. TDP-43 proteinopathy has also been associated with both FTLD and amyotrophic lateral sclerosis, which suggests these are two processes on a disease continuum (Neumann et al. 2006). Elevated levels of TDP-43 in the CSF and plasma are seen in FTLD, amyotrophic lateral sclerosis, and AD; plasma levels of phosphorylated TDP-43 may be more specific for FTLD (Foulds et al. 2009) (option D). Tau elevations can be found in conditions such as FTLD and Parkinson-plus syndromes (option B). Hsich et al. (1996) described an immunoassay for the detection of the 14-3-3 protein in CSF that had a specificity of 99% and a sensitivity of 96% for the diagnosis of CJD among patients with dementia (option A). In patients with AD and MCI due to AD (option C), CSF levels of β-amyloid peptide 1–42 are reduced, whereas levels of p-tau and t-tau are increased (Blennow et al. 2010; Hansson et al. 2006). **(pp. 112–113)**

5.10 Testing for which biomarker is recommended by the American Academy of Neurology for confirming or rejecting the diagnosis of Creutzfeldt-Jakob disease (CJD) in clinically appropriate circumstances?

A. TDP-43 assay.
B. Progranulin (PGRN).
C. 14-3-3 protein assay.
D. β-Amyloid peptide 1–42.

The correct response is option C: 14-3-3 protein assay.

The American Academy of Neurology recommends testing for CSF 14-3-3 protein (option C) for confirming or rejecting the diagnosis of CJD in clinically appropriate circumstances (Knopman et al. 2001). Hsich et al. (1996) described an immunoassay for the detection of the 14-3-3 protein in CSF that had a specificity of 99% and a sensitivity of 96% for the diagnosis of CJD among patients with dementia. Two promising assays for FTLD include the measurement of plasma levels of PGRN (option B) and TDP-43 (option A). In patients with AD and MCI due to AD, CSF levels of β-amyloid peptide 1–42 are reduced (option D). **(pp. 112–113)**

5.11 Tricyclic antidepressant use in the elderly has the potential to cause which of these cardiovascular effects?

A. Shortened PR and QRS intervals.
B. Atrioventricular block.
C. Decreased QT intervals.
D. Sinoatrial block.

The correct response is option B: Atrioventricular block.

Tricyclic antidepressants are associated with atrioventricular block (option B); they are also associated with increased PR and QRS intervals (option A) and increased QT intervals (option C). Lithium is associated with sick sinus syndrome and sinoatrial block (option D). **(Table 5–3, "Common electrocardiographic abnormalities associated with psychotropic medications," p. 114)**

5.12 Which neuroimaging method can differentiate between acute and chronic infarcts?

A. Diffusion-weighted imaging (DWI).
B. Computed tomography (CT).

C. Magnetic resonance imaging (MRI).

D. Plain film radiograph.

The correct response is option A: Diffusion-weighted imaging (DWI).

A limitation of CT (option B) and MRI (option C) is that neither can differentiate between acute and chronic lesions. DWI (option A) overcomes this difficulty. DWI is based on the capacity of fast MRI to detect a signal related to the movement of water molecules between two closely spaced radio frequency pulses (diffusion). This technique can detect abnormalities due to ischemia within 3–30 minutes of onset, whereas conventional MRI and CT images would still appear normal. Therefore, DWI is helpful in defining the clinically appropriate infarct when multiple subcortical infarcts of various ages are present. Plain film radiographs (option D) remain an integral piece of the diagnostic imaging performed in geriatric psychiatry. Such techniques are most commonly used to detect lung pathology that may contribute to mental status changes or to detect bone fractures. Plain film radiographs are critical for individuals who have both severe dementia and either a recent history of falls or newly developed limb immobility. **(pp. 115, 117–118)**

5.13   When the clinical diagnosis is unclear, which imaging technique can be useful to distinguish Alzheimer's disease (AD) from frontotemporal dementia (FTD)?

A. MRI.

B. ^{18}Fluorodeoxyglucose positron emission tomography (FDG-PET).

C. Diffusion-weighted imaging (DWI).

D. Computed tomography (CT).

The correct response is option B: ^{18}Fluorodeoxyglucose positron emission tomography (FDG- PET).

FDG-PET imaging can be useful in distinguishing AD from FTD when the clinical diagnosis is unclear (option B). On FDG-PET imaging, AD causes hypometabolism predominantly in posterior temporoparietal association and posterior cingulate cortices, whereas FTD causes hypometabolism in the frontal lobes and anterior temporal and anterior cingulate cortices. CT (option D) is particularly useful for demonstrating bone abnormalities (such as skull fractures), areas of hemorrhage (such as a subdural hematoma), and the mass effect from various lesions. It can also display atrophy or ventricular enlargement. However, CT is not very useful for visualizing posterior fossa or brain stem structures because of surrounding bone. In the psychiatric workup of a geriatric patient, MRI (option A) should be considered when the clinician suspects small lesions in regions difficult to visualize—for example, to obtain evidence of midbrain hemorrhage in a patient with suspected Wernicke's encephalopathy, or to confirm a suspected pituitary tumor in a patient with hyperprolactinemia. DWI (option C) is helpful in defining the clinically appropriate infarct when multiple subcortical infarcts of various ages are present. **(pp. 116–118)**

5.14   A 56-year-old man presents with a rapidly progressive dementia, leading to memory loss and hallucinations. The treatment team suspects Creutzfeldt-Jakob disease (CJD), and an electroencephalogram (EEG) is requested. What EEG pattern would you expect if CJD is the correct diagnosis?

A. Periodic sharp-wave complexes.
B. Slowing of the normal background activity.
C. Slowing of the posterior dominant rhythm.
D. Increased generalized slow-wave activity.

The correct response is option A: Periodic sharp-wave complexes.

CJD is a rare, rapidly progressive prion disease characterized by dementia and neurological signs that may include gait disturbances and myoclonus. Electroencephalography may play an important role in diagnosing this disease: periodic sharp-wave complexes (option A) are strongly associated with CJD, with a sensitivity of 67% and a specificity of 86%. In delirium, except that caused by alcohol or sedative-hypnotic withdrawal, electroencephalograms typically display slowing of the posterior dominant rhythm (option C) and increased generalized slow-wave activity (option D). Kowalski et al. (2001) reported that the degree of EEG change (slowing of normal background activity) (option B) is correlated with cognitive impairment. **(pp. 119–120)**

5.15   Which omics technology examines proteins, including posttranslational modifications such as phosphorylation, ubiquination, and glycosylation?

A. Epigenomics.
B. Metabolomics.
C. Transcriptomics.
D. Proteomics.

The correct response is option D: Proteomics.

Proteomics (option D) examines proteins, including posttranslational modifications such as phosphorylation, ubiquination, and glycosylation, that can affect the proteins' functioning. Epigenomics (option A) examines epigenetic changes (including DNA methylation and histone modification) that affect whether parts of the DNA sequences can be transcribed. Metabolomics (option B) examines metabolic content of cell or organism (including changes in protein, nucleic acid, carbohydrates, and lipids). Transcriptomics (option C) examines RNA transcripts, namely, the expression of genomic material, including microRNAs, which can negatively regulate or degrade transcripts. **(Table 5–5, "Omics technologies," p. 123)**

References

Blennow K, Hampel H, Weiner M, Zetterberg H: Cerebrospinal fluid and plasma biomarkers in Alzheimer disease. Nat Rev Neurol 6(3):131–144, 2010 20157306

Foulds PG, Davidson Y, Mishra M, et al: Plasma phosphorylated-TDP-43 protein levels correlate with brain pathology in frontotemporal lobar degeneration. Acta Neuropathol 118(5):647–658, 2009 19823856

Hansson O, Zetterberg H, Buchhave P, et al: Association between CSF biomarkers and incipient Alzheimer's disease in patients with mild cognitive impairment: a follow-up study. Lancet Neurol 5(3):228–234, 2006 16488378

Hsich G, Kenney K, Gibbs CJ, et al: The 14-3-3 brain protein in cerebrospinal fluid as a marker for transmissible spongiform encephalopathies. N Engl J Med 335(13):924–930, 1996 8782499

Klee GG, Hay ID: Biochemical testing of thyroid function. Endocrinol Metab Clin North Am 26(4):763–775, 1997 9429859

Knopman DS, DeKosky ST, Cummings JL, et al: Practice parameter: diagnosis of dementia (an evidence-based review). Report of the Quality Standards Subcommittee of the American Academy of Neurology. Neurology 56(9):1143–1153, 2001 11342678

Kowalski JW, Gawel M, Pfeffer A, Barcikowska M: The diagnostic value of EEG in Alzheimer disease: correlation with the severity of mental impairment. J Clin Neurophysiol 18(6):570–575, 2001 11779971

Neumann M, Sampathu DM, Kwong LK, et al: Ubiquitinated TDP-43 in frontotemporal lobar degeneration and amyotrophic lateral sclerosis. Science 314(5796):130–133, 2006 17023659

CHAPTER 6

Neuropsychological Assessment of Late-Life Cognitive Disorders

6.1   Which of the following is true regarding neuropsychological testing?

A. It is useful only in detecting moderate to severe cognitive impairment.
B. It does not help differentiate among cognitive disorders.
C. It is sensitive but not reliable in diagnosing cognitive disorders.
D. It can be useful in establishing baseline cognitive function and monitoring treatment response.

The correct response is option D: It can be useful in establishing baseline cognitive function and monitoring treatment response.

Neuropsychological testing can be used to establish an objective baseline for purposes of tracking changes in mentation over time (option D); this baseline is useful in clarifying diagnostic assignments due to neurodegenerative diseases such as Alzheimer's disease (AD) in which the establishment of progression is essential. The neuropsychological examination in this context can also be used to monitor treatment response. Neuropsychological assessment continues to play a central role in the diagnosis of neurocognitive disorders, in the detection of mild neurocognitive disorders likely to transition to a more fully expressed syndrome (Gomar et al. 2011) (option A), and in the differentiation among the plethora of cognitive disorders that can interfere with functional ability and quality of life (Knopman et al. 2001; Weintraub et al. 2012) (option B). The neuropsychological assessment offers a sensitive, reliable (option C), and noninvasive approach to early symptom verification as well as a potentially cost-effective means for managing patients with memory disorders (Welsh-Bohmer et al. 2003). **(pp. 127–128)**

6.2   Which of the following is a neuropsychological test commonly used to assess orientation and global mental status?

A. Wechsler Adult Intelligence Scale, 4th Edition (WAIS-IV).
B. Mini-Mental State Examination.
C. Trail Making Test.
D. Boston Naming Test.

The correct response is option B: Mini-Mental State Examination.

The Mini-Mental State Examination (option B) is frequently used to test orientation and global mental status. Other tests of global mental status include the Montreal Cognitive Assessment and Alzheimer's Disease Assessment Scale—Cognitive. WAIS-IV (option A) tests intellect, the Trail Making Test (option C) assesses executive function, and the Boston Naming Test (option D) assesses language. **(Table 6–1, "Common neuropsychological tests used in geriatric assessment," pp. 130–131)**

6.3   The Wisconsin Card Sorting Test examines which cognitive domain?

A. Executive function.
B. Attention/concentration.
C. Memory.
D. Visuoperception.

The correct response is option A. Executive function.

The Wisconsin Card Sorting Test is a test of executive function (option A). It does not test attention/concentration (option B), memory (option C), or visuoperception (option D). **(Table 6–1, "Common neuropsychological tests used in geriatric assessment," pp. 130–131)**

6.4   Which neuropsychological test is used to assess visuoperception?

A. Grooved Pegboard.
B. Judgment of Line Orientation Test.
C. Minnesota Multiphasic Personality Inventory—2.
D. Color Trail Making Test.

The correct response is option B: Judgment of Line Orientation Test.

The Judgment of Line Orientation Test (option B) assesses visuoperception. The Grooved Pegboard test (option A) assesses sensorimotor abilities, the Minnesota Multiphasic Personality Inventory—2 (option C) tests personality and behavior, and the Color Trail Making Test (option D) assesses executive function. **(Table 6–1, "Common neuropsychological tests used in geriatric assessment," pp. 130–131)**

6.5   Which of the following cognitive changes is typical of normal aging?

A. Deficits in cued recall.
B. Deficits in delayed recognition.
C. Decreased speed and efficiency of information processing.
D. Significant impairment in visuospatial skills.

The correct response is option C: Decreased speed and efficiency of information processing.

Compared with young adults, older individuals show selective losses in functions related to speed and efficiency of information processing (option C). Particularly vulnerable are memory retrieval abilities, attentional capacity, executive skills, and divergent thinking such as working memory and multitasking (Samson and Barnes 2013; Salthouse 1996; van Hooren et al. 2007). On formal neuropsychological testing, memory measures involving delayed free recall are typically affected (Craik and Rose 2012), although not to the pronounced extent found in AD (Welsh et al. 1991). Unlike individuals with neurocognitive disorder due to AD, older adults without neurocognitive disorders typically demonstrate intact memory ability on tests such as cued recall (option A) and delayed recognition (option B). In addition to having a decline in memory, normal older adults also show some decrements compared with younger cohorts on tests of visuoperceptual, visuospatial, and constructional functions. These modest declines (option D) are seen on tests involving visual analysis and integration, such as the Block Design subtest of the WAIS-IV (Wechsler 2009), and similar integrative tests involving visual processing. **(pp. 132–133)**

6.6   Marked impairment of recent memory with rapid forgetting after a brief delay is characteristic of which neurocognitive disorder?

A. Alzheimer's disease (AD).
B. Huntington's disease.
C. Frontotemporal neurocognitive disorder.
D. Geriatric depression.

The correct response is option A: Alzheimer's disease (AD).

On formal neuropsychological testing, the memory problem of AD (option A) is manifest as a rapid forgetting of new information after very brief delays of 5 minutes or more (Welsh et al. 1991). Patients with Huntington's disease (option B) have difficulties in memory retrieval and benefit from retrieval supports. Patients with frontotemporal neurocognitive disorder (option C) typically present with pronounced executive impairments and less obvious memory impairments. Geriatric depression (option D) is characterized by memory retrieval difficulties that improve with cueing, and patients also demonstrate difficulties in attention and concentration and exhibit poor motivation. **(p. 134; Table 6–2, "Clinical neurocognitive syndromes and associated neuropsychological profiles," pp. 135–138)**

6.7   Which of the following cognitive deficit patterns is characteristic of major vascular neurocognitive disorder?

A. Marked impairment in recent memory with rapid forgetting after brief delays.
B. Fluctuations in alertness and acute confusional state.
C. Prominent personality or behavior change.
D. Multifocal "patchy" impairments.

The correct response is option D: Multifocal "patchy" impairments.

Multi-infarct dementia, arising from multiple large- and small-vessel strokes, will demonstrate a pattern of multifocal impairments (option D) on testing that respect the cerebral territories involved by the infarctions (Chui et al. 1992; Román et al. 1993). In disorders attributed to diffuse small-vessel disease (e.g., Binswanger's disease), the pattern shown on testing reflects the disruption in the dorsolateral prefrontal and subcortical circuitry (Kramer et al. 2002). Memory is involved, but the deficits are often patchy in nature (option D). Patients may show impaired recollection of some recent event but show a surprising memory of some other occurrence transpiring within the same time frame. Pronounced impairment in recent memory processing with rapid forgetting of new information after very brief delays (option A) describes memory impairments of AD. Fluctuations in alertness (option B) can be seen in neurocognitive disorder with Lewy bodies. Prominent personality or behavioral change (option C) is typical of frontotemporal neurocognitive disorder. **(pp. 134, 139; Table 6–2, "Clinical neurocognitive syndromes and associated neuropsychological profiles," pp. 135–138)**

6.8   Which neurocognitive disorder is often characterized by behavioral disinhibition or apathy with early loss of insight?

A. Alzheimer's disease (AD).
B. Major vascular neurocognitive disorder.
C. Frontotemporal lobar degeneration (FTLD).
D. Major neurocognitive disorder with Lewy bodies.

The correct response is option C: Frontotemporal lobar degeneration (FTLD).

The neuropsychological profile of FTLD (option C) is distinct from that of AD or any other form of major neurocognitive disorder (Weintraub et al. 2012). There are typically prominent early changes in behavior, personality, or language as opposed to impairments in memory and other aspects of cognition. Disinhibition or its converse, behavioral apathy and inertia (option C), frequently occurs. Insight into impairment and into personality change is also affected, and this capacity commonly is disturbed early in the course of FTLD (Rankin et al. 2005). This behavior pattern contrasts with that of AD (option A), in which insight is generally lost later in the neurodegenerative process (Salmon et al. 2008). Behavioral disinhibition and apathy are not typical of major vascular neurocognitive disorder (option B) or major neurocognitive disorder with Lewy bodies (option D). **(p. 140)**

6.9   Frontotemporal lobar degeneration (FTLD) is marked by pronounced impairment in which cognitive domain?

A. Attention.
B. Visuoperception.
C. Executive function.
D. Memory.

The correct response is option C: Executive function.

In FTLD, there is impairment in executive function (option C). The dysexecutive syndrome of FTLD is characterized by slow information processing, cognitive rigidity, diminished abstract reasoning, poor response inhibition, and impaired planning. Clinically, from the outset, the neuropsychological profile of FTLD is distinct from that of AD or any other form of major neurocognitive disorder (Weintraub et al. 2012). There are typically prominent early changes in behavior, personality, or language as opposed to impairments in memory (option D) and other aspects of cognition (options A and B). **(p. 140)**

6.10   Which neurocognitive disorder is characterized by extrapyramidal motor symptoms, visual hallucinations, and fluctuations in cognition and attention?

A. Major neurocognitive disorder with Lewy bodies.
B. Major neurocognitive disorder due to Parkinson's disease.
C. Huntington's disease.
D. Creutzfeldt-Jakob disease (CJD).

The correct response is option A: Major neurocognitive disorder with Lewy bodies.

Major neurocognitive disorder with Lewy bodies (option A) is characterized by early fluctuations in cognition and attention, recurrent and persistent visual hallucinations, and extrapyramidal motor symptoms. In major neurocognitive disorder due to Parkinson's disease (option B), the prevailing features are parkinsonism, akinetic rigidity, and generalized slowing in motor movement/initiation and thought processes (bradykinesia and bradyphrenia, respectively). Huntington's disease (option C) is characterized by early age at onset, choreiform movements, and bradyphrenia. CJD (option D) is characterized by rapid onset and course, neurocognitive disorder with pyramidal and extrapyramidal signs, and transient spikes on electroencephalogram. **(p. 142; Table 6–2, "Clinical neurocognitive syndromes and associated neuropsychological profiles," pp. 135–138)**

6.11   Which of the following best differentiates neurocognitive disorder due to Parkin-
        son's disease and neurocognitive disorder with Lewy bodies?

        A. Neuropsychological test results alone.
        B. Clinical history and examination.
        C. Neuroimaging alone.
        D. Cerebrospinal fluid studies.

The correct response is option B: Clinical history and examination.

Differentiating Parkinson's disease dementia (PDD) from dementia with Lewy
bodies (DLB) rests on the relative occurrence of dementia with respect to the extrapyramidal motor symptoms. In PDD the symptoms of dementia emerge in the
context of a previously established diagnosis of Parkinson's disease, whereas in
DLB the symptoms of cognitive and functional impairments either predate or follow the onset of parkinsonian symptoms within a 1-year time interval. The integration of the clinical examination findings (which includes history and review of
systems, motor examination, cognitive findings, behavioral ratings, psychiatric
interview, and supportive laboratory studies such as neuroimaging) (option B) is
necessary to clarify these disorders from one another and to make an accurate diagnosis early in the process (Litvan et al. 2012). In this context, particular attention
to the history of symptoms (e.g., fluctuations in ability throughout the day) and
to the presence or absence of defined behavioral impairments is crucial to the diagnosis (Geser et al. 2005; Pillon et al. 1991). On neuropsychological evaluation
(option A), the cognitive impairments of PDD and DLB are similar, but the profiles can be differentiated from those typically observed in AD (Tröster 2008;
Welsh-Bohmer and Warren 2006). Both PDD and DLB are characterized by a pattern of memory retrieval problems and mild dysexecutive disturbances, which
early in the course are less dramatic and globally impairing than the cognitive
deficits of AD (Hamilton et al. 2004). Neuroimaging (option C) and laboratory
studies alone (option D) do not differentiate these two disorders. **(p. 142)**

6.12   Which of the following neurocognitive disorders is characterized by deficits in at-
        tention, memory retrieval difficulties that improve with cues, and poor effort on
        tasks?

        A. Alzheimer's disease (AD).
        B. Major vascular neurocognitive disorder.
        C. Neurocognitive disorder with Lewy bodies.
        D. Neurocognitive disorder associated with geriatric depression.

**The correct response is option D: Neurocognitive disorder associated with ge-
riatric depression.**

Neurocognitive disorder associated with geriatric depression (option D) is characterized by a neuropsychological profile of impaired attention and concentration, difficulties with memory retrieval that improve with cueing/recognition,

and poor motivation. The neuropsychological profile of AD (option A) reveals impaired memory consolidation with rapid forgetting. Other features of AD include diminished executive skills, impaired semantic fluency and naming, and impaired visuospatial analysis and praxis. Major vascular neurocognitive disorder (option B) can present with language/memory retrieval difficulties that benefit from structural supports/cueing, but poor effort on tasks and impairments in attention are more typical of geriatric depression. Neurocognitive disorder with Lewy bodies (option C) is marked by memory impairment of AD but with some partial saving. Apraxia and visuospatial difficulties are pronounced in this disorder. **(Table 6–2, "Clinical neurocognitive syndromes and associated neuropsychological profiles," pp. 135–138)**

6.13   What percentage of adults ages 65 years and over experience symptoms of depression?

A. 1%–5%.
B. 20%–30%.
C. 50%–60%.
D. More than 80%.

The correct response is option B: 20%–30%.

The problem of geriatric depression is fairly common, with some epidemiologically based studies suggesting that nearly one-third (28%) (option B) of elderly individuals older than 65 years exhibit prominent affective syndromes (Lyketsos et al. 2001). Depression also frequently co-occurs in the context of a range of medical disorders, including AD, stroke and cerebrovascular conditions, and Parkinson's disease, complicating the diagnosis of these disorders and exacerbating functional loss associated with these disorders. **(p. 143)**

6.14   Cognitive impairment associated with geriatric depression is due to dysfunction in which brain area?

A. Temporal lobe.
B. Parietal lobe.
C. Occipital lobe.
D. Frontal lobe.

The correct response is option D: Frontal lobe.

On formal neuropsychological testing, depressed patients show impairments on tests sensitive to frontal lobe function (option D; options A, B, and C are incorrect). Difficulties can be readily seen on tests of selective and sustained attention, verbal fluency, inhibitory control, and set shifting (Boone et al. 1994, 1995; Lockwood et al., 2002). The neurocognitive profile tends to be one of a dysexecutive syndrome with impairments in planning, organization, initiation, sequencing, working memory, and behavioral shifting in response to feedback. Short-term memory and visuospatial skills are also disturbed, in part because of the attentional and organizational compromises. **(p. 143)**

6.15 Which of the following neuropsychological testing profiles distinguishes the memory impairment of Alzheimer's disease (AD) from that associated with geriatric depression?

A. Impaired free recall but better preserved recognition memory in depression.
B. Impaired recognition memory in depression.
C. Impaired acquisition in AD.
D. Poor effort on testing in AD.

The correct response is option A: Impaired free recall but better preserved recognition memory in depression.

In geriatric depression, memory is impaired on both acquisition and recall, leading to a profile characterized by a flattened learning curve and impaired free recall of previously learned information after brief delays (Hart et al. 1987) (option A). Recognition memory is better preserved but can be characterized by false-negative tendencies (not recognizing previous target material) (option B). The memory disturbance of depression is distinguished from AD by the impaired acquisition and recognition elements. In AD, acquisition is relatively better preserved (option C), whereas recognition is characterized by false-positive tendencies (recognizing foils incorrectly as previously presented targets). In depressed patients there is often a heightened tendency to abandon effortful tests (option D). **(p. 143)**

References

Boone KB, Lesser I, Miller B, et al: Cognitive functioning in a mildly to moderately depressed geriatric sample: relationship to chronological age. J Neuropsychiatry Clin Neurosci 6(3):267–272, 1994 7950350

Boone KB, Lesser I, Miller B, et al: Cognitive functioning in older depressed outpatients: relationship of presence and severity of depression on neuropsychological test scores. Neuropsychology 9:390–398, 1995

Chui HC, Victoroff JI, Margolin D, et al: Criteria for the diagnosis of ischemic vascular dementia proposed by the State of California Alzheimer's Disease Diagnostic and Treatment Centers. Neurology 42(3 Pt 1):473–480, 1992 1549205

Craik FIM, Rose NS: Memory encoding and aging: a neurocognitive perspective. Neurosci Biobehav Rev 36(7):1729–1739, 2012 22155274

Geser F, Wenning GK, Poewe W, McKeith I: How to diagnose dementia with Lewy bodies: state of the art. Mov Disord 20(Suppl 12):S11–S20, 2005 16092075

Gomar JJ, Bobes-Bascaran MT, Conejero-Goldberg C, et al; Alzheimer's Disease Neuroimaging Initiative: Utility of combinations of biomarkers, cognitive markers, and risk factors to predict conversion from mild cognitive impairment to Alzheimer disease in patients in the Alzheimer's disease neuroimaging initiative. Arch Gen Psychiatry 68(9):961–969, 2011 21893661

Hamilton JM, Salmon DP, Galasko D, et al: A comparison of episodic memory deficits in neuropathologically-confirmed Dementia with Lewy bodies and Alzheimer's disease. J Int Neuropsychol Soc 10(5):689–697, 2004 15327716

Hart RP, Kwentus JA, Taylor JR, Harkins SW: Rate of forgetting in dementia and depression. J Consult Clin Psychol 55(1):101–105, 1987 3571646

Knopman DS, DeKosky ST, Cummings JL, et al: Practice parameter: diagnosis of dementia (an evidence-based review). Report of the Quality Standards Subcommittee of the American Academy of Neurology. Neurology 56(9):1143–1153, 2001 11342678

Kramer JH, Reed BR, Mungas D, et al: Executive dysfunction in subcortical ischaemic vascular disease. J Neurol Neurosurg Psychiatry 72(2):217–220, 2002 11796772

Litvan I, Goldman JG, Tröster AI, et al: Diagnostic criteria for mild cognitive impairment in Parkinson's disease: Movement Disorder Society Task Force guidelines. Mov Disord 27(3):349–356, 2012 22275317

Lockwood KA, Alexopoulos GS, van Gorp WG: Executive dysfunction in geriatric depression. Am J Psychiatry 159(7):1119–1126, 2002 12091189

Lyketsos CG, Sheppard JM, Steinberg M, et al: Neuropsychiatric disturbance in Alzheimer's disease clusters into three groups: the Cache County study. Int J Geriatr Psychiatry 16(11):1043–1053, 2001 11746650

Pillon B, Dubois B, Agid Y: Severity and specificity of cognitive impairment in Alzheimer's, Huntington's, and Parkinson's diseases and progressive supranuclear palsy. Ann N Y Acad Sci 640:224–227, 1991 1837977

Rankin KP, Baldwin E, Pace-Savitsky C, et al: Self awareness and personality change in dementia. J Neurol Neurosurg Psychiatry 76(5):632–639, 2005 15834018

Román GC, Tatemichi TK, Erkinjuntti T, et al: Vascular dementia: diagnostic criteria for research studies. Report of the NINDS-AIREN International Workshop. Neurology 43(2):250–260, 1993 8094895

Salmon E, Perani D, Collette F, et al: A comparison of unawareness in frontotemporal dementia and Alzheimer's disease. J Neurol Neurosurg Psychiatry 79(2):176–179, 2008 17898032

Salthouse TA: The processing-speed theory of adult age differences in cognition. Psychol Rev 103(3):403–428, 1996 8759042

Samson RD, Barnes CA: Impact of aging brain circuits on cognition. Eur J Neurosci 37(12):1903–1915, 2013 23773059

Tröster AI: Neuropsychological characteristics of dementia with Lewy bodies and Parkinson's disease with dementia: differentiation, early detection, and implications for "mild cognitive impairment" and biomarkers. Neuropsychol Rev 18(1):103–119, 2008 18322801

van Hooren SA, Valentijn AM, Bosma H, et al: Cognitive functioning in healthy older adults aged 64-81: a cohort study into the effects of age, sex, and education. Neuropsychol Dev Cogn B Aging Neuropsychol Cogn 14(1):40–54, 2007 17164189

Wechsler D: Wechsler Intelligence Scale, 4th Edition. San Antonio, TX, Psychological Corporation, 2009

Weintraub S, Wicklund AH, Salmon DP: The neuropsychological profile of Alzheimer disease. Cold Spring Harb Perspect Med 2(4):a006171, 2012 22474609

Welsh K, Butters N, Hughes J, et al: Detection of abnormal memory decline in mild cases of Alzheimer's disease using CERAD neuropsychological measures. Arch Neurol 48(3):278–281, 1991 2001185

Welsh-Bohmer KA, Warren LH: Neurodegenerative dementias, in Geriatric Neuropsychology: Assessment and Intervention. Edited by Attix DK, Welsh-Bohmer KA. New York, Guilford, 2006, pp 56–88

Welsh-Bohmer KA, Koltai DC, Mason DJ: The clinical utility of neuropsychological evaluation of patients with known or suspected dementia, in Demonstrating Utility and Cost Effectiveness in Clinical Neuropsychology. Edited by Prigatano G, Pliskin N. Philadelphia, PA, Psychology Press-Taylor and Francis Group, 2003, pp 177–200

CHAPTER 7

Delirium

7.1 It has been noted that differentiating dementia from delirium can be particularly difficult. Which of the following is a key diagnostic feature that aids in differentiating these two conditions?

A. An acute and rapid onset.
B. Laboratory tests that are pathognomonic for delirium.
C. No alterations in attention.
D. There is no need to differentiate the two conditions.

The correct response is option A: An acute and rapid onset.

It is important not to underestimate the waxing and waning periods of delirium, because periods of lucidity and reversal of symptoms can often be deceiving. Impairment in attention, a hallmark feature of delirium, is clinically manifested through the patient's difficulty in focusing on the task at hand, maintaining or following a conversation, and/or shifting of attention, often leading to perseveration on a previous topic or task (option C). Patients with dementia who develop a superimposed delirium experience a more rapid progression of cognitive dysfunction and worse long-term prognosis (Fick and Foreman 2000; Jackson et al. 2004). The key diagnostic feature that aids in distinguishing these two conditions is that delirium has an acute and rapid onset, whereas dementia is much more gradual in progression (option A). Differentiating among diagnoses is critical because delirium carries a more serious prognosis without proper evaluation and management (option D). No specific laboratory tests currently exist that will aid in the definitive identification of delirium (option B). The laboratory evaluation for delirium is intended to identify contributing factors that will need to be addressed, and the approach should be guided by astute clinical judgment and tailored to the individual situation. **(pp. 160–163)**

7.2 What is the recommended use of neuroimaging in evaluating a patient with delirium?

A. All patients presenting with delirium should get a head computed tomography (CT) or magnetic resonance imaging (MRI) scan.

B. Neuroimaging is recommended for the evaluation of chronic focal neurological symptoms.

C. Neuroimaging is recommended if there is suspected or evident trauma or injury.

D. Neuroimaging is recommended for the routine evaluation of fever.

The correct response is option C: Neuroimaging is recommended if there is suspected or evident trauma or injury.

In general, the routine use of neuroimaging in delirium is not recommended (option A) because the overall diagnostic yield is low, and the findings from neuroimaging change the management of patients in less than 10% of cases (Hirao et al. 2006). Brain imaging techniques—CT, positron emission tomography (PET), single photon emission computed tomography (SPECT), and MRI—have low diagnostic yield in unselected patients but are recommended in cases of head trauma or injury (option C), for evaluation of new focal neurological symptoms (option B), for assessment for suspected encephalitis, or for evaluation of fever of unknown origin (option D). **(p. 163)**

7.3   What is the most frequently considered pathophysiological mechanism of delirium?

A. Cholinergic dysfunction.

B. Release of tumor necrosis factor (TNF-α).

C. Genetic factors such as toll-like receptor 4.

D. Hypercapnia.

The correct response is option A: Cholinergic dysfunction.

Although many neurotransmitters are implicated in delirium (Gaudreau and Gagnon 2005), the most frequently considered mechanism of delirium is dysfunction in the cholinergic system (option A). Acetylcholine plays a key role in mediating consciousness and attentional process. Given that delirium is manifested by an acute confusional state, often with alterations of consciousness, it is likely to have a cholinergic basis. Evidence for the cholinergic connection includes findings that anticholinergic drugs can induce delirium in humans and animals and that serum anticholinergic activity is increased in patients with delirium (Hshieh et al. 2008; Lauretani et al. 2010). Also, cholinesterase inhibitors have been found to reduce symptoms of delirium in some studies (Gleason 2003; Wengel et al. 1998). Release of pro-inflammatory markers such as TNF-α (option B), genetic factors such as toll-like receptor 4 (option C), and hypercapnia (option D) are all hypothetical pathophysiological contributors to delirium (see Table 7–6), but they do not yet have human studies available to support the mechanism (Inouye et al. 2014). **(p. 163; Table 7–6, "Potential pathophysiological contributors to delirium," p. 164)**

7.4   Which medication or drug class poses the greatest risk for causing or precipitating delirium in older adults?

A. Sedative-hypnotic drugs.
B. Narcotics.
C. Anticholinergic drugs.
D. St. John's wort.

The correct response is option C: Anticholinergic drugs.

Medication use contributes to delirium in more than 40% of cases (Inouye 1994; Inouye and Charpentier 1996). The Beers Criteria by the American Geriatrics Society (2012) lists medications that cause or exacerbate delirium. The medications most frequently associated with delirium are those with psychoactive effects such as sedative-hypnotics, anxiolytics, narcotics, and histamine type 2 blockers. Drugs with anticholinergic effects, including antipsychotics, antihistamines, antidepressants, antiparkinsonian agents, and anticonvulsants, are also commonly associated with delirium. Sedative-hypnotic drugs are associated with a 3- to 12-fold increased risk of delirium (option A), narcotics with a threefold risk (option B), and anticholinergic drugs with a 5- to 12-fold risk (option C) (Agostini and Inouye 2003; Foy et al. 1995; Schor et al. 1992). A systematic review of prospective studies identified opioids, benzodiazepines, dihydropyridines, and antihistamines as increasing the risk of delirium (Clegg and Young 2011). Some homeopathic or herbal therapies, especially those used for mood disorders (e.g., St. John's wort, kava kava), may increase the risk of delirium (option D), especially when used in combination with prescribed psychoactive medications. **(pp. 165–166; Table 7–8, "Drugs to avoid in delirium: Beers Criteria," p. 168)**

7.5   In a general medicine service, which predisposing factor poses the greatest relative risk for delirium?

A. Alcohol abuse.
B. Dementia.
C. Vision impairment.
D. Older age.

The correct response is option A: Alcohol abuse.

Of the predisposing factors for delirium listed in Table 7–7, alcohol abuse (option A) poses a relative risk of 5.7, dementia (option B) 2.3–4.7, vision impairment (option C) 2.1–3.5, and older age (option D) 4.0. **(Table 7–7, "Risk factors for delirium from validated predictive models," p. 167)**

7.6 What were the clinical highlights of using haloperidol versus placebo in a randomized controlled trial of 457 noncardiac surgery patients by Wang et al. (2012)?

A. Decreased length of hospital stay.
B. Decreased incidence of delirium.
C. Fewer postoperative complications.
D. Decreased mortality.

The correct response is option B: Decreased incidence of delirium.

A randomized controlled trial of haloperidol versus placebo in 457 noncardiac surgery patients in the intensive care unit (ICU) showed reduced incidence of delirium (haloperidol 15.3% vs. placebo 23.2%, $P=0.03$) (option B) but no difference in length of hospital stay (option A), postoperative complications (option C), or mortality (option D) (Wang et al. 2012). **(p. 168)**

7.7 According to the Beers Criteria, which of the following drugs should be avoided in the treatment of delirium?

A. Rivastigmine.
B. Olanzapine.
C. Haloperidol.
D. Sedative-hypnotics.

The correct response is option D: Sedative-hypnotics.

Of the four options, only sedative-hypnotics (option D) are listed in Beers Criteria as drugs that should be avoided in delirium. Rivastigmine (option A) has been associated with longer delirium duration and increased mortality (van Eijk et al. 2010) but is not listed in the Beers Criteria. Olanzapine (option B) has shown reduced incidence of delirium compared with placebo in 400 patients following hip replacement but resulted in greater duration and severity of delirium (Larsen et al. 2010). A randomized controlled trial of haloperidol (option C) versus placebo in 457 noncardiac surgery patients in the ICU showed reduced incidence of delirium (haloperidol 15.3% vs. placebo 23.2%, $P=0.03$) but no difference in length of hospital stay, postoperative complications, or mortality (Wang et al. 2012). **(p. 168)**

7.8 Which of the following is the most effective for alleviating symptoms associated with delirium?

A. Rivastigmine.
B. Olanzapine.
C. Primary prevention.
D. Haloperidol.

The correct response is option C: Primary prevention.

Primary prevention (option C)—that is, preventing delirium before it develops—is the most effective strategy to alleviate symptoms associated with delirium. The Hospital Elder Life Program (HELP; www.hospitalelderlifeprogram.org) utilizes a multicomponent targeted intervention approach to aid in preventing delirium and is the most widely disseminated approach to delirium prevention (Inouye et al. 1999, 2006). In one trial, treatment with rivastigmine (option A) resulted in higher delirium duration and mortality in 104 ICU patients (van Eijk et al. 2010). In another trial, treatment with olanzapine (option B) reduced incidence of delirium compared with placebo in 400 patients following hip replacement but resulted in greater duration and severity of delirium (Larsen et al. 2010). In a randomized controlled trial, haloperidol (option D) showed reduced incidence of delirium versus placebo but no difference in length of hospital stay, postoperative complications, or mortality (Wang et al. 2012). **(pp. 168–169)**

7.9   What is the first-line treatment of delirium?

A. Nonpharmacological approaches.
B. Physical restraints.
C. Normalization of sleep-wake cycle.
D. Pharmacological management.

The correct response is option A: Nonpharmacological approaches.

Nonpharmacological approaches (option A), such as those used in the HELP protocols (www.hospitalelderlifeprogram.org), should be implemented as the first-line treatment of delirium. Nonpharmacological treatment approaches include reorientation (e.g., using orientation boards, clocks, calendars), behavioral interventions, encouraging the presence of family members, and transferring a disruptive patient to a private room or closer to the nurse's station for increased supervision. Consistent and compassionate staff are essential in facilitating contact and communication with the patient through frequent verbal reorienting strategies, clear instructions, frequent eye contact, and the inclusion of patients as much as possible in all decision making regarding their daily and medical care. Sensory deficits should be assessed and then corrected by ensuring that all assistive devices, such as eyeglasses and hearing aids, are readily available, functioning, and being used properly by the patient. The use of physical restraints (option B) should be minimized due to their role in prolonging delirium, worsening agitation, and increasing complications such as strangulation (Inouye et al. 2007). Normalization of sleep-wake cycle (option C) is only part of the initial management of delirium. Daytime napping should be discouraged, the patient should be exposed to bright light, and uninterrupted period for sleep at night should be facilitated. Pharmacological management (option D), such as haloperidol 0.25–0.5 mg twice daily or atypical antipsychotics, should be reserved for patients with severe agitation or severe psychotic symptoms. **(p. 169; Table 7–9, "Initial management of delirium," p. 170)**

7.10   What is the most common cause of delirium?

A. Underlying dementia.
B. Multifactorial causes.
C. Anticholinergic medications.
D. Antihistamines.

The correct response is option B: Multifactorial causes.

Underlying dementia (option A) and cognitive impairment are the leading risk factors for development of delirium but are not the most common cause of it. Although a single factor may lead to delirium, more commonly delirium is multifactorial in older persons (option B). Anticholinergic medications (option C) and antihistamines (option D) are also commonly associated with delirium as noted by the Beers Criteria, but usually with other concomitant factors. **(p. 165; Table 7–7, "Risk factors for delirium from validated predictive models," p. 167; Table 7–8, "Drugs to avoid in delirium: Beers Criteria," p. 168)**

7.11   In an intensive care unit, which of the following precipitating factors poses the greatest relative risk for delirium?

A. Elevated serum urea.
B. Metabolic acidosis.
C. Infection.
D. Use of sedative-hypnotics.

The correct response is option D: Use of sedative-hypnotics.

Use of sedative-hypnotic medication (option D) poses a relative risk of 4.5, followed by infection (option C) with a relative risk of 3.1, metabolic acidosis (option B) with a relative risk of 1.4, and elevated serum urea (option A) with a relative risk of 1.1. **(Table 7–7, "Risk factors for delirium from validated predictive models," p. 167)**

7.12   In noncardiac surgical patients, which of the following predisposing factors poses the greatest relative risk for delirium?

A. Older age (≥75 years).
B. History of delirium.
C. Hearing impairment.
D. Dementia.

The correct response is option A: Older age (≥75 years).

Older age (option A) poses a relative risk of 3.3–6.6, followed by history of delirium (option B) with a relative risk of 3.0, dementia (option D) with a relative risk of 2.8, and hearing impairment (option C) with a relative risk of 1.3. **(Table 7–7, "Risk factors for delirium from validated predictive models," p. 167)**

7.13   What is the clinical setting with the highest incidence of delirium?

A. Geriatric unit.
B. Palliative care setting.
C. Nursing home/postacute care.
D. Intensive care unit (ICU).

The correct response is option D: Intensive care unit (ICU).

The highest incidence rates have been observed in the ICU (option D) with an incidence range of 19%–82%. Palliative care (option B) settings have a 47% incidence of delirium. Nursing homes and postacute care settings (option C) have an incidence of delirium of 20%–22%. Geriatric units (option A) have an incidence of delirium of 20%–29%. **(Table 7–1, "Incidence, prevalence, and outcomes of delirium," p. 157)**

7.14   As a clinician, which approach would be most helpful in avoiding the common mistake of not recognizing delirium?

A. Performing a comprehensive psychiatric evaluation and supporting the findings with a Confusion Assessment Method (CAM).
B. Performing a thorough medical evaluation and running a Delirium Observation Screening Scale.
C. Combining insightful clinical judgment with a thorough medical evaluation.
D. Performing a thorough medical and psychiatric evaluation and measuring symptoms with the Delirium Rating Scale.

The correct response is option C: Combining insightful clinical judgment with a thorough medical evaluation.

Delirium goes unrecognized by clinicians in up to 70% of patients who develop this condition (Inouye et al. 2001); therefore, careful clinical assessment for this condition is imperative. Identification of delirium relies on insightful clinical judgment combined with a thorough medical evaluation (option C). The clinician should assess for recent changes or updates in medication regimen, new infections, or recent development of medical illnesses that may contribute to delirium. Sudden and acute onset, fluctuating course, and alteration in attention are the central features of delirium. Therefore, it is important to establish a patient's level of baseline cognitive functioning and the course of cognitive change when evaluating for the presence of delirium. A detailed and in-depth background interview with a proxy informant, such as a family member, caregiver, or medical professional who knows the patient, proves invaluable when documenting change in a patient's mental status. Over 24 delirium instruments have been used in published studies (Adamis et al. 2010), but they cannot replace the importance of clinical judgment and medical evaluation. The Confusion Assessment Method (CAM; Inouye et al. 1990) (option A) is the most widely used instrument for the identification of delirium and provides a simple diagnostic algorithm (Wei et al.

2008; Wong et al. 2010). Several behavioral checklists for symptoms of delirium that are used, particularly in nursing-based studies, include the Delirium Observation Screening Scale (Schuurmans et al. 2003) (option B), the Nursing Delirium Screening Checklist (Gaudreau et al. 2005), and the NEECHAM Confusion Scale (Neelon et al. 1996). Delirium severity is most widely measured using the Delirium Rating Scale (Trzepacz et al. 1988, 2001) (option D) and the Memorial Delirium Assessment Scale (Breitbart et al. 1997). **(pp. 156–160)**

References

Adamis D, Sharma N, Whelan PJ, Macdonald AJ: Delirium scales: a review of current evidence. Aging Ment Health 14(5):543–555, 2010 20480420

Agostini JV, Inouye SK: Delirium, in Principles of Geriatric Medicine and Gerontology, 5th Edition. New York, McGraw-Hill, 2003, pp 647–658

American Geriatrics Society: American Geriatrics Society updated Beers Criteria for potentially inappropriate medication use in older adults. J Am Geriatr Soc 60:616–631, 2012 22376048

Breitbart W, Rosenfeld B, Roth A, et al: The Memorial Delirium Assessment Scale. J Pain Symptom Manage 13(3):128–137, 1997 9114631

Clegg A, Young JB: Which medications to avoid in people at risk of delirium: a systematic review. Age Ageing 40(1):23–29, 2011 21068014

Fick D, Foreman M: Consequences of not recognizing delirium superimposed on dementia in hospitalized elderly individuals. J Gerontol Nurs 26(1):30–40, 2000 10776167

Foy A, O'Connell D, Henry D, et al: Benzodiazepine use as a cause of cognitive impairment in elderly hospital inpatients. J Gerontol A Biol Sci Med Sci 50(2):M99–M106, 1995 7874596

Gaudreau JD, Gagnon P: Psychotogenic drugs and delirium pathogenesis: the central role of the thalamus. Med Hypotheses 64(3):471–475, 2005 15617851

Gaudreau JD, Gagnon P, Harel F, et al: Fast, systematic, and continuous delirium assessment in hospitalized patients: the Nursing Delirium Screening Scale. J Pain Symptom Manage 29(4):368–375, 2005 15857740

Gleason OC: Donepezil for postoperative delirium. Psychosomatics 44(5):437–438, 2003 12954923

Hirao K, Ohnishi T, Matsuda H, et al: Functional interactions between entorhinal cortex and posterior cingulate cortex at the very early stage of Alzheimer's disease using brain perfusion single-photon emission computed tomography. Nucl Med Commun 27(2):151–156, 2006 16404228

Hshieh TT, Fong TG, Marcantonio ER, Inouye SK: Cholinergic deficiency hypothesis in delirium: a synthesis of current evidence. J Gerontol A Biol Sci Med Sci 63(7):764–772, 2008 18693233

Inouye SK: The dilemma of delirium: clinical and research controversies regarding diagnosis and evaluation of delirium in hospitalized elderly medical patients. Am J Med 97(3):278–288, 1994 8092177

Inouye SK, Charpentier PA: Precipitating factors for delirium in hospitalized elderly persons. Predictive model and interrelationship with baseline vulnerability. JAMA 275(11):852–857, 1996 8596223

Inouye SK, van Dyck CH, Alessi CA, et al: Clarifying confusion: the confusion assessment method. A new method for detection of delirium. Ann Intern Med 113(12):941–948, 1990 2240918

Inouye SK, Bogardus ST Jr, Charpentier PA, et al: A multicomponent intervention to prevent delirium in hospitalized older patients. N Engl J Med 340(9):669–676, 1999 10053175

Inouye SK, Foreman MD, Mion LC, et al: Nurses' recognition of delirium and its symptoms: comparison of nurse and researcher ratings. Arch Intern Med 161(20):2467–2473, 2001 11700159

Inouye SK, Baker DI, Fugal P, Bradley EH; HELP Dissemination Project: Dissemination of the hospital elder life program: implementation, adaptation, and successes. J Am Geriatr Soc 54(10):1492–1499, 2006 17038065

Inouye SK, Zhang Y, Jones RN, et al: Risk factors for delirium at discharge: development and validation of a predictive model. Arch Intern Med 167(13):1406–1413, 2007 17620535

Inouye SK, Westendorp RG, Saczynski JS: Delirium in elderly people. Lancet 383(9920):911–922, 2014 23992774

Jackson JC, Gordon SM, Hart RP, et al: The association between delirium and cognitive decline: a review of the empirical literature. Neuropsychol Rev 14(2):87–98, 2004 15264710

Larsen KA, Kelly SE, Stern TA, et al: Administration of olanzapine to prevent postoperative delirium in elderly joint-replacement patients: a randomized, controlled trial. Psychosomatics 51(5):409–418, 2010 20833940

Lauretani F, Ceda GP, Maggio M, et al: Capturing side-effect of medication to identify persons at risk of delirium. Aging Clin Exp Res 22(5-6):456–458, 2010 21422797

Neelon VJ, Champagne MT, Carlson JR, Funk SG: The NEECHAM Confusion Scale: construction, validation, and clinical testing. Nurs Res 45(6):324–330, 1996 8941300

Schor JD, Levkoff SE, Lipsitz LA, et al: Risk factors for delirium in hospitalized elderly. JAMA 267(6):827–831, 1992 1732655

Schuurmans MJ, Shortridge-Baggett LM, Duursma SA: The Delirium Observation Screening Scale: a screening instrument for delirium. Res Theory Nurs Pract 17(1):31–50, 2003 12751884

Trzepacz PT, Baker RW, Greenhouse J: A symptom rating scale for delirium. Psychiatry Res 23(1):89–97, 1988 3363018

Trzepacz PT, Mittal D, Torres R, et al: Validation of the Delirium Rating Scale-revised-98: comparison with the delirium rating scale and the cognitive test for delirium. J Neuropsychiatry Clin Neurosci 13(2):229–242, 2001 11449030

van Eijk MM, Roes KC, Honing ML, et al: Effect of rivastigmine as an adjunct to usual care with haloperidol on duration of delirium and mortality in critically ill patients: a multicentre, double-blind, placebo-controlled randomised trial. Lancet 376(9755):1829–1837, 2010 21056464

Wang W, Li HL, Wang DX, et al: Haloperidol prophylaxis decreases delirium incidence in elderly patients after noncardiac surgery: a randomized controlled trial. Crit Care Med 40(3):731–739, 2012 22067628

Wei LA, Fearing MA, Sternberg EJ, Inouye SK: The Confusion Assessment Method: a systematic review of current usage. J Am Geriatr Soc 56(5):823–830, 2008 18384586

Wengel SP, Roccaforte WH, Burke WJ: Donepezil improves symptoms of delirium in dementia: implications for future research. J Geriatr Psychiatry Neurol 11(3):159–161, 1998 9894735

Wong CL, Holroyd-Leduc J, Simel DL, Straus SE: Does this patient have delirium?: value of bedside instruments. JAMA 304(7):779–786, 2010 20716741

CHAPTER 8

Dementia and Mild Neurocognitive Disorders

8.1 Which of the following is the most common neuropsychiatric symptom in a patient presenting with a diagnosis of Parkinson's disease (PD)?

A. Depression.
B. Sleep fragmentation.
C. Visual hallucinations.
D. Rapid eye movement sleep behavior disorders.

The correct response is option C: Visual hallucinations.

Neuropsychiatric symptoms are common in PD both with and without dementia. These symptoms include depression, psychosis, anxiety, impulse control disorders, disorders of sleep and wakefulness, and apathy (Weintraub and Burn 2011). Visual hallucinations can be seen in up to 50% of patients (option C). Depression can be seen in up to 40% of patients (option A). Sleep disorders occur in up to 30% of patients and include rapid eye movement sleep behavior disorders (option D), nightmares, sleep fragmentation (option B), and daytime sleepiness. Persecutory delusions are also quite common. Many medications used to treat PD, such as anticholinergic agents, amantadine, dopaminergic agents, and catechol O-methyltransferase inhibitors, can exacerbate visual hallucinations and delusions. **(p. 204)**

8.2 Which of the following laboratory studies is recommended by the American Academy of Neurology and the National Institute for Health and Care Excellence for the basic workup of a patient with dementia?

A. Electrocardiogram
B. Toxicology.
C. Thyroid function tests.
D. Urinalysis.

The correct response is option C: Thyroid function tests.

A basic dementia screen typically involves laboratory studies and brain imaging. The American Academy of Neurology (Knopman et al. 2001) and the National Institute for Health and Care Excellence (2011) recommend obtaining a metabolic panel, liver function test, complete blood count, thyroid function studies (option C), vitamin B_{12} levels, and folate levels. In at-risk populations or if the clinical picture indicates, the clinician may consider additional tests, such as heavy metal screen, HIV, syphilis serology, toxicology (option B), electrocardiogram (option A), and chest radiograph, to determine possible underlying pathology. Electroencephalography is not part of a routine dementia workup unless frontotemporal lobar degeneration, Creutzfeldt-Jakob disease, or delirium is suspected. Urinalysis (option D) is useful when the clinician suspects delirium as part of the differential diagnosis. **(pp. 186–187)**

8.3   A stepwise progression with variable rates of decline is a hallmark feature in which of the following causes of dementia?

A. Lewy body disorders.
B. Cerebrovascular disease.
C. Alzheimer's disease (AD).
D. Frontotemporal lobar degeneration.

The correct response is option B: Cerebrovascular disease.

A stepwise progression with variable rates of decline is a hallmark feature of cerebrovascular disease (option B). Lewy body disorders (option A) have a progressive cognitive decline with fluctuating cognition. AD (option C) is characterized by a slow progressive cognitive and functional decline. Frontotemporal lobar degeneration (option D) has a progressive change in personality, behavior, and language and a more rapid rate of decline than with AD. **(Table 8–6, "The most common causes of dementia," p. 190)**

8.4   A 68-year-old man presents with early dementia, fluctuating level of consciousness, parkinsonism, and visual hallucinations. Which of the following is the most likely diagnosis?

A. Dementia due to Alzheimer's disease (AD).
B. Dementia with Lewy bodies (DLB).
C. Dementia due to frontotemporal lobar degeneration.
D. Parkinson disease dementia (PDD).

The correct response is option B: Dementia with Lewy bodies (DLB).

The early deficits in DLB are in attention, executive, and visuospatial abilities. Core features include fluctuating cognition with variations in attention and levels of alertness, recurrent well-formed visual hallucinations, and parkinsonian features. Suggestive features include rapid eye movement sleep behavior disorder, severe sensitivity to neuroleptics, and low dopamine transporter uptake in the basal ganglia as demonstrated on positron emission tomography or single-photon emission computed tomography imaging. The diagnostic criteria for probable DLB require one of the following:

- The presence of dementia plus at least two core features
- The presence of dementia plus one core feature and one suggestive feature

If dementia and parkinsonism coexist, the differential diagnosis is sorted out by examining the relative course of the cognitive and motor symptoms. The emergence of dementia after many years of motor symptoms supports a diagnosis of PDD (option D). In contrast, the early presence of dementia in a patient with motor parkinsonism supports a diagnosis of DLB (option B). Researchers use a 1-year interval between onset of PD and onset of dementia to differentiate PDD from DLB. A typical clinical pattern in a patient with AD (option A) displays loss of memory occurring fairly early, followed by the development of agnosia, apraxia, and aphasia. Patients also follow predictable progression in functional impairments and, in later stages, universally develop problems with mobility and continence. Neuropsychiatric symptoms are nearly universal. The most common presentation of frontotemporal lobar degeneration (option C) is the behavioral variant (bvFTLD) (Kertesz et al. 2007). It is characterized by progressive changes in personality and behavior, as well as cognitive dysfunction. Cognitive tests, such as the Mini-Mental State Examination, may not be able to reveal cognitive deficits early in the course of bvFTLD. Motor impairment syndromes co-occur. **(pp. 193, 195, 201, 202, 204; Table 8–6, "The most common causes of dementia," p. 190)**

8.5   Which of the following medications has been approved by the U.S. Food and Drug Administration for the treatment of cognitive symptoms in all stages of Alzheimer's disease (AD)?

A. Memantine.
B. Donepezil.
C. Galantamine.
D. Tacrine.

The correct response is option B: Donepezil.

Donepezil, rivastigmine, and galantamine are all approved for the treatment of mild to moderate AD. Donepezil and the patch preparation of rivastigmine are approved for the treatment of severe AD (option B; option C is incorrect). Memantine (option A) is approved for the treatment of moderate to severe AD. Tacrine (option D), the first agent approved for use in AD, is no longer available in the United States because it can cause hepatotoxicity, specifically a transient and reversible transaminitis. **(p. 217)**

8.6   Which of the following is an effective treatment modality for Alzheimer's disease (AD)?

A. Antihypertensive medications.
B. Folate.

C. *Ginkgo biloba.*
D. Anti-inflammatory agents.

The correct response is option A: Antihypertensive medications.

One of the most effective therapies for AD is the aggressive management of associated vascular risk factors such as blood pressure (particularly keeping systolic blood pressure below 160 mm Hg) (option A), high cholesterol, diabetes, obesity, and sedentary lifestyle (Mielke et al. 2007). As articulated in the principles of care of the American Association for Geriatric Psychiatry (Lyketsos et al. 2006), estrogen, anti-inflammatory agents (e.g., prednisone, nonsteroidal anti-inflammatory drugs) (option D), and *Ginkgo biloba* (option C) are not effective treatments for AD. Under investigation are the usefulness of other antioxidants (vitamins C and D), folate (option B) to reduce homocystinemia, and dietary modifications. **(p. 213)**

8.7 Which of the following medications, used for the treatment of cognitive symptoms of Alzheimer's dementia, is the least likely to cause bradycardia as a side effect?

A. Donepezil.
B. Galantamine.
C. Rivastigmine.
D. Memantine.

The correct response is option D: Memantine.

Nausea, vomiting, diarrhea, anorexia, weight loss, dyspepsia, insomnia, and vagotonic effects leading to bradycardia and heart block are common side effects of donepezil (option A), rivastigmine (option C), and galantamine (option B). Bradycardia is not a common side effect of memantine (option D); common side effects of memantine include dizziness, headache, confusion, constipation, and fatigue. **(Table 8–8, "FDA-approved medications available in the United States for the treatment of cognitive symptoms in Alzheimer's dementia," p. 218)**

8.8 Rivastigmine has been approved by the U.S. Food and Drug Administration (FDA) for the treatment of cognitive symptoms of Alzheimer's dementia. In what other condition causing dementia has the FDA approved the use of rivastigmine?

A. Vascular dementia.
B. Frontotemporal lobar degeneration
C. Parkinson's disease dementia (PDD).
D. Dementia with Lewy bodies (DLB).

The correct response is option C: Parkinson's disease dementia (PDD).

Although clinical trials have suggested that cholinesterase inhibitors may be of value in treating vascular dementia, none has been approved by the FDA for that purpose. The National Institute for Health and Care Excellence (2012) recommends that cholinesterase inhibitors and memantine should not be prescribed clinically for the treatment of cognitive decline in individuals with vascular dementia (option A). Although no cholinesterase inhibitors have demonstrated value in treating cognitive deficits in patients with frontotemporal lobar degeneration (option B), a medication trial is reasonable when the underlying cause of dementia is unclear. Both oral and transdermal preparations of rivastigmine have been approved for the treatment of mild to moderate dementia in PDD (option C). Cholinesterase inhibitors have been effective in treating cognitive impairment in DLB (option D), although this is considered an off-label use. **(p. 220)**

8.9   What antipsychotic medication is least likely to cause extrapyramidal side effects in a patient with dementia with Lewy bodies (DLB)?

A. Risperidone.
B. Clozapine.
C. Haloperidol.
D. Olanzapine.

The correct response is option B: Clozapine.

Patients with DLB present an additional challenge to antipsychotic therapy because they are extremely sensitive to the extrapyramidal side effects of all antipsychotics except clozapine (option B). Adverse events range from parkinsonism to acute dystonia to neuroleptic malignant syndrome. Clinicians should avoid use of conventional antipsychotics (options A, C, and D) in patients with DLB. **(pp. 226–227)**

8.10   Which of the following behaviors in a patient with dementia is most likely to benefit from the use of antipsychotic medications?

A. Agitation in the context of hallucinations.
B. Nighttime wakefulness and wandering.
C. Refusal of care.
D. Urinating in the trash.

The correct response is option A: Agitation in the context of hallucinations.

Antipsychotic medications are the core treatments of agitation (option A) and psychosis. In the Clinical Antipsychotic Trial of International Effectiveness—Alzheimer's Disease, risperidone and olanzapine showed the most, albeit modest, benefit of symptom reduction as assessed by various rating scales. Antipsychotics had no effect on other outcomes such as cognition, functioning, or quality of life (Sultzer et al. 2008). Psychotropic medications are unlikely to affect poor self-care or refusal of care (option C), memory problems, inattention, unfriendliness, repetitive verbalizations or questioning, shadowing, or wandering (option B) (Kales et al. 2014). They are also unlikely to improve behaviors that can ultimately be attributed to apraxia or agnosia (e.g., urinating in a trash can because it resembles a toilet bowl) (option D). **(pp. 223, 226)**

8.11   What agent has shown the best evidence for improving dementia-related apathy?

A. Antidepressants.
B. Antiepileptics.
C. Stimulants.
D. Cholinesterase inhibitors.

The correct response is option D: Cholinesterase inhibitors.

Cholinesterase inhibitors (option D) have the best evidence for improving or stabilizing apathy, with no clear indication that any one cholinesterase inhibitor is superior to the other (Berman et al. 2012). There is some evidence for modest benefits of memantine, mixed evidence for benefits of atypical antipsychotics, and no good evidence to support using antidepressants (option A), antiepileptics (option B), or traditional antipsychotics to treat apathy (Berman et al. 2012). Despite a perception that apathy is treatable with stimulants (option C), only a handful of small eligible trials of methylphenidate since 1975 have shown significant improvement. **(p. 229)**

References

Berman K, Brodaty H, Withall A, Seeher K: Pharmacologic treatment of apathy in dementia. Am J Geriatr Psychiatry 20(2):104–122, 2012 21841459

Kales HC, Gitlin LN, Lyketsos CG; Detroit Expert Panel on Assessment and Management of Neuropsychiatric Symptoms of Dementia: Management of neuropsychiatric symptoms of dementia in clinical settings: recommendations from a multidisciplinary expert panel. J Am Geriatr Soc 62(4):762–769, 2014 24635665

Kertesz A, Blair M, McMonagle P, Munoz DG: The diagnosis and course of frontotemporal dementia. Alzheimer Dis Assoc Disord 21(2):155–163, 2007 17545742

Knopman DS, DeKosky ST, Cummings JL, et al: Practice parameter: diagnosis of dementia (an evidence-based review). Report of the Quality Standards Subcommittee of the American Academy of Neurology. Neurology 56(9):1143–1153, 2001 11342678

Lyketsos CG, Colenda CC, Beck C, et al; Task Force of American Association for Geriatric Psychiatry: Position statement of the American Association for Geriatric Psychiatry regarding principles of care for patients with dementia resulting from Alzheimer disease. Am J Geriatr Psychiatry 14(7):561–572, 2006 16816009

Mielke MM, Rosenberg PB, Tschanz J, et al: Vascular factors predict rate of progression in Alzheimer disease. Neurology 69(19):1850–1858, 2007 17984453

National Institute for Health and Care Excellence: Donepezil, galantamine, rivastigmine and memantine for the treatment of Alzheimer's disease. Review of NICE technology appraisal guidance 117, 2011. Available at: http://guidance.nice.org.uk/TA217/Guidance/pdf/English. Accessed February 2014.

National Institute for Health and Care Excellence: Dementia: supporting people with dementia and their carers in health and social care. Clinical Guideline 42, 2012. Available at: http://publications.nice.org.uk/dementia-cg42/guidance#diagnosis-and-assessment-of-dementia. Accessed December 2013.

Sultzer DL, Davis SM, Tariot PN, et al; CATIE-AD Study Group: Clinical symptom responses to atypical antipsychotic medications in Alzheimer's disease: phase 1 outcomes from the CATIE-AD effectiveness trial. Am J Psychiatry 165(7):844–854, 2008 18519523

Weintraub D, Burn DJ: Parkinson's disease: the quintessential neuropsychiatric disorder. Mov Disord 26(6):1022–1031, 2011 21626547

CHAPTER 9

Depressive Disorders

9.1   Which of the following medications is considered first line of treatment for mild to moderate forms of depression?

A. Bupropion.
B. Trazodone.
C. Citalopram.
D. Nortriptyline.

The correct response is option C: Citalopram.

Citalopram (option C), escitalopram, fluoxetine, paroxetine, and sertraline have been shown to be effective in treating geriatric depression. These agents have become the drugs of first choice for treating mild to moderate forms of depression. Trazodone (option B) and bupropion (option A) are alternatives in patients who cannot tolerate tricyclic antidepressants (TCAs), selective serotonin reuptake inhibitors (SSRIs), or mixed agents like venlafaxine. TCAs (option D) are the agents of choice for some patients with more severe forms of major depression who can tolerate the side effects and do not respond to other medications. **(pp. 264, 265)**

9.2   Which of the following is the best modality of treatment for an older adult with psychotic depression?

A. Low dose of a stimulant.
B. Electroconvulsive therapy (ECT).
C. Antidepressant only.
D. St. John's wort.

The correct response is option B: Electroconvulsive therapy (ECT).

Meyers et al. (1984) studied the prevalence of delusions in 50 patients hospitalized for endogenous major depression. Individuals with delusional depression tended to be older and to respond to ECT (option B), as opposed to TCAs. Antidepressants (option C), specifically SSRIs, have become the drugs of first choice for treating mild to moderate forms of depression. Some clinicians prescribe low morning doses of stimulant medications (option A), such as 5 mg of methylphenidate, to improve mood in the apathetic older adult. St. John's wort (*Hypericum perforatum*) (option D) shows some antidepressant properties (Kasper et al. 2006) but has not been studied in elderly population. **(pp. 259, 264, 266, 628)**

9.3   Which of the following has proven to be the most robust predictor of late-life depression?

A. Religious involvement.
B. Perceived social support.
C. Personality pathology.
D. Cognitive distortions.

The correct response is option B: Perceived social support.

Social support is a multifactorial construct that includes perception, structure of the social network, and tangible help and assistance (Turner and Turner 1999). Perceived social support has proved to be the most robust predictor of late-life depressive symptoms (Bruce 2002) (option B). Investigators from Hong Kong, in a community study, found that depressive symptoms were associated with impaired social support (including network size, network composition, social contact frequency, satisfaction with social support, and instrumental-emotional support (Chi and Chou 2001). Personality pathology (option C) is a measurable phenomenon that is known to affect the outcome of major depression (Weissman et al. 1978). Unfortunately, there are no published reports of personality as a predictor of major depression outcome in elderly patients. Psychological factors, such as personality attributes, neuroticism, cognitive distortions (option D), and emotional control, may contribute to the onset of late-life depression but are not specific to the origins of depression in older individuals. Religious involvement (option A) also appears to be a predictor of faster recovery from depression in both community-dwelling and clinical samples of older adults (Braam et al. 1997; Koenig 2007; Koenig et al. 1998). **(pp. 248–249, 254, 256)**

9.4   Which one of the following stressors was more related to severe depressive symptoms in older adults in a community survey?

A. Death of a spouse.
B. Physical illness.
C. Divorce.
D. Difficulty with the law.

The correct response is option B: Physical illness.

Using a community survey, investigators at Duke University Medical Center attempted to untangle the different subtypes of depression in late life (Blazer et al. 1987). More than 1,300 older adults in urban and rural communities who were age 60 or older were screened for depressive symptomatology. Of the 27% reporting depressive symptoms, 19% had mild dysphoria only. Persons with symptomatic depression—that is, subjects with more severe depressive symptoms—made up 4% of the population. These individuals were primarily experiencing stressors, such as physical illness (option B) and stressful life events. Stressful events that are predictable or "on-time" events often cause less depression in older adults than in younger adults. Older adults, in contrast to younger adults, recognize that death of a spouse is expected (by observing their peers) and have actually rehearsed the event, such as by considering what they might do if a spouse dies (option A). Events that can lead to depression, such as divorce (option C) and difficulties with the law (option D), are more frequent early in life than in late life. In one study, significant difficulty with the law (something more serious than a traffic violation) was reported during the preceding year by 9% of younger adults but less than 1% of older individuals (Hughes et al. 1988). **(pp. 245, 255–256)**

9.5 Which of the following is a risk factor for the emergence of Alzheimer's disease in a depressed patient?

A. Frailty.
B. Poor social support.
C. Functional limitation.
D. Mild cognitive impairment.

The correct response is option D: Mild cognitive impairment.

Early depressive symptoms associated with mild cognitive impairment (option D) may represent a risk for impending Alzheimer's disease or vascular dementia (Li et al. 2001). Factors predicting partial remission were similar to those predicting no remission, and poor social support (option B) and functional limitations (option C) increased the risk for poor outcome (Hybels et al. 2005) but are not considered a risk for impending Alzheimer's disease. Frailty (option A), leading to profound weight loss, can contribute to clinically important depressive symptoms (Fried 1994). **(pp. 246–247)**

9.6 Which of the following medications is most associated with agitation in older adults?

A. Trazodone.
B. Doxepin.
C. Bupropion.
D. Fluoxetine.

The correct response is option C: Bupropion.

Bupropion can be effective in treating depression in elderly people but generally is used once other medications have proved ineffective. Bupropion therapy should be initiated at 75 mg twice daily, with an increase to 150 mg twice daily (not to exceed 150 mg in a single dose). Agitation is the most common side effect that troubles older adults (option C). For a significant number of older adults, SSRIs (option D) cause unacceptable effects, including excessive activation and disturbance of sleep, tremor, headache, significant gastrointestinal side effects, hyponatremia, and weight loss. Important advantages of the use of these drugs in treating elderly patients are the lack of anticholinergic, orthostatic, and cardiac side effects; lack of sedation; and safety in overdose. Trazodone (option A) has advantages over TCAs (option B) in that it is virtually free of anticholinergic effects, and it has advantages over the newer antidepressants in that it has strong sedative effects. Nevertheless, the drug is not without side effects, including excessive daytime sedation, priapism (occasionally), and significant orthostatic hypotension. **(pp. 264–265)**

9.7   Which of the following is the most common type of delusion in an older adult with a psychotic depression?

A. Nihilistic delusion.
B. Delusion of having an incurable disease.
C. Delusion of grandiosity.
D. Delusion of guilt.

The correct response is option B: Delusion of having an incurable disease.

Delusions of persecution or of having an incurable illness (option B) are more common than delusions associated with guilt (option D). Nihilistic delusions (delusions of nothingness) (option A) may occur more commonly in late life, but they are not the most common type of delusion. Delusions of grandiosity (option C) are associated more with bipolar disorder (manic episode) than with depression. **(pp. 258, 259)**

9.8   Which of the following adverse effects with electroconvulsive therapy is a risk for an older woman with osteoporosis?

A. Confusion.
B. Compression fractures.
C. Hypotension.
D. Amnesia.

The correct response is option B: Compression fractures.

In elderly patients, cardiovascular effects are of greatest concern and include premature ventricular contractions, ventricular arrhythmias, and transient systolic hypertension (option C). Confusion (option A) and amnesia (option D) often result after a treatment, but the duration of this confusional episode is brief. Compression fractures (option B) are a particular risk in older women because of high incidence of osteoporosis in the postmenopausal population. **(p. 268)**

9.9 Which of the following predictors of recovery is considered to predict faster recovery from depression for a community-dwelling patient?

A. Religious involvement.
B. Absence of substance abuse.
C. Current or recent employment.
D. Absence of major life events and serious medical illness.

The correct response is option A: Religious involvement.

Religious involvement (option A) appears to be a predictor of faster recovery from depression in both community-dwelling and clinical samples of older adults (Braam et al. 1997; Koenig 2007; Koenig et al. 1998). Other factors associated with improved outcome in late-life depression include a history of recovery from previous episodes, a family history of depression, female gender, extroverted personality, current or recent employment (option C), absence of substance abuse (option B), no history of major psychiatric disorder, less severe depressive symptomatology, and absence of major life events and serious medical illness (option D) (Baldwin and Jolley 1986; Cole et al. 1999; Post 1972). **(pp. 248–249)**

9.10 Which of the following tests is not indicated in the workup of a depressed older adult?

A. Thyroid-stimulating hormone.
B. Magnetic resonance imaging (MRI).
C. Vitamin B_{12}.
D. Biological markers.

The correct response is option D: Biological markers.

The laboratory workup of the depressed older adult is important. It should include a thyroid panel and determination of thyroid-stimulating hormone levels (option A). Because both depressive and cognitive symptoms can result from deficits in vitamin B_{12} (option C) or folate, it is important to obtain levels of these vitamins. No biological markers (option D) or tests are available to confirm the diagnosis of depression, yet some tests may assist in identifying subtypes of depression; for example, MRI scans (option B) for subcortical white matter hyperintensities can confirm the presence of vascular depression (Krishnan et al. 1988). **(p. 262)**

References

Baldwin RC, Jolley DJ: The prognosis of depression in old age. Br J Psychiatry 149(5):574–583, 1986 3814949

Blazer D, Hughes DC, George LK: The epidemiology of depression in an elderly community population. Gerontologist 27(3):281–287, 1987 3609795

Braam AW, Beekman AT, Deeg DJ, et al: Religiosity as a protective or prognostic factor of depression in later life; results from a community survey in the Netherlands. Acta Psychatr Scand 96(3):199–205, 1997 9296551

Bruce ML: Psychosocial risk factors for depressive disorders in late life. Biol Psychiatry 52(3):175–184, 2002 12182924

Chi I, Chou KL: Social support and depression among elderly Chinese people in Hong Kong. Int J Aging Hum Dev 52(3):231–252, 2001 11407488

Cole MG, Bellavance F, Mansour A: Prognosis of depression in elderly community and primary care populations: a systematic review and meta-analysis. Am J Psychiatry 156(8):1182–1189, 1999 10450258

Fried L: Frailty, in Principles of Geriatric Medicine and Gerontology, 3rd Edition. Edited by Hazzard W, Bierman E, Blas J, et al. New York, McGraw-Hill, 1994, pp 1149–1156

Hughes DC, Blazer DG, George LK: Age differences in life events: a multivariate controlled analysis. Int J Aging Hum Dev 27(3):207–220, 1988 3243654

Hybels CF, Blazer DG, Steffens DC: Predictors of partial remission in older patients treated for major depression: the role of comorbid dysthymia. Am J Geriatr Psychiatry 13(8):713–721, 2005 16085788

Kasper S, Anghelescu IG, Szegedi A, et al: Superior efficacy of St John's wort extract WS 5570 compared to placebo in patients with major depression: a randomized, double-blind, placebo-controlled, multi-center trial [ISRCTN77277298]. BMC Med 4:14, 2006 16796730

Koenig HG: Religion and remission of depression in medical inpatients with heart failure/pulmonary disease. J Nerv Ment Dis 195(5):389–395, 2007 17502804

Koenig HG, George LK, Peterson BL: Religiosity and remission of depression in medically ill older patients Am J Psychiatry 155(4):536–542, 1998 9546001

Krishnan KR, Goli V, Ellinwood EH, et al: Leukoencephalopathy in patients diagnosed as major depressive. Biol Psychiatry 23(5):529–533, 1988 3345325 [Erratum in: Biol Psychiatry 25(6)]

Li YS, Meyer JS, Thornby J: Longitudinal follow-up of depressive symptoms among normal versus cognitively impaired elderly. Int J Geriat Psychiatry 16(7):718–727, 2001 11466752

Lustman PJ, Griffith LS, Freedland KE, et al: Cognitive behavior therapy for depression in type 2 diabetes mellitus. A randomized, controlled trial. Ann Intern Med 129(8):613–621, 1998 9786808

Meyers BS, Kalayam B, Mei-Tal V: Late-onset delusional depression: a distinct clinical entity? J Clin Psychiatry 45(8):347–349, 1984 6746580

Post F: The management and nature of depressive illnesses in late life: a follow-through study. Br J Psychiatry 121(563):393–404, 1972 4342641

Turner R, Turner J: Social integration and support, in Handbook of Sociology of Mental Health. Edited by Aneshensel C, Phelan J. New York, Kluwer Academic, 1999, pp 301–319

Weissman MM, Prusoff BA, Klerman GL: Personality and the prediction of long-term outcome of depression. Am J Psychiatry 135(7):797–800, 1978 665790

CHAPTER 10

Bipolar and Related Disorders

10.1 Which of the following episodes must a patient experience to be diagnosed with bipolar I disorder?

A. Both depressed and manic episodes.
B. Depressed episode.
C. Hypomanic episode.
D. Manic episode.

The correct response is option D: Manic episode.

For a diagnosis of bipolar I disorder, the patient must have experienced at least one manic episode (option D)—that is, an alteration in mood that is euphoric, expansive, or irritable and is associated with increased energy. These changes must last for at least 1 week and be accompanied by three of the seven associated symptoms listed in DSM-5 (e.g., decreased need for sleep, racing thoughts, pressured speech, increased behaviors that may have high likelihood for bad outcome). It is not necessary for a patient to have experienced a depressive episode (options A and B) to be diagnosed with a bipolar disorder, although the vast majority of patients with bipolar disorders have experienced depression and many report it to be the most commonly experienced mood problem. For a diagnosis of bipolar II disorder, the patient must have experienced one or more major depressive episodes and at least one hypomanic episode (option C). **(pp. 283–284)**

10.2 How does the community prevalence of bipolar disorder in late life compare with the prevalence among younger cohorts?

A. The community prevalence of bipolar disorder in older cohorts is higher than that in younger cohorts.
B. The community prevalence of bipolar disorder in older cohorts is lower than that in younger cohorts.

C. The community prevalence of bipolar disorder in older cohorts is the same as that in younger cohorts.

D. The community prevalence of bipolar disorder in older cohorts has not been studied.

The correct response is option B: The community prevalence of bipolar disorder in older cohorts is lower than that in younger cohorts.

The Epidemiologic Catchment Area (ECA) study found that bipolar disorder for adults ages 65 years and older had a 1-year prevalence range of 0.0%–0.5%, with a cross-site mean of 0.1%. This was markedly lower than the prevalence among young (ages 18–44 years; 1.4%) and middle-age (ages 45–64 years; 0.4%) adults (option B; options A, C, and D are incorrect). Similarly, a large health maintenance organization administrative database review containing almost 300,000 unique individuals found a prevalence of 0.25% for bipolar disorder in persons ages 65 years and older and a prevalence rate of 0.46% in adults ages 40–64 years (Unützer et al. 1998). Additional studies (Chou et al. 2011; Hirschfeld et al. 2003; Klap et al. 2003) also revealed findings suggesting that the prevalence of bipolar disorder declines with age or in aging cohorts. Most of the large-scale prevalence surveys have excluded patients who were institutionalized in hospitals, nursing homes, or other residential treatment centers, likely resulting in underestimates. **(p. 285)**

10.3 Which of the following comorbid conditions has been identified as a risk factor for late-life mania?

A. Anxiety disorder.
B. Eating disorder.
C. Neurological illness.
D. Substance abuse.

The correct response is option C: Neurological illness.

Psychiatric comorbidity is frequently seen in patients with bipolar disorder and has been a major point of discussion in the literature on bipolar disorder, yet there is very little information about its presence in late-life bipolar disorder. There are no published reports on comorbid eating disorders (option B) or attention disorders. In a review of the national Veterans Health Administration database (Sajatovic et al. 2006) to examine the prevalence of dementia, posttraumatic stress disorder (PTSD), and anxiety disorders in older patients with bipolar disorder, 5.4% had PTSD and 9.4% had an anxiety disorder. In a separate study from the Netherlands of a cohort of elderly patients with bipolar disorder, comorbid anxiety disorders were relatively rare (e.g., 6-month prevalence of generalized anxiety disorder, 5%) (Dols et al. 2014) (option A). Comorbid lifetime alcohol dependence and abuse (option D) were 24.8% and 13.9% among those with bipolar disorder. In another study of bipolar patients hospitalized in a state psychiatric facility (Cassidy et al. 2001), nearly 60% had some history of lifetime substance abuse, but in the patients older than age 60, only 29% had a history of lifetime substance abuse. There have been more studies assessing the presence of comorbid medical problems than studies assessing psychiatric problems in late-life bipolar disorder. Depp and Jeste (2004) noted that the sample-weighted prevalence of comorbid neurological illness was 23.1%. Shulman et al. (1992) compared 50 geriatric patients hospitalized for mania with 50 age-matched patients hospitalized for unipolar depression. They found that the rates of neurological illness in manic patients were significantly higher (36% vs. 8%), suggesting that neurological disease (option C) is a risk factor for development of mania in late life. **(pp. 286–287)**

10.4 Which of the following psychiatric conditions is associated with the highest rate of type II diabetes?

A. Bipolar disorder in older psychiatric inpatients.
B. Bipolar disorder in mixed-age psychiatric inpatients.
C. Schizophrenia in older psychiatric inpatients.
D. Unipolar depression in older psychiatric inpatients.

The correct response is option A: Bipolar disorder in older psychiatric inpatients.

In a study of older psychiatric inpatients (Regenold et al. 2002), type II diabetes was present in 26% of those with bipolar disorder (option A), which is a much higher rate than in patients with unipolar depression (option D), patients with schizophrenia (option C), and inpatients with bipolar disorder in other studies (9.9% in mixed-age inpatient sample; Cassidy et al. 1999) (option B). Moreover, in another study (Dols et al. 2014), elderly patients with bipolar disorder had an average of 1.7 medical comorbid conditions, predominately hypertension (27.8%), arthrosis (29.1%), allergies (25.6%), and peripheral atherosclerotic disease (18.8%). Only 21.8% had no somatic illnesses. Metabolic syndrome was found in 28.7% of patients. **(p. 287)**

10.5 When comparing older and younger patients with bipolar disorder, which of the following is more common in younger patients?

A. Dementia.
B. Diabetes.
C. Medical comorbidity.
D. Substance abuse.

The correct response is option D: Substance abuse.

Dementia has become an increasing concern for older adults in general and possibly a special concern for older adults with bipolar disorder. Kocsis et al. (1993) followed 38 elderly patients with bipolar disorder treated with lithium and found that rates of cognitive and functional impairment (option A) were much higher than in the general population. Regenold et al. (2002) found that type II diabetes (option B) was present in 26% of older inpatients with bipolar disorder versus 9.9% in mixed-age inpatient sample (Cassidy et al. 1999). Medical comorbidity (option C) is also higher in older adults with bipolar disorder (Beyer et al. 2005), with special concern about neurological illness and diabetes. Cassidy et al. (2001) reviewed rates of substance abuse (option D) in patients hospitalized at a state psychiatric facility for bipolar disorder. Nearly 60% had some history of lifetime substance abuse, but in the patients older than age 60, only 29% had a history of lifetime substance abuse. **(pp. 286–288)**

10.6   How does the mortality rate for elderly patients with bipolar disorder compare with the mortality rate for elderly patients with unipolar depression?

A. The mortality rate for bipolar disorder is approximately a quarter of the mortality rate for unipolar depression.
B. The mortality rate for bipolar disorder is approximately half of the mortality rate for unipolar depression.
C. The mortality rate for bipolar disorder is approximately the same as the mortality rate for unipolar depression.
D. The mortality rate for bipolar disorder is approximately twice the mortality rate for unipolar depression.

The correct response is option D: The mortality rate for bipolar disorder is approximately twice the mortality rate for unipolar depression.

Ramsey et al. (2013) found that odds of mortality for patients with lifetime manic spectrum episodes were much higher (odds ratio 1.4) than for those with no lifetime manic spectrum episodes. Shulman et al. (1992) found that the mortality rate over a 10- to 15-year follow-up for elderly hospitalized patients with bipolar disorder was significantly higher than that of elderly hospitalized unipolar depressed patients (50% vs. 20%) (option D; options A, B, and C are incorrect), suggesting that mania appears to have a poorer prognosis and to be a more severe form of affective illness than unipolar depression. Dementia and poorer cognitive performance on neurological testing are possibly increased, or apparent earlier, in older adults with bipolar disorder. Medical comorbidity is also higher in older adults with bipolar disorder (Beyer et al. 2005), with special concern about neurological illness and diabetes. All of these problems may contribute to higher mortality rates for patients with bipolar disorder than for individuals without psychiatric illness and for unipolar depressed patients. **(p. 288)**

10.7   Which course for bipolar disorder is more frequently experienced in older adults compared with younger adults?

A. Depressive episode followed by a long latency period of 10–20 years before onset of mania.
B. Depressive episode followed by a short latency period of 1–2 years before onset of mania.
C. Manic episode followed by a long latency period of 10–20 years before onset of depression.

D. Manic episode followed by a short latency period of 1–2 years before onset of depression.

The correct response is option A: Depressive episode followed by a long latency period of 10–20 years before onset of mania.

Goodwin and Jamison (1990) reported that depression was the initial episode more often in older adults than in younger patients (options C and D). Various investigators have described a latency period of 10–20 years between first depressed episode and onset of mania (Broadhead and Jacoby 1990; Shulman and Post 1980; Shulman et al. 1992; Snowdon 1991; Stone 1989) (option A; option B is incorrect). Kessing (2006), in a study of Denmark's health care utilization, found that first psychiatric hospitalizations for older adults with bipolar disorder were much more likely to be for depressive episodes than for manic episodes. Furthermore, older adults with bipolar disorder appear to experience more mixed symptoms than the classic manic presentation (Post 1968; Spar et al. 1979). **(p. 288)**

10.8 Which cognitive functions are *least* affected by bipolar disorder?

A. Executive function.
B. Language.
C. Processing speed.
D. Verbal memory.

The correct response is option B: Language.

Cognitive dysfunctions are increasingly recognized as a core feature of bipolar disorder. The affected abilities are most often noted in assessments of executive function, verbal memory, and processing speed (option B; options A, C, and D are incorrect). These dysfunctions are not solely related to residual mood effects, drug effects, or other confounding factors but rather appear to be related to illness severity. They are also apparent in first-degree relatives. These findings have suggested that bipolar disorder may be associated with various neurobiological factors that may reflect a neurodegenerative process. Studies of older adults with bipolar disorder have found patterns similar to that of younger adults with bipolar disorder: deficits in executive functioning, working memory, verbal memory, attention, construction, and processing speed. **(p. 291)**

10.9 Which of the following neuroimaging findings has been most consistently associated with older patients with bipolar disorder?

A. Cortical atrophy on head computed tomography.
B. Hyperintensities on T_2-weighted magnetic resonance imaging (MRI).
C. Left-sided temporal lobe lesions on neuroimaging.
D. Smaller cortical sulcal widening on MRI.

The correct response is option B: Hyperintensities on T$_2$-weighted magnetic resonance imaging (MRI).

"Hyperintense" signals viewed on T$_2$-weighted MRI have been one of the earliest and most consistent neuroimaging findings in the study of bipolar disorder. The presence of hyperintensities not only is more common among patients with bipolar disorder than among control subjects (Dupont et al. 1995) but remains significantly more common when medical risk factors (e.g., hypertension, vascular disease) are controlled for (Altshuler et al. 1995; Hickie et al. 1995; McDonald et al. 1999). Specific studies of bipolar disorder in late life have consistently found a higher presence of hyperintensities in individuals with bipolar disorder than in control subjects (option B). Volumetric studies of total brain volumes for patients with bipolar disorder have shown only limited changes. Young et al. (1999) compared 30 geriatric manic patients with control subjects but did not find any difference in the ventricular-brain ratios (option A). They did note that subjects with bipolar disorder had greater cortical sulcal widening (option D). Research suggests that development of mania after right-sided lesions occurs more often when the basal region of the right temporal lobe is involved (Starkstein et al. 1990) (option C). **(pp. 292–294)**

10.10 For older patients presenting with new onset of mania, which of the following evaluations would be *least* likely to help inform etiology?

A. Family history.
B. Laboratory studies.
C. Medical and neurological examinations.
D. Review of medications.

The correct response is option A: Family history.

Because the onset of bipolar disorder in late life is relatively uncommon, every patient who presents with a new onset of mania should undergo a good medical evaluation, with special emphasis on the neurological examination (option C). Because older adults may be receiving a higher number of medications, these should be reviewed for possible temporal association (option D). A laboratory workup consisting of a thyroid panel and basic tests should also be completed (option B). Finally, consideration should be given to neuroimaging, especially if the presentation is associated with psychosis. Patients with early-onset illness may have an increased prevalence of close family members with affective disorders compared with patients who had later-onset illness (option A). **(pp. 290, 294)**

10.11 In a trial comparing lithium and valproate for treating late-life mania, how did lithium and valproate perform?

A. Lithium was not well tolerated.
B. Lithium led to greater reduction in mania scores.
C. Valproate was not well tolerated.
D. Valproate led to greater reduction in mania scores.

The correct response is option B: Lithium led to greater reduction in mania scores.

The National Institute for Mental Health commissioned a study to evaluate the efficacy and tolerability of lithium and valproate in late-life mania. Young et al. (2012) conducted a blinded trial of 224 patients with mania over age 60 who were administered either lithium or valproate. They found that both lithium and valproate were well tolerated (options A and C) and efficacious, but lithium was associated with greater reduction in mania scores (option B; option D is incorrect). **(p. 295)**

10.12 An older patient with bipolar disorder who has been maintained on lithium for many years presents to the emergency department with symptoms of lithium toxicity and a lithium level of 1.3. Which of the following is the most likely cause of the elevated lithium level?

A. The patient's lisinopril was discontinued.
B. The patient's naproxen was increased.
C. The patient's renal clearance increased with age.
D. The patient's theophylline was increased.

The correct response is option B: The patient's naproxen was increased.

Several factors can affect lithium levels. With aging, the renal clearance of lithium decreases (option C) and the elimination half-life increases (Foster 1992; Shulman et al. 1987; Sproule et al. 2000). Medications commonly prescribed to the elderly, such as thiazide diuretics, nonsteroidal anti-inflammatory agents (option B), and angiotensin-converting enzyme inhibitors (option A), can increase lithium concentrations. Other medications, such as theophylline, can decrease lithium concentrations (option D). **(p. 295)**

10.13 Which of the following symptoms is associated with commonly reported adverse effects of lithium in the elderly?

A. Cognitive impairment.
B. New onset of psoriasis.
C. Urinary retention.
D. Weight loss.

The correct response is option A: Cognitive impairment.

Commonly reported adverse effects of lithium in the elderly include cognitive impairment (option A), ataxia, urinary frequency (option C), weight gain (option D), edema, tremor, and worsening of psoriasis (option B) and arthritis. Because of adverse effects (including neurotoxicity) that can occur even at therapeutic levels, appropriate lithium serum levels in the elderly are largely determined by medical status, frailty, and conservative dosing (Sajatovic et al. 2005b; Young et al. 2004). **(p. 295)**

10.14 Which medication is the most prescribed medication treatment for elderly persons with bipolar disorder?

A. Carbamazepine.
B. Lamotrigine.
C. Lithium.
D. Valproate.

The correct response is option D: Valproate.

Since 2000 there has been a marked increase in the prescription of valproate for bipolar disorder, especially for elderly patients. Prescriptions for valproate for elderly patients with bipolar disorder increased while prescriptions of lithium decreased, so that valproate is now the most prescribed medication treatment for elderly persons with bipolar disorder (option D; options A, B, and C are incorrect). **(p. 296)**

10.15 An older patient will be starting valproate to treat mania. The patient is also on warfarin for atrial fibrillation and lamotrigine for seizure disorder. What should be considered for management of this patient when starting valproate?

A. As patients age, the free fraction of plasma valproate decreases.
B. The lamotrigine dose should be increased.
C. The warfarin dose should be increased.
D. Coagulation parameters should be monitored.

The correct response is option D: Coagulation parameters should be monitored.

As patients age, the elimination half-life of valproate may be prolonged and the free fraction of plasma valproate increases (option A). Valproate may affect other medications' effects. It can inhibit the metabolism of lamotrigine so that the dose of lamotrigine may need to be lowered to minimize side effects (option B). Valproate also may increase the unbound fraction of warfarin (option C); coagulation parameters should therefore be monitored in patients undergoing anticoagulation therapy (option D). **(p. 296)**

10.16 An elderly Hispanic woman with bipolar disorder has previously tried lithium and valproate with suboptimal response and tolerability. You are considering a trial of carbamazepine. Which laboratory test would not be a crucial part of the workup prior to starting carbamazepine in an older Hispanic woman?

A. Complete blood cell count.
B. Electrolytes.
C. Genetic blood test.
D. Liver enzymes.

The correct response is option C: Genetic blood test.

Before initiating carbamazepine, the physician should check liver enzymes (option D), electrolytes (option B), and complete blood cell count (option A). Because carbamazepine can also affect the heart's rhythm, an electrocardiogram should be considered. The U.S. Food and Drug Administration (2007) (FDA) has recommended that patients of Asian ancestry have a genetic blood test to identify an inherited variant of the human leukocyte antigen allele *HAL-B*1502* (found almost exclusively in people of Asian ancestry) before starting therapy (option C). Patients testing positive should not be treated with carbamazepine. **(pp. 296–297)**

10.17 Which of the following anticonvulsants may be associated with fewer cognitive side effects in older bipolar patients?

A. Carbamazepine.
B. Lamotrigine.
C. Topiramate.
D. Valproate.

The correct response is option B: Lamotrigine.

It has been suggested that lamotrigine (option B) may have fewer negative effects on cognition than other anticonvulsant medications (options A, C, and D), which may be important for some geriatric patients (Aldenkamp et al. 2003). **(pp. 297–298)**

10.18 When compared with lithium, lamotrigine has been demonstrated to significantly delay the time to intervention for any mood episode. In which type of mood recurrences specifically is lamotrigine most effective?

A. Depressive recurrences.
B. Manic recurrences.
C. Depressive recurrences in patients with depression associated with low cardiometabolic risk factors.
D. Depressive recurrences in patients with high level of manic symptoms.

The correct response is option A: Depressive recurrences.

Lamotrigine was approved by the FDA in 2003 for the maintenance phase of bipolar disorder. Sajatovic et al. (2005a) found that lamotrigine significantly delayed the time to intervention for any mood episode, whereas lithium and placebo did not. In a subanalysis of the type of mood episode that was more likely to recur, the authors found that lamotrigine was significantly more effective than lithium and placebo at increasing time to intervention for depressive recurrences (option A), but lithium performed much better in increasing time to intervention for manic episodes (option B). In a follow-up analysis evaluating clinical correlates of treatment response, Gildengers et al. 2012) noted that lamotrigine worked best in depressed patients with high cardiometabolic risk factors (option C) and a low level of manic symptoms with their depression (option D). **(p. 297)**

10.19 Which of the following antidepressants is more likely to induce mania in late life?

A. Amitriptyline.
B. Bupropion.
C. Citalopram.
D. Trazodone.

The correct response is option A: Amitriptyline.

In a retrospective study of elderly inpatients who had antidepressant-induced mania, Young et al. (2003) found that tricyclic antidepressants (option A) were more likely than other antidepressants (options B, C, and D) to induce manias in late life, suggesting that the use of selective serotonin reuptake inhibitors may be preferable in elderly patients. **(p. 298)**

10.20 Which of the following atypical antipsychotic agents has the most data to support its use in acute bipolar mania in late life?

A. Aripiprazole.
B. Clozapine.
C. Olanzapine.
D. Ziprasidone.

The correct response is option C: Olanzapine.

Beyer et al. (2001) reported on a pooled subanalysis of three double-blind, placebo-controlled acute bipolar mania clinical trials with olanzapine, focusing on subjects older than age 50 years. In comparison with placebo, olanzapine (option C) was found to be efficacious for the treatment of acute mania without any significant change in the side-effect profile. Information on quetiapine, risperidone, clozapine (option B), ziprasidone (option D), aripiprazole (option A), and asenapine is much more limited. Case reports and open-label studies in geriatric bipolar patient treatment are published for quetiapine, risperidone, clozapine, and asenapine. No published reports are currently available for ziprasidone or aripiprazole. **(pp. 298–299)**

References

Aldenkamp AP, De Krom M, Reijs R: Newer antiepileptic drugs and cognitive issues. Epilepsia 44(Suppl 4):21–29, 2003 12823566

Altshuler LL, Curran JG, Hauser P, et al: T2 hyperintensities in bipolar disorder: magnetic resonance imaging comparison and literature meta-analysis. Am J Psychiatry 152(8):1139–1144, 1995 7625460

Beyer JL, Siegal A, Kennedy JS, et al: Olanzapine, divalproex, and placebo treatment non-head-to-head comparisons of older adult acute mania. Presented at the annual meeting of the International Psychogeriatric Association, Nice, France, September 2001

Beyer J, Kuchibhatla M, Gersing K, Krishnan KR: Medical comorbidity in a bipolar outpatient clinical population. Neuropsychopharmacology 30(2):401–404, 2005 15536492

Broadhead J, Jacoby R: Mania in old age: a first prospective study. Int J Geriatr Psychiatry 5:215–222, 1990

Cassidy F, Ahearn E, Carroll BJ: Elevated frequency of diabetes mellitus in hospitalized manic-depressive patients. Am J Psychiatry 156(9):1417–1420, 1999 10484954

Cassidy F, Ahearn EP, Carroll BJ: Substance abuse in bipolar disorder. Bipolar Disord 3(4):181–188, 2001 11552957

Chou KL, Mackenzie CS, Liang K, Sareen J: Three-year incidence and predictors of first-onset of DSM-IV mood, anxiety, and substance use disorders in older adults: results from Wave 2 of the National Epidemiologic Survey on Alcohol and Related Conditions. J Clin Psychiatry 72(2):144–155, 2011 21382305

Depp CA, Jeste DV: Bipolar disorder in older adults: a critical review. Bipolar Disord 6(5):343–367, 2004 15383127

Dols A, Rhebergen D, Beekman A, et al: Psychiatric and medical comorbidities: results from a bipolar elderly cohort study. Am J Geriatr Psychiatry 22(11):1066–1074, 2014 24495405

Dupont RM, Jernigan TL, Heindel W, et al: Magnetic resonance imaging and mood disorders. Localization of white matter and other subcortical abnormalities. Arch Gen Psychiatry 52(9):747–755, 1995 7654126

Foster JR: Use of lithium in elderly psychiatric patients: a review of the literature. Lithium 3:77–93, 1992

Gildengers A, Tatsuoka C, Bialko C, et al: Correlates of treatment response in depressed older adults with bipolar disorder. J Geriatr Psychiatry Neurol 25(1):37–42, 2012 22467845

Goodwin FK, Jamison KR: Manic-Depressive Illness. New York, Oxford University Press, 1990

Hickie I, Scott E, Mitchell P, et al: Subcortical hyperintensities on magnetic resonance imaging: clinical correlates and prognostic significance in patients with severe depression. Biol Psychiatry 37(3):151–160, 1995 7727623

Hirschfeld RM, Lewis L, Vornik LA: Perceptions and impact of bipolar disorder: how far have we really come? Results of the national depressive and manic-depressive association 2000 survey of individuals with bipolar disorder. J Clin Psychiatry 64(2):161–174, 2003 12633125

Kessing LV: Diagnostic subtypes of bipolar disorder in older versus younger adults. Bipolar Disord 8(1):56–64, 2006 16411981

Klap R, Unroe KT, Unützer J: Caring for mental illness in the United States: a focus on older adults. Am J Geriatr Psychiatry 11(5):517–524, 2003 14506085

Kocsis JH, Shaw ED, Stokes PE, et al: Neuropsychologic effects of lithium discontinuation. J Clin Psychopharmacol 13(4):268–275, 1993 8376614

McDonald WM, Tupler LA, Marsteller FA, et al: Hyperintense lesions on magnetic resonance images in bipolar disorder. Biol Psychiatry 45(8):965–971, 1999 10386178

Post F: The factor of ageing in affective illness, in Recent Developments in Affective Disorders, Special Publication 2. Edited by Coppen A, Walk A. London, Royal Medico-Psychological Association, 1968, pp 105–116

Ramsey CM, Spira AP, Mojtabai R, et al: Lifetime manic spectrum episodes and all-cause mortality: 26-year follow-up of the NIMH Epidemiologic Catchment Area Study. J Affect Disord 151(1):337–342, 2013 23835104

Regenold WT, Thapar RK, Marano C, et al: Increased prevalence of type 2 diabetes mellitus among psychiatric inpatients with bipolar I affective and schizoaffective disorders independent of psychotropic drug use. J Affect Disord 70(1):19–26, 2002 12113916

Sajatovic M, Gyulai L, Calabrese JR, et al: Maintenance treatment outcomes in older patients with bipolar I disorder. Am J Geriatr Psychiatry 13(4):305–311, 2005a 15845756

Sajatovic M, Madhusoodanan S, Coconcea N: Managing bipolar disorder in the elderly: defining the role of the newer agents. Drugs Aging 22(1):39–54, 2005b 15663348

Sajatovic M, Blow FC, Ignacio RV: Psychiatric comorbidity in older adults with bipolar disorder. Int J Geriatr Psychiatry 21(6):582–587, 2006 16783798

Shulman K, Post F: Bipolar affective disorder in old age. Br J Psychiatry 136:26–32, 1980 7357218

Shulman KI, Mackenzie S, Hardy B: The clinical use of lithium carbonate in old age: a review. Prog Neuropsychopharmacol Biol Psychiatry 11(2-3):159–164, 1987 3114827

Shulman KI, Tohen M, Satlin A, et al: Mania compared with unipolar depression in old age. Am J Psychiatry 149(3):341–345, 1992 1536272

Snowdon J: A retrospective case-note study of bipolar disorder in old age. Br J Psychiatry 158:485–490, 1991 2054563

Spar JE, Ford CV, Liston EH: Bipolar affective disorder in aged patients. J Clin Psychiatry 40(12):504–507, 1979 500573

Sproule BA, Hardy BG, Shulman KI: Differential pharmacokinetics of lithium in elderly patients. Drugs Aging 16(3):165–177, 2000 10803857

Starkstein SE, Mayberg HS, Berthier ML, et al: Mania after brain injury: neuroradiological and metabolic findings. Ann Neurol 27(6):652–659, 1990 2360802

Stone K: Mania in the elderly. Br J Psychiatry 155:220–224, 1989 2597918

Unützer J, Simon G, Pabiniak C, et al: The treated prevalence of bipolar disorder in a large staff-model HMO. Psychiatr Serv 49(8):1072–1078, 1998 9712215

U.S. Food and Drug Administration: Carbamazepine prescribing information to include recommendation of genetic test for patients with Asian ancestry. FDA News, December 12, 2007. Available at http://www.fda.gov/bbs/topics/NEWS/2007/NEW01755.html. Accessed February 17, 2008.

Young RC, Nambudiri DE, Jain H, et al: Brain computed tomography in geriatric manic disorder. Biol Psychiatry 45(8):1063–1065, 1999 10386193

Young RC, Jain H, Kiosses DN, Meyers BS: Antidepressant-associated mania in late life. Int J Geriatr Psychiatry 18(5):421–424, 2003 12766919

Young RC, Gyulai L, Mulsant BH, et al: Pharmacotherapy of bipolar disorder in old age: review and recommendations. Am J Geriatr Psychiatry 12(4):342–357, 2004 15249272

Young RC, Mulsant BH, Sajatovic M, et al: GERI-BD: A randomized, double-blind controlled trial of lithium and divalproex in the treatment of mania in older patients with bipolar disorder, Session presentation at the American Association of Geriatric Psychiatrists, San Antonio, TX, 2012

CHAPTER 11

Schizophrenia Spectrum and Other Psychotic Disorders

11.1 When Alzheimer's disease (AD) patients with psychosis are compared with those without psychosis, which of the following is most likely to be found?

A. More rapid cognitive decline in those with psychosis.
B. Lower rates of agitation in those with psychosis.
C. A family history of dementia in those with psychosis.
D. A family history of prior psychiatric illness in those with psychosis.

The correct response is option A: More rapid cognitive decline in those with psychosis.

AD patients with psychosis and those without psychosis differ in several important ways. Neuropsychologically, AD patients with psychosis have shown greater impairment in executive functioning, more rapid cognitive decline (Jeste et al. 1992; Stern et al. 1994) (option A), and greater prevalence of extrapyramidal symptoms (Stern et al. 1994). Patients with psychosis of AD tend to have a greater risk of agitation (option B) and greater likelihood of being institutionalized than patients with AD without psychosis. Some studies found a significant association between psychosis and age, age at onset of AD, and illness duration; however, gender, education, and family history of dementia (option C) or psychiatric illness (option D) showed weak or inconsistent relationships with psychosis. **(pp. 315–316, 324)**

11.2 Which of the following neurocognitive disorders is least likely to be associated with psychotic symptoms?

A. Lewy body dementia.
B. Parkinson's disease.
C. Vascular dementia.
D. Normal pressure hydrocephalus.

The correct response is option D: Normal pressure hydrocephalus.

Psychosis is common in several neurocognitive disorders. Visual hallucinations and secondary delusions are common in Lewy body disease (option A), and vascular neurocognitive disorder (option C) may also be accompanied by delusions or hallucinations (Schneider 1999). Naimark et al. (1996) found psychotic symptoms in approximately one-third of a sample of patients with Parkinson's disease (option B), with hallucinations being more common than delusions. Patients with normal pressure hydrocephalus (option D) most commonly present with memory impairment, gait disturbance, and urinary incontinence and rarely present with predominant psychotic symptoms. **(p. 317; Table 6–2, "Clinical neurocognitive syndromes and associated neuropsychological profiles," p. 137)**

11.3   Recommended adjunctive psychosocial treatment for elderly individuals with schizophrenia includes which of the following?

A. Sensory enhancement.
B. Daily structured activities.
C. Cognitive-behavioral social skills training.
D. Social contact.

The correct response is option C: Cognitive-behavioral social skills training.

Over the past decade, effective psychosocial interventions for older adults with chronic psychotic disorders have been developed. Granholm et al. (2005) conducted a randomized controlled trial to examine the effects of adding cognitive-behavioral social skills training (CBSST) to treatment as usual for 76 middle-aged and elderly stable outpatients with schizophrenia. The investigators found that CBSST (option C) led to significantly increased frequency of social functioning activities, greater cognitive insight (more objectivity in reappraising psychotic symptoms), and greater skill mastery. Sensory enhancement (option A), social contact (option D), and daily structured activities (option B) are recommended as adjunctive treatment for patients with psychosis of AD rather than elderly individuals with schizophrenia. **(p. 320; Table 11–2, "Comparison of psychosis of Alzheimer's disease (AD) with schizophrenia in older patients," p. 316)**

11.4   Which of the following is a distinguishing factor for late-onset schizophrenia as compared with early-onset illness?

A. Increased likelihood of first-degree relatives with a psychotic spectrum disorder.
B. Greater portion of women affected as compared to men.
C. Higher average antipsychotic dose requirement.
D. Increased severity of positive symptoms including hallucinations and delusions.

The correct response is option B: Greater portion of women affected as compared to men.

Risk factors and clinical presentation associated with late-onset schizophrenia are similar to those associated with early-onset schizophrenia, including a family history of schizophrenia (Brodaty et al. 1999; Jeste et al. 1995) (option A). Distinguishing factors of patients with late-onset illness (onset after age 40 years) include lower average severity of positive symptoms (option D) and lower average antipsychotic dose requirement (option C). Women are overrepresented among the late-onset patients (option B). It has been speculated that estrogen may serve as an endogenous antipsychotic, masking schizophrenic symptoms in vulnerable women until after menopause (Seeman 1996). **(pp. 311–313, 323)**

11.5   In choosing a medication to treat hallucinations due to neurocognitive disorders, why might a provider choose olanzapine over haloperidol?

A. Olanzapine has a U.S. Food and Drug Administration (FDA) indication for psychosis caused by Alzheimer's disease.
B. Olanzapine has a lower risk of extrapyramidal side effects compared with haloperidol.
C. Olanzapine has a lower risk of mortality compared with treatment with haloperidol.
D. There is no increased risk of stroke with use of olanzapine.

The correct response is option B: Olanzapine has a lower risk of extrapyramidal side effects compared with haloperidol.

Atypical antipsychotics have for the most part replaced conventional antipsychotics in treating psychosis, aggression, and agitation in patients with neurocognitive disorders because of greater perceived tolerability, lower risk for acute extrapyramidal symptoms (option B), and comparatively lower risk of tardive dyskinesia. Most antipsychotics that are prescribed for older adults are for behavioral disturbances associated with neurocognitive disorders, despite their lacking this FDA-approved indication (Weiss et al. 2000) (option A). However, the use of atypical antipsychotics in elderly patients with dementia has been associated with both cerebrovascular adverse events (option D) and death (option C), leading to black box warnings by the FDA. **(pp. 321–322)**

11.6   Compared with patients with early- or late-onset schizophrenia, patients with very-late-onset schizophrenia-like psychosis (VLOSLP) are characterized by which of the following factors?

A. Increased predominance of negative symptoms.
B. Onset after 50 years of age.
C. Decreased risk of tardive dyskinesia.
D. Decreased early childhood maladjustment.

The correct response is option D: Decreased early childhood maladjustment.

VLOSLP represents a heterogeneous clinical condition with psychotic symptoms beginning after age 60 (option B). Factors distinguishing individuals with VLOSLP from "true" schizophrenia include a smaller genetic load, less evidence of early childhood maladjustment (option D), a relative lack of thought disorder and negative symptoms (including blunted affect) (option A), a greater risk of tardive dyskinesia (option C), and evidence of a neurodegenerative rather than a neurodevelopmental process (Andreasen 1999; Howard et al. 1997). **(pp. 313, 324)**

11.7   A 65-year-old woman with no prior psychiatric history and intact cognitive function develops a delusion that neighbors are poisoning her garden. Which of the following is true about older patients with delusional disorder?

A. There is higher prevalence of illness among men than among women.
B. Average age of onset is between ages 30 and 40 years.
C. Social functioning is typically preserved.
D. There is an increased risk with family history of schizoid personality disorder.

The correct response is option D: There is an increased risk with family history of schizoid personality disorder.

The patient described is likely suffering from a delusional disorder of the persecutory type. There are no significant gender differences in the prevalence of delusional disorder (option A), and the average age at onset is 40–49 years for men and 60–69 years for women (option B). When delusional disorder arises in late life, basic personality features, intellectual performance, and occupational function are preserved, but social functioning is compromised (option C). Risk factors for delusional disorder include a family history of schizophrenia or avoidant, paranoid, or schizoid personality disorder (option D). Immigration and low socioeconomic status may be risk factors for development of delusional disorder. **(pp. 314–315)**

11.8   Current treatment guidelines recommend what treatment as a first-line approach for an 85-year-old woman with major neurocognitive disorder whose family complains she is hallucinating and seeing little children in the room?

A. Atypical antipsychotic.
B. Typical antipsychotic.
C. Behavioral intervention.
D. Selective serotonin reuptake inhibitor.

The correct response is option C: Behavioral intervention.

Because of the concerns about safety and effectiveness of antipsychotic medications (options A and B) and the lack of alternative FDA-approved pharmacotherapies (option D) for treating psychosis in patients with dementia, most current treatment guidelines recommend nonpharmacological treatment of symptoms (option C) as a first-line approach to management of these symptoms unless more aggressive management is deemed necessary to preserve safety. **(p. 323)**

11.9   Which of the following is associated with poorer functional capacity in older patients with schizophrenia?

A. High education level.
B. Positive symptoms.
C. Negative symptoms.
D. Good performance on neuropsychological testing.

The correct response is option C: Negative symptoms.

Among community-dwelling older outpatients with schizophrenia, cognitive functioning seems to remain relatively stable, other than the changes expected from normal aging (Heaton et al. 2001). In general, worse neuropsychological test performance (option D), lower educational level (option A), and negative symptoms (option C) but not positive symptoms (option B) are associated with poorer functional capacity in older outpatients with schizophrenia (Evans et al. 2003). **(pp. 310–311)**

11.10   What is the prevalence of schizophrenia among elderly individuals?

A. 0.1%–0.5%.
B. 2.5%.
C. 5.5%.
D. 10.1%.

The correct response is option A: 0.1%–0.5%.

Delusions, hallucinations, and other psychotic symptoms can accompany a number of conditions in late life. These symptoms may be more common than previously thought; Swedish investigators found that in a sample of 85-year-old people, the prevalence of psychotic symptoms was 10.1% (option D), with 6.9% experiencing hallucinations, 5.5% having delusions, and 6.9% experiencing paranoid ideation (Ostling and Skoog 2002). The prevalence of schizophrenia is approximately 0.6% among adults ages 45–64 and 0.1%–0.5% among elderly individuals (option A) (Castle and Murray 1993; Copeland et al. 1998; Keith et al. 1991). According to DSM-5, the lifetime prevalence of delusional disorder is estimated to be 0.2% and the most common subtype is persecutory. In the landmark Epidemiologic Catchment Area study conducted in the 1980s, the 1-month estimate of the prevalence of affective disorders in persons ages 65 years and older was 2.5% (option B) compared with 6.4% for persons ages 25–44 years (Regier et al. 1988). All disorders, with the exception of cognitive impairment, were more prevalent in younger or middle-aged adults than in older adults. Of those ages 65 and older, the two most prevalent disorders in this age group were any anxiety disorder (5.5%) (option C) and severe cognitive impairment (4.9%) (Regier et al. 1988). **(pp. 6, 8, 309, 310, 314)**

11.11 The FDA issued a black box warning for elderly patients with dementia treated with antipsychotics because of an increased risk of what compared with those treated with placebo?

A. Death.
B. Metabolic syndrome.
C. Fractures.
D. Aggression.

The correct response is option A: Death.

In May 2004, the FDA issued a black box warning that elderly patients with dementia treated with atypical antipsychotic drugs are at an increased risk for death (option A) compared with those treated with placebo. Data from a study by Jin et al. (2012) raise serious concerns about the longer-term safety and effectiveness of atypical antipsychotics in middle-aged and older adults, showing a high 1-year cumulative incidence of metabolic syndrome (36% in 1 year), but there is no black box warning for this (option B). In older adults serotonergic agents are associated with adverse events, including fractures, but there is no black box warning (option C). Atypical antipsychotics are used to help treat aggression in patients with neurocognitive disorder (option D). Because of the risk of use of antipsychotics in elderly patients with neurocognitive disorders, using the lowest effective dose and attempting dose reduction is recommended. **(pp. 227, 319, 322)**

11.12 Studies have found poorer self-assessed quality of life in persons with schizophrenia to be associated with all but which of the following?

A. Poor social skills.
B. Depression.
C. Lack of negative symptoms.
D. Financial instability.

The correct response is option C: Lack of negative symptoms.

Self-appraisal is considered to be essential in studies of quality of life for patients with schizophrenia. Several studies have found poorer self-assessed quality of life to be associated with depression (option B), positive and negative symptoms (option C), cognitive deficits, financial strain (option D), poor social support, and poor social skills (option A) (Vahia et al. 2007). These findings suggest that a multimodal approach to management of these patients is necessary to improve quality of life. **(p. 311)**

11.13 Compared with younger adults, how does pharmacotherapy of older adults with chronic psychotic disorders differ?

A. There are no randomized controlled trials conducted in older adults.
B. Maintenance pharmacotherapy should be avoided.

C. Recommended starting and maintenance doses are lower than doses in younger adults.

D. The risk of side effects with antipsychotics is equal in both younger and older adults.

The correct response is option C: Recommended starting and maintenance doses are lower than doses in younger adults.

Pharmacotherapy for older adults with chronic psychotic disorders can be challenging. A few randomized, placebo-controlled, double-blind clinical trials have been conducted in this population (option A). Maintenance pharmacotherapy is usually required for older patients with schizophrenia due to risk of relapse (option B). Because older patients are at higher risk of adverse antipsychotic effects (option D), due to age-related pharmacokinetic and pharmacodynamic factors (Hämmerlein et al. 1998), coexisting medical illnesses, and concomitant medications, the recommended starting and maintenance doses of antipsychotics in older adults are much lower than the usual doses in younger adults (option C). Patients with late-onset schizophrenia respond well to low-dose antipsychotic medication, requiring about 50% of the dose typically taken by older patients with early-onset schizophrenia and 25%–33% of the dose used in younger patients with schizophrenia. **(pp. 317–318)**

11.14 What makes the use of typical antipsychotics problematic in older adults?

A. There is a higher incidence of tardive dyskinesia in older patients compared with younger patients.

B. Higher dose of medication should be used for treatment.

C. There is a higher incidence of metabolic side effects compared with atypical antipsychotics.

D. They are less efficacious than atypical antipsychotics.

The correct response is option A: There is a higher incidence of tardive dyskinesia in older patients compared with younger patients.

Use of conventional or typical antipsychotics in older adults is problematic because of the higher incidence of tardive dyskinesia in older patients (option A). Aging appears to be the most important risk factor for the development of tardive dyskinesia (American Psychiatric Association 2000; Yassa and Jeste 1992). Other side effects of conventional neuroleptics include sedation, anticholinergic effects, cardiovascular effects including orthostatic hypotension, parkinsonian reactions, and neuroleptic malignant syndrome. Patients with late-onset schizophrenia respond well to low-dose antipsychotic medication (option B). Compared with typical antipsychotics, atypical antipsychotics have a less favorable side-effect profile in terms of metabolic function (option C). However, atypical antipsychotics carry a much lower risk of tardive dyskinesia than conventional neuroleptics, even when taken by very high-risk patients such as middle-aged and older adults with borderline tardive dyskinesia (Dolder and Jeste 2003; Jeste et al. 1999). Few efficacy comparisons have been done of conventional antipsychotics versus atypical antipsychotics in patients with schizophrenia over age 65. In a study of 42 elderly inpatients, Howanitz et al. (1999) found that clozapine (≤300 mg/day) and chlorpromazine (≤600 mg/day) had similar efficacy (option D). The National Institute of Mental Health's Clinical Antipsychotic Trials of Intervention Effectiveness (CATIE) study (Lieberman et al. 2005), which included adults age 18-65, found no significant differences in effectiveness between the conventional antipsychotic perphenazine and the atypical antipsychotics risperidone, olanzapine, quetiapine, or ziprasidone but it is unknown how these findings would translate to patients older than age 65. **(pp. 318–319)**

11.15 Which antipsychotic does not have evidence supporting the reduction of tardive dyskinesia in patients with preexisting tardive dyskinesia?

A. Clozapine.
B. Risperidone.
C. Olanzapine.
D. Quetiapine.

The correct response is option D: Quetiapine.

Atypical antipsychotics carry a much lower risk of tardive dyskinesia than conventional neuroleptics, even when taken by very high-risk patients such as middle-aged and older adults with borderline tardive dyskinesia (Dolder and Jeste 2003; Jeste et al. 1999). Clozapine (option A) has shown efficacy in reducing tardive dyskinesia in patients with existing tardive dyskinesia (Kane et al. 1993; Lieberman et al. 1999; Simpson et al. 1978; Small et al. 1987). A beneficial effect of other atypical agents, specifically risperidone (option B) and olanzapine (option C), on preexisting tardive dyskinesia has also been reported (Jeste et al. 1997; Kinon et al. 2004; Littrell et al. 1998; Street et al. 2000). Quetiapine (option D) was not found to be efficacious in patients with tardive dyskinesia in two double-blind trials (Kurlan et al. 2007; Rabey et al. 2007). **(pp. 318, 550)**

References

American Psychiatric Association: Diagnostic and Statistical Manual of Mental Disorders, 4th Edition, Text Revision. Washington, DC, American Psychiatric Association, 2000

Andreasen NC: I don't believe in late-onset schizophrenia, in Late-Onset Schizophrenia. Edited by Howard R, Rabins PV, Castle DJ. Philadelphia, PA, Wrightson Biomedical, 1999, pp 111–123

Brodaty H, Sachdev P, Rose N, et al: Schizophrenia with onset after age 50 years, I: phenomenology and risk factors. Br J Psychiatry 175:410–415, 1999 10789270

Castle DJ, Murray RM: The epidemiology of late-onset schizophrenia. Schizophr Bull 19(4):691–700, 1993 8303220

Copeland JRM, Dewey ME, Scott A, et al: Schizophrenia and delusional disorder in older age: community prevalence, incidence, comorbidity, and outcome. Schizophr Bull 24(1):153–161, 1998 9502553

Dolder CR, Jeste DV: Incidence of tardive dyskinesia with typical versus atypical antipsychotics in very high risk patients. Biol Psychiatry 53(12):1142–1145, 2003 12814866

Evans JD, Heaton RK, Paulsen JS, et al: The relationship of neuropsychological abilities to specific domains of functional capacity in older schizophrenia patients. Biol Psychiatry 53(5):422–430, 2003 12614995

Granholm E, McQuaid JR, McClure FS, et al: A randomized, controlled trial of cognitive behavioral social skills training for middle-aged and older outpatients with chronic schizophrenia. Am J Psychiatry 162(3):520–529, 2005 15741469

Hämmerlein A, Derendorf H, Lowenthal DT: Pharmacokinetic and pharmcodynamic changes in the elderly. Clinical implications. Clin Pharmacokinet 35(1):49–64, 1998 9673834

Heaton RK, Gladsjo JA, Palmer BW, et al: Stability and course of neuropsychological deficits in schizophrenia. Arch Gen Psychiatry 58(13):24–32, 2001 11146755

Howard RJ, Graham C, Sham P, et al: A controlled family study of late-onset non-affective psychosis (late paraphrenia). Br J Psychiatry 170:511–514, 1997 9330015

Howanitz E, Pardo M, Smelson DA, et al: The efficacy and safety of clozapine versus chlorpromazine in geriatric schizophrenia. J Clin Psychiatry 60(1):41–44, 1999 10074877

Jeste DV, Wragg RE, Salmon DP, et al: Cognitive deficits of patients with Alzheimer's disease with and without delusions. Am J Psychiatry 149(2):184–189, 1992 1734737

Jeste DV, Harris MJ, Krull A, et al: Clinical and neuropsychological characteristics of patients with late-onset schizophrenia. Am J Psychiatry 152(5):722–730, 1995 7726312

Jeste DV, Klausner M, Brecher M, et al: A clinical evaluation of risperidone in the treatment of schizophrenia: a 10-week, open-label, multicenter trial. ARCS Study Group. Assessment of Risperdal in a Clinical Setting. Psychopharmacology (Berl) 131:239–247, 1997 9203234

Jeste DV, Lacro JP, Bailey A, et al: Lower incidence of tardive dyskinesia with risperidone compared with haloperidol in older patients. J Am Geriatr Soc 47(6):716–719, 1999 10366172

Jin H, Shih PA, Golshan S, et al: Comparison of longer-term safety and effectiveness of 4 atypical antipsychotics in patients over age 40: a trial using equipoise-stratified randomization. J Clin Psychiatry 74(1):10–18, 2012 23218100

Kane JM, Woerner MG, Pollack S, et al: Does clozapine cause tardive dyskinesia? J Clin Psychiatry 54(9):327–330, 1993 8104929

Keith SJ, Regier DA, Rae DS: Schizophrenic disorders, in Psychiatric Disorders in America: the Epidemiologic Catchment Area Study. Edited by Robins LN, Regier DA. New York, Free Press, 1991, pp 33–52

Kinon BJ, Jeste DV, Kollack-Walker S, et al: Olanzapine treatment for tardive dyskinesia in schizophrenia patients: a prospective clinical trial with patients randomized to blinded dose reduction periods. Biol Psychiatry 28(6):985–996, 2004 15380859

Kurlan R, Cummings J, Raman R, Thal L; Alzheimer's Disease Cooperative Study Group: Quetiapine for agitation or psychosis in patients with dementia and parkinsonism. Neurology 68(17):1356–1363, 2007 17452579

Lieberman JA, Saltz BL, Johns CA, et al: The effects of clozapine on tardive dyskinesia. Br J Psychiatry 158:503–510, 1999 1675900

Lieberman JA, Stroup TS, McEvoy JP, et al: Effectiveness of antipsychotic drugs in patients with chronic schizophrenia. N Engl J Med 353(12):1209–1223, 2005 16172203

Littrell KH, Johnson CG, Littrell S, Peabody CD: Marked reduction of tardive dyskinesia with olanzapine. Arch Gen Psychiatry 55(3):279–280, 1998 9510225

Naimark D, Jackson E, Rockwell E, Jeste DV: Psychotic symptoms in Parkinson's disease patients with dementia. J Am Geriatr Soc 44(3):296–299, 1996 8600200

Ostling S, Skoog I: Psychotic symptoms and paranoid ideation in a nondemented population-based sample of the very old. Arch Gen Psychiatry 59(1):53–59, 2002 11779282

Rabey JM, Prokhorov T, Miniovitz A, et al: Effect of quetiapine in psychotic Parkinson's disease patients: a double-blind labeled study of 3 months' duration. Mov Disord 22(3):313–318, 2007 17034006

Regier DA, Boyd JH, Burke JD Jr, et al: One-month prevalence of mental disorders in the United States. Based on five Epidemiologic Catchment Area sites. Arch Gen Psychiatry 45(11):977–986, 1988 3263101

Schneider LS: Pharmacologic management of psychosis in dementia. J Clin Psychiatry 60(suppl 8):54–60, 1999 10335671

Seeman MV: The role of estrogen in schizophrenia. J Psychiatry Neurosci 21(3):123–127, 1996 8820178

Simpson GM, Lee JH, Shrivastava RK, et al: Clozapine in tardive dyskinesia. Psychopharmacology (Berl) 56(1):75–80, 1978 415329

Small JG, Milstein V, Marhenke JD, et al: Treatment outcome with clozapine in tardive dyskinesia, neuroleptic sensitivity, and treatment-resistant psychosis. J Clin Psychiatry 48(7):263–267, 1987 2885310

Stern Y, Albert M, Brandt J, et al: Utility of extrapyramidal signs and psychosis as predictors of cognitive and functional decline, nursing home admission, and death in Alzheimer's disease: prospective analyses from the Predictors Study. Neurology 44(12):2300–2307, 1994 7991116

Street JS, Tollefson GD, Tohen M, et al: Olanzapine for psychotic conditions in the elderly. Psychiatric Ann 30:191–196, 2000

Vahia I, Bankole AO, Reyes P, et al: Schizophrenia in later life. Aging Health 3:383–396, 2007

Weiss E, Hummer M, Killer D, et al: Off-label use of antipsychotic drugs. J Clin Psychopharmacol 20(6):605–698, 2000 11106144

Yassa R, Jeste DV: Gender differences in tardive dyskinesia: a critical review of the literature. Schizophr Bull 18(4):701–715, 1992 1359633

CHAPTER 12

Anxiety, Obsessive-Compulsive, and Trauma-Related Disorders

12.1 Which of the following is a new diagnosis in DSM-5?

A. Posttraumatic stress disorder (PTSD).
B. Hoarding disorder.
C. Obsessive-compulsive disorder (OCD).
D. Panic disorder with agoraphobia.

The correct response is option B: Hoarding disorder.

PTSD (option A) was reclassified as a trauma- and stressor-related disorder, and OCD (option C) was reclassified as one of the obsessive-compulsive and related disorders. Hoarding disorder (option B), a relatively common problem in older adults, has been added in DSM-5 (also as one of the obsessive-compulsive and related disorders). Panic disorder and agoraphobia (option D) are now diagnosed separately. Panic disorder diagnosis is unchanged. **(p. 334; Table 12–1, "DSM-5 changes of most relevance to older adults: anxiety, obsessive-compulsive, and trauma-related disorders," p. 335)**

12.2 What is the prevalence of anxiety disorders in the elderly?

A. The prevalence of late-life anxiety is currently unknown.
B. All of the anxiety disorders are less common in older adults.
C. If present, anxiety disorders are typically comorbid conditions stemming from depression and/or cognitive decline.
D. Anxiety disorders are the most prevalent disorders in older adults.

The correct response is option A: The prevalence of late-life anxiety is currently unknown.

Prevalence estimates are limited by the well-known challenges in identifying anxiety disorders in this age group (Wolitzky-Taylor et al. 2010). Chief among these challenges is that older adults are less able as a group than younger adults to accurately identify anxiety symptoms (Wetherell et al. 2009). Furthermore, avoidance and the "excessive" nature of anxiety, which are two distinguishing features in DSM-IV, are quite challenging to detect in older people. Additionally, anxiety conditions germane to elderly persons—such as anxiety in the context of dementia (Starkstein et al. 2007), anxiogenic medical conditions such as heart disease (Todaro et al. 2007), fear of falling (Gagnon et al. 2005), and hoarding syndrome (Saxena 2007)—may not be discerned by standard epidemiological assessments or methodology. Thus, the prevalence and significance of such conditions are currently unknown (option A; options B, C, and D are incorrect). **(pp. 334–335)**

12.3 Aging may be protective from anxiety, and some reports have noted a decline in the propensity for negative affect from adulthood to "early" elderly years. What is one of the likely explanations for the protective effect of aging?

A. Older adults may be more resilient to stressors because of increased ability to regulate their emotions.
B. Aging may reduce the propensity for anxiety because of degeneration in the hippocampus.
C. The onset of anxiety disorders is in childhood or early adulthood, and symptoms of anxiety disorders rarely persist beyond three to five decades.
D. Many prescription medications used in the elderly reduce anxiety.

The correct response is option A: Older adults may be more resilient to stressors because of increased ability to regulate their emotions.

Aging provides the opportunity to inoculate against the anxiety-producing nature of stressors and to practice emotion regulation (Jarvik and Russell 1979) (option A). Aging may reduce the propensity for anxiety because of degeneration in anxiety-producing brain regions, such as the locus coeruleus (Flint 1994) (option B). The largest epidemiological study to specifically examine the question of incident mental disorders in elderly found that late-onset anxiety disorders are not rare (Chou et al. 2011). Aging is associated with a number of new stressors, such as chronic illness and disability that may be particularly anxiogenic. Also, age-related degeneration in brain regions associated with adaptive responses to anxiety (e.g., the dorsolateral prefrontal cortex) may reduce the ability of some to manage anxiogenic situations; findings of poststroke generalized anxiety disorder (GAD; Aström 1996) and cerebral lesions associated with late-onset OCD (Swoboda and Jenike 1995) are congruent with this assertion (option C). Many prescription medications can induce anxiety (e.g., anticholinergics, psychostimulants, steroids) (option D), and this possibility should be a part of any differential diagnosis of new-onset anxiety in an elderly person. **(pp. 337–339)**

12.4 Which anxiety diagnosis is easiest to detect in an older adult?

A. Panic disorder.
B. Specific phobia (e.g., fear of falling).
C. Agoraphobia.
D. Generalized anxiety disorder (GAD).

The correct response is option D: Generalized anxiety disorder (GAD).

Most studies have found a low prevalence of panic disorder (option A) in older adults in the community. Late-onset panic disorder appears to be rare and may often be a prodrome of a medical or neurological problem. When panic disorder does occur in elderly persons, it tends to be associated with less severe or less frequent panic attacks than in young adults, who frequently have daily attacks (Sheikh et al. 2004). Phobia (option B) may be difficult to detect in an older adult—particularly if the phobia has been lifelong—because of lifestyle accommodation around it (e.g., avoiding social situations in the case of social phobia). The difficulty of diagnosing phobias is exemplified by fear of falling, a common problem in elderly persons. Under DSM-IV criteria, this condition usually could not be diagnosable as a phobia, in part because individuals who fear falling typically do not feel their fear to be excessive or unreasonable (Gagnon et al. 2005). Agoraphobia (option C) can present within the context of panic attacks but frequently does not do so in elderly persons (McCabe et al. 2006). It can appear de novo in the context of a stroke or other medical event, in which case it can be highly disabling, leading to inhibition of activities necessary for restoration after the event (Burvill et al. 1995). The condition itself may lead to decreased ability to detect it; accordingly, studies of adults who are homebound or receiving home-based aging services have found high rates of anxiety symptoms (Gum et al. 2009; Jayasinghe et al. 2013). GAD (option D) is a common and impairing disorder in older adults; it is highly comborbid with personality, mood, and other anxiety disorders (Mackenzie et al. 2011). **(pp. 341–344, 346)**

12.5 Which symptom in older adults is common to all of the most common anxiety disorders and related conditions: specific phobias (including social phobia), panic disorder, obsessive-compulsive disorder (OCD), hoarding disorder, generalized anxiety disorder (GAD), and posttraumatic stress disorder (PTSD)?

A. Situational fear.
B. Situational avoidance.
C. Anticipatory worry.
D. Autonomic arousal.

The correct response is option C. Anticipatory worry.

Situational fear (option A) and situational avoidance (option B) are present in specific phobias (including social phobia), panic disorder, OCD, and PTSD but not in GAD or hoarding disorder. Autonomic arousal (option D) is present in specific phobias (including social phobia), panic disorder, and PTSD but not in GAD, OCD, or hoarding disorder. Anticipatory worry (option C) is common to all of the above conditions (specific phobia, panic disorder, GAD, OCD, hoarding disorder, and PTSD). **(Table 12–4, "Shared and distinct clinical features of anxiety disorders and related conditions," p. 340)**

12.6 A 75-year-old woman goes to her internist for a regular appointment to follow up on management of hypertension and diabetes. She appears preoccupied and keyed up and responds to her doctor's questions about the nature of her preoccupations as worries about her husband, who was just hospitalized for treatment of angina. The woman reveals that she has been having more worries as she has gotten older. Her worrying may occur as often as every day, when there are precipitants such as her family members being ill or her own health problems. She usually tries to occupy herself with either home chores or going out for a walk. Generally, this strategy works well for her. She denies any problems with her functioning and continues to be socially engaged with her friends. She also continues to enjoy her family and hobbies, such as reading and crossword puzzles. What is the most likely condition with which this woman struggles?

A. Panic disorder.
B. Generalized anxiety disorder (GAD).
C. Normal aging.
D. Specific phobia.

The correct response is option C: Normal aging.

All of the anxiety disorders cause clinically significant distress or impairment in social, occupational, or other important areas of functioning. Panic disorder tends to be associated with less severe or less frequent panic attacks in elderly persons than in young adults. Nevertheless, because the disability due to panic disorder tends to be related to the behavioral avoidance rather than the frequency of attacks themselves, panic disorder can still be a highly disabling condition in elderly persons. Recurrent unexpected panic attacks (option A) are characterized by an abrupt surge of intense fear or intense discomfort that reaches a peak within minutes and includes symptoms of autonomic arousal. Worry in DSM-5-diagnosed GAD (option B) must be excessive, be difficult to control, and cause distress. Associated features of GAD are muscle tension, restlessness (or feeling keyed up or on edge), sleep difficulties, concentration problems (often thought by older adults to be memory problems), fatigue, and irritability. Late-life GAD is associated with impaired quality of life but low levels of professional help seeking in mental health settings (Mackenzie et al. 2011). Elderly persons with GAD often present to primary care or specialty medical care with these associated symptoms, which then become the targets of treatment. The actual content of worry in late-life GAD has been noted to be similar to that in older adults without GAD—that is, concerns about health or disability, family relationships, or finances (Diefenbach et al. 2001). The patient does not meet the criteria for specific phobia (option D); her worry is within normal range—it is not excessive to the point that she cannot distract herself or cannot function or enjoy her life—and it cannot be described as "out of proportion to the actual danger." She also does not report any of the various criteria for an anxiety disorder: situational fear, situational avoidance, autonomic arousal, anticipatory worry, obsessions and compulsions, or panic attacks. Therefore, considering that the patient has worries that are common to older age and does not meet criteria for any of the anxiety disorders, her condition is normal for her age (option C). **(pp. 344–346; Table 12–4, "Shared and distinct features of anxiety disorders and related conditions," p. 340; Table 12–5, "DSM-5 diagnostic criteria for specific phobia," p. 342; Table 12–8, "DSM-5 diagnostic criteria for panic disorder," p. 345)**

12.7   What is the least helpful factor to consider when making a diagnosis of generalized anxiety disorder (GAD) in older adults?

A. The amount of worry.
B. The difficulty the individual has in stopping the worry.
C. The degree of distress or functional impairment related to worrying.
D. The degree to which the worry is realistic versus excessive.

The correct response is option D: The degree to which the worry is realistic versus excessive.

The objects of worry for elderly persons with GAD are largely the same as those for older adults without GAD: health, disability in self or spouse, and finances (Diefenbach et al. 2001). Because these are often realistic sources of concern in aging, older adults with GAD may be unlikely to feel that their worry is excessive or is about minor issues, as required by the GAD criteria. In working with older individuals, clinicians need to consider the amount of worry (option A), the difficulty the individual has in stopping it (option B), and the degree of distress or functional impairment related to worrying (option C), rather than the degree to which the worry is realistic versus excessive (option D). **(pp. 347–348)**

12.8   Which characteristic of the fear of falling has prevented incorporation of this condition into DSM-5?

A. Many older patients lack the insight into the excessiveness of the fear.
B. The individuals affected by the fear of falling do not avoid activities or going out of their home.
C. Fear of falling is uncommon.
D. Fear of falling is not sufficiently impairing.

The correct response is option A: Many older patients lack the insight into the excessiveness of the fear.

Fear of falling is a common syndrome in community-dwelling older adults; estimates are 7%–14% (option C). Fear of falling consists of moderate to severe fear with avoidance of multiple situations and activities (e.g., approximately 3% of older adults avoid leaving their houses or yards as a result of fear of falling; Arfken et al.

1994). The fear of falling is frequently excessive relative to objective fall risk. However, fear of falling does not map well onto the pre–DSM-5 requirement of insight into excessiveness of the fear, which many older patients lack (option A). For example, Gagnon et al. (2005) found that only 1 of 48 subjects with moderate or severe fear of falling considered their fear to be unreasonable, even though the fear frequently resulted in the individuals' avoidance of activities, in some cases to the point of their being housebound (Flint 2005) (options B and D). **(p. 352)**

12.9 The comorbidity of anxiety disorders and related conditions with late-life depression can be described by which of the following characteristics?

   A. About a quarter of elderly patients with major depressive disorder (MDD) also have an anxiety disorder or significant anxiety symptoms.
   B. Depressive symptoms are more stable than those of anxiety, lasting longer and precipitating anxiety conditions.
   C. There is an overlap of symptoms of anxiety disorders and MDD.
   D. Elderly patients with depression and anxiety experience greater suicidal ideation but not greater risk of suicide.

The correct response is option C: There is an overlap of symptoms of anxiety disorders and MDD.

The Longitudinal Aging Study Amsterdam (LASA) study found that 48% of elderly persons with MDD also had a current comorbid anxiety disorder, whereas approximately one-fourth of those with anxiety disorders had MDD (Beekman et al. 2000) (option A). The comorbidity is not surprising given the extensive symptomatic overlap of anxiety disorders and related conditions (particularly GAD and PTSD) with MDD. While classified in separate categories in DSM-5, MDD, persistent depressive disorder (dysthymia), PTSD, and GAD are all centrally defined by distress from negative affect (option C). Symptomatically, anxiety symptoms are more stable than those of depression and more likely to lead to depressive symptoms than vice versa (Wetherell et al. 2001). As a result, anxiety disorders might be a risk factor for late-life depression (Hettema et al. 2006). When depression precedes or coexists with the anxiety disorder, anxiety symptoms often persist after remission of depression and increase risk for depressive relapse (Dombrovski et al. 2007; Flint and Rifat 1997) (option B). Depressed elderly patients with comorbid anxiety have greater somatic symptoms, greater suicidal ideation (Jeste et al. 2006; Lenze et al. 2000), and a higher risk of suicide (Allgulander and Lavori 1993) (option D). **(p. 355)**

12.10 An 86-year-old woman has a 6-year history of generalized anxiety disorder (GAD) as well as a fear of falling. She recently had an increase in intensity of her anxiety symptoms, along with the onset of mild cognitive impairment. What is the most likely explanation of her symptoms?

   A. The patient has a separate anxiety disorder that is now co-occurring with either stable mild cognitive impairment or early dementia.

B. The patient likely had a prodromal anxiety disorder (diagnosed as GAD) that manifested before symptoms of dementia were recognized, and anxiety is now exacerbated by the presence of cognitive impairment.

C. All of the patient's anxiety symptoms are a direct result of the patient's age.

D. The patient's mild cognitive impairment is a direct result of years of experiencing anxiety symptoms.

The correct response is option B: The patient likely had a prodromal anxiety disorder (diagnosed as GAD) that manifested before symptoms of dementia were recognized, and anxiety is now exacerbated by the presence of cognitive impairment.

When anxiety symptoms have occurred for a long time (>10 years) before the cognitive decline, this suggests a separate anxiety disorder (not a prodrome) (option A). When anxiety symptoms and cognitive difficulties begin approximately concurrently, the anxiety may either be result of the disease course that gives rise to the cognitive decline or be due to cognitive problems stemming from the anxiety and its neurobiological consequences. Age alone is not the etiology of anxiety symptoms (option C). Because anxiety symptoms can be a prodromal manifestation of dementia, new-onset anxiety with mild cognitive impairment (or even subjective complaints) may portend a developing disease process (option B). Seignourel et al. (2008) reported that if patients with dementia have insight into their mental decline (likely in the early stages), then anxiety is more likely to be present. Bryant et al. (2013) found that as dementia becomes more severe, instead of anxiety, agitation is more likely to be present. Studies examining links between negative affect with cognitive impairment and decline consistently find that worry has the largest effect (Andreescu et al. 2014; Pietrzak et al. 2012; Rosenberg et al. 2013; Wilson et al. 2011). This observational research is not able to discern whether anxiety is the cause or consequence of cognitive decline; to our knowledge, no studies are under way to dissect this complex and possibly bidirectional relationship (option D). **(pp. 357–359)**

12.11 What is the best approach to treatment of generalized anxiety disorder (GAD) in older adults?

A. An antidepressant, particularly a selective serotonin reuptake inhibitor (SSRI).

B. Psychotherapy, especially cognitive-behavioral therapy (CBT).

C. Combination of benzodiazepine and CBT.

D. Combination of SSRI and CBT.

The correct response is option D: Combination of SSRI and CBT.

To date, the proven treatments for late-life anxiety disorders are simply the same treatments demonstrated to be effective in young adults. There is evidence that older adults with GAD can learn new skills in CBT and use them effectively over time (Wetherell et al. 2005). The question of whether medication or psychotherapy is better remains unresolved, but a more clinically salient question may be whether further enhancements or a sequential approach of using medications and CBT would be more effective in older adults (options A and B). Addressing this issue, Wetherell et al. (2013) found that augmenting SSRI treatment with CBT improved worry symptoms and reduced relapse rates in older adults with GAD. This report suggests that a combination of pharmacotherapy and psychotherapy approaches may provide the greatest benefits for patients with this disorder (option D). Some studies have found that benzodiazepines are efficacious in reducing anxiety symptoms in late-life anxiety (Bresolin et al. 1988; Koepke et al. 1982). However, these medications increase the risk of falls (e.g., Landi et al. 2005; Lenze et al. 2009) and cognitive impairment (Billioti de Gage et al. 2014) (option C). **(pp. 359–361)**

References

Allgulander C, Lavori PW: Causes of death among 936 elderly patients with "pure" anxiety neurosis in Stockholm County, Sweden, and in patients with depressive neurosis or both diagnoses. Compr Psychiatry 34(5):299–302, 1993 8306638

Andreescu C, Teverovsky E, Fu B, et al: Old worries and new anxieties: behavioral symptoms and mild cognitive impairment in a population study. Am J Geriatr Psychiatry 22(3):274–284, 2014 23759435

Arfken CL, Lach HW, Birge SJ, Miller JP: The prevalence and correlates of fear of falling in elderly persons living in the community. Am J Public Health 84(4):565–570, 1994 8154557

Aström M: Generalized anxiety disorder in stroke patients. A 3-year longitudinal study. Stroke 27(2):270–275, 1996 8571422

Beekman ATF, de Beurs E, van Balkom AJLM, et al: Anxiety and depression in later life: co-occurrence and communality of risk factors. Am J Psychiatry 157(1):89–95, 2000 10618018

Billioti de Gage S, Moride Y, Ducruet T, et al: Benzodiazepine use and risk of Alzheimer's disease: case-control study. BMJ 349:g5205, 2014 25208536

Bresolin N, Monza G, Scarpini E, et al: Treatment of anxiety with ketazolam in elderly patients. Clin Ther 10(5):536–542, 1988 2908803

Bryant C, Mohlman J, Gum A, et al: Anxiety disorders in older adults: looking to DSM5 and beyond. Am J Geriatr Psychiatry 21(9):872–876, 2013 23567396

Burvill PW, Johnson GA, Jamrozik KD, et al: Anxiety disorders after stroke: results from the Perth Community Stroke Study. Br J Psychiatry 166(3):328–332, 1995 7788124

Chou KL, Mackenzie CS, Liang K, Sareen J: Three-year incidence and predictors of first-onset of DSM-IV mood, anxiety, and substance use disorders in older adults: results from Wave 2 of the National Epidemiologic Survey on Alcohol and Related Conditions. J Clin Psychiatry 72(2):144–155, 2011 21382305

Diefenbach GJ, Stanley MA, Beck JG: Worry content reported by older adults with and without generalized anxiety disorder. Aging Ment Health 5(3):269–274, 2001 11575066

Dombrovski AY, Mulsant BH, Houck PR, et al: Residual symptoms and recurrence during maintenance treatment of late-life depression. J Affect Disord 103(1-3):77–82, 2007 17321595

Flint AJ: Epidemiology and comorbidity of anxiety disorders in the elderly. Am J Psychiatry 151(5):640–649, 1994 8166303

Flint AJ: Anxiety and its disorders in late life: moving the field forward. Am J Geriatr Psychiatry 13(1):3–6, 2005 15653934

Flint AJ, Rifat SL: Two-year outcome of elderly patients with anxious depression. Psychiatry Res 66(1):23–31, 1997 9061801

Gagnon N, Flint AJ, Naglie G, Devins GM: Affective correlates of fear of falling in elderly persons. Am J Geriatr Psychiatry 13(1):7–14, 2005 15653935

Gum AM, Petkus A, McDougal SJ, et al: Behavioral health needs and problem recognition by older adults receiving home-based aging services. Int J Geriatr Psychiatry 24(4):400–408, 2009 18836987

Hettema JM, Kuhn JW, Prescott CA, Kendler KS: The impact of generalized anxiety disorder and stressful life events on risk for major depressive episodes. Psychol Med 36(6):789–795, 2006 16515735

Jarvik LF, Russell D: Anxiety, aging and the third emergency reaction. J Gerontol 34(2):197–200, 1979 438473

Jayasinghe N, Rocha LP, Sheeran T, et al: Anxiety symptoms in older home health care recipients: prevalence and associates. Home Health Care Serv Q 32(3):163–177, 2013 23937710

Jeste ND, Hays JC, Steffens DC: Clinical correlates of anxious depression among elderly patients with depression. J Affect Disord 90(1):37–41, 2006 16325261

Koepke HH, Gold RL, Linden ME, et al: Multicenter controlled study of oxazepam in anxious elderly outpatients. Psychosomatics 23(6):641–645, 1982 6750675

Landi F, Onder G, Cesari M, et al; Silver Network Home Care Study Group: Psychotropic medications and risk for falls among community-dwelling frail older people: an observational study. J Gerontol A Biol Sci Med Sci 60(5):622–626, 2005 15972615

Lenze EJ, Mulsant BH, Shear MK, et al: Comorbid anxiety disorders in depressed elderly patients. Am J Psychiatry 157(5):722–728, 2000 10784464

Lenze EJ, Iaboni A, Wetherell J: Benzodiazepines in older adults: definite harms, doubtful benefits (letter). BMJ 349:g5205, 2009, http://www.bmj.com/content/349/bmj.g5205/rr/777842, accessed December 4, 2014.

Mackenzie CS, Reynolds K, Chou KL, et al: Prevalence and correlates of generalized anxiety disorder in a national sample of older adults. Am J Geriatr Psychiatry 19(4):305–315, 2011 21427639

McCabe L, Cairney J, Veldhuizen KS, et al: Prevalence and correlates of agoraphobia in older adults. Am J Geriatr Psychiatry 14(6):515–522, 2006 16731720

Pietrzak RH, Maruff P, Woodward M, et al: Mild worry symptoms predict decline in learning and memory in healthy older adults: a 2-year prospective cohort study. Am J Geriatr Psychiatry 20(3):266–275, 2012 22354117

Rosenberg PB, Mielke MM, Appleby BS, et al: The association of neuropsychiatric symptoms in MCI with incident dementia and Alzheimer disease. Am J Geriatr Psychiatry 21(7):685–695, 2013 23567400

Saxena S: Is compulsive hoarding a genetically and neurobiologically discrete syndrome? Implications for diagnostic classification. Am J Psychiatry 164(3):380–384, 2007 17329459

Seignourel PJ, Kunik ME, Snow L, et al: Anxiety in dementia: a critical review. Clin Psychol Rev 28(7):1071–1082, 2008 18555569

Sheikh JI, Swales PJ, Carlson EB, Lindley SE: Aging and panic disorder: phenomenology, comorbidity, and risk factors. Am J Geriatr Psychiatry 12(1):102–109, 2004 14729565

Starkstein SE, Jorge R, Petracca G, Robinson RG: The construct of generalized anxiety disorder in Alzheimer disease. Am J Geriatr Psychiatry 15(1):42–49, 2007 17194814

Swoboda KJ, Jenike MA: Frontal abnormalities in a patient with obsessive-compulsive disorder: the role of structural lesions in obsessive-compulsive behavior. Neurology 45(12):2130–2134, 1995 8848180

Todaro JF, Shen BJ, Raffa SD, et al: Prevalence of anxiety disorders in men and women with established coronary heart disease. J Cardiopulm Rehabil Prev 27(2):86–91, 2007 17558244

Wetherell JL, Gatz M, Pedersen NL: A longitudinal analysis of anxiety and depressive symptoms. Psychol Aging 16(2):187–195, 2001 11405307

Wetherell JL, Hopko DR, Diefenbach GJ, et al: Cognitive-behavioral therapy for late-life generalized anxiety disorder: who gets better? Behav Ther 36:147–156, 2005

Wetherell JL, Petkus AJ, McChesney K, et al: Older adults are less accurate than younger adults at identifying symptoms of anxiety and depression. J Nerv Ment Dis 197(8):623–626, 2009 19684501

Wetherell JL, Petkus AJ, White KS, et al: Antidepressant medication augmented with cognitive-behavioral therapy for generalized anxiety disorder in older adults. Am J Psychiatry 170(7):782–789, 2013 23680817

Wilson RS, Begeny CT, Boyle PA, et al: Vulnerability to stress, anxiety, and development of dementia in old age. Am J Geriatr Psychiatry 19(4):327–334, 2011 21427641

Wolitzky-Taylor KB, Castriotta N, Lenze EJ, et al: Anxiety disorders in older adults: a comprehensive review. Depress Anxiety 27(2):190–211, 2010 20099273

CHAPTER 13

Somatic Symptom and Related Disorders

13.1 Which of the following disorders is no longer classified under somatic symptom and related disorders in DSM-5?

A. Illness anxiety disorder.
B. Factitious disorder.
C. Conversion disorder.
D. Body dysmorphic disorder.

The correct response is option D: Body dysmorphic disorder.

The seven disorders encompassed in the DSM-5 category of somatic symptom and related disorders are somatic symptom disorder, illness anxiety disorder (option A), conversion disorder (functional neurological symptom disorder) (option C), psychological factors affecting other medical conditions, factitious disorder (option B), other specified somatic symptom and related disorder, and unspecified somatic symptom and related disorder. DSM-IV disorders that are subsumed under this new nomenclature include somatization disorder, undifferentiated somatoform disorder, hypochondriasis, pain disorder, and factitious disorders (which appeared in their own separate category in DSM-IV). Body dysmorphic disorder (option D) is not included in the new somatic symptom disorder category and is now classified as one of the other specified obsessive-compulsive and related disorders. **(p. 373)**

13.2 Which of the following symptoms is unlikely to be associated with somatic symptom and related disorders in older adults?

A. Depression.
B. Delusional thinking.
C. Anxiety.
D. Substance abuse.

The correct response is option B: Delusional thinking.

Somatoform symptoms in late life are often obscured by comorbid physical and psychiatric illnesses. In particular, these disorders have been strongly associated with stress, depression (option A), anxiety (option C), psychological trauma, substance abuse (option D), and personality disorders (de Waal et al. 2004; Haftgoli et al. 2010; Hasin and Katz 2007; Sack et al. 2007; Tomenson et al. 2012) but not delusional thinking (option B). **(p. 374)**

13.3 Which of the following features is commonly seen across somatic symptom and related disorders?

A. Reduced pain sensitivity.
B. Absence of functional disability.
C. Excessive fears about health status.
D. Attenuated sensitivity to somatic sensations.

The correct response is option C: Excessive fears about health status.

Three important factors associated with all of the somatic symptom and related disorders are high sensitivity to somatic sensations and pain (options A and D); catastrophizing, in which there are excessive and unrealistic fears regarding one's health status (option C); and excess functional disability associated with the symptoms (option B) (Bortz 2008; Egloff et al. 2014). **(p. 374)**

13.4 Which of the following DSM-5 disorders is a more common somatic symptom and related disorder in the elderly?

A. Body dysmorphic disorder.
B. Conversion disorder.
C. Factitious disorder.
D. Unspecified somatic symptom and related disorder.

The correct response is option B: Conversion disorder.

The seven disorders encompassed in the DSM-5 category of somatic symptom and related disorders are somatic symptom disorder, illness anxiety disorder, conversion disorder (functional neurological symptom disorder), psychological factors affecting other medical conditions, factitious disorder, other specified somatic symptom and related disorder, and unspecified somatic symptom and related disorder (option D). The somatic symptom and related disorder diagnostic categories of primary relevance to the older patient are somatic symptom disorder, illness anxiety disorder, and conversion disorder (option B). Body dysmorphic disorder (option A) is no longer considered a somatic symptom disorder, and like factitious disorder (option C), it is rare in the elderly. **(p. 375)**

13.5 A 68-year-old woman with hypertension, type 2 diabetes mellitus, and hyperlipidemia presents for psychiatric evaluation on referral from the emergency department, where she has presented six times in the last year because of her concern that she has pancreatic cancer. She reports generalized abdominal discomfort that "comes and goes." A thorough medical workup, including imaging and evaluation by a gastroenterologist, is negative. She is anxious and complains of poor sleep due to her concerns about her health. She has no other psychiatric symptoms or prior history. Which of the following somatic symptom and related disorders is the most likely diagnosis?

A. Malingering.
B. Illness anxiety disorder, care-seeking type.
C. Conversion disorder.
D. Delusional disorder.

The correct response is option B: Illness anxiety disorder, care-seeking type.

The DSM-5 category of illness anxiety disorder (option B) incorporates the essence of what was previously labeled *hypochondriasis*. It is characterized by an excessive preoccupation with having or acquiring a serious illness, despite the fact that somatic symptoms are either not present or, if present, are very mild in intensity. Key to this preoccupation is a high level of anxiety about one's health associated with excessive health-related behaviors such as checking one's body for signs of illness or maladaptive avoidance of medical appointments or settings (American Psychiatric Association 2013). It is believed that misinterpretation of normal bodily sensations as indicative of severe illness is the main dynamic underlying health anxiety disorder (Krautwurst et al. 2014). Conversion disorder (option C), also labeled *functional neurological symptom disorder* in DSM-5, is characterized by one or more symptoms of altered voluntary motor or sensory function, which do not appear compatible with recognized neurological or medical conditions. The symptoms may involve weakness or paralysis, abnormal movements (e.g., tremor), swallowing or speech symptoms, pseudoseizures, or sensory loss. Unlike malingering (option A), the somatic symptom disorders do not represent intentional, conscious attempts by patients to present physical symptoms in order to achieve a specific goal (e.g., to get out of work). Delusional disorder (option D) is not a somatic symptom and related disorder. **(pp. 374–377)**

13.6 Which of the following symptoms is most common in elderly persons with somatic symptom disorder?

A. Depression.
B. Substance abuse.
C. Insomnia.
D. Pain.

The correct response is option D: Pain.

Pain (option D) is the most common medical complaint in elderly persons, with pain due to musculoskeletal disease (e.g., osteoarthritis, back pain, headache) being the most common type (Deen 2008; Leveille et al. 2001). Close to 50% of elderly individuals have chronic pain, and the percentage approaches 70% for those in long-term care (Otis and McGeeney 2000). Up to 17% suffer from substantial daily pain (Sawyer et al. 2007). Persistent pain is associated with significant functional and social impairment (Scudds and Ostbye 2001), as well as comorbid psychiatric symptoms, including depression (option A), insomnia (option C), and substance abuse (option B) (Karp and Weiner 2011). **(pp. 376–377)**

13.7   Which of the following symptoms is more common in younger versus older persons with conversion disorder?

A. Pseudoseizures.
B. Paralysis.
C. Swallowing difficulty.
D. Weakness.

The correct response is option A: Pseudoseizures.

Conversion disorder, also labeled *functional neurological symptom disorder* in DSM-5, is characterized by one or more symptoms of altered voluntary motor or sensory function, which do not appear compatible with recognized neurological or medical conditions. The symptoms cause significant distress and/or impairment in important areas of functioning, and may involve weakness (option D) or paralysis (option B), abnormal movements (e.g., tremor), swallowing (option C) or speech symptoms, pseudoseizures, or sensory loss. Psychogenic nonepileptic seizures (PNESs), sometimes referred to as pseudoseizures (option A), represent one type of conversion symptom. They are characterized by behavioral spells that mimic various forms of seizures but are not associated with electroencephalographic findings and have a presumed psychological etiology (D'Alessio et al. 2006; Mari et al. 2006). PNESs are more frequent in young women and are seen in 5%–20% of outpatients with epilepsy, often in combination with an actual seizure disorder (Chabolla et al. 1996); however, they have also been diagnosed in individuals older than age 60 years (Behrouz et al. 2006). **(pp. 377–378)**

13.8   The prevalence of which of the following somatic symptom and related disorders is associated with increased age?

A. Somatic symptom disorder.
B. Illness anxiety disorder.
C. Alexithymia.
D. Dissociative amnesia.

The correct response is option B: Illness anxiety disorder.

The prevalence of somatic symptom and related disorders has not been associated with increased age, with the exception of hypochondriasis (option B; option A is incorrect). Options C and D are factors associated with somatic symptom and related disorders. **(p. 380; Table 13–4, "Factors associated with somatic symptom and related disorders," p. 380)**

References

American Psychiatric Association: Diagnostic and Statistical Manual of Mental Disorders, 5th Edition, DSM-5. Washington, DC, American Psychiatric Association, 2013

Behrouz R, Heriaud L, Benbadis SR: Late-onset psychogenic nonepileptic seizures. Epilepsy Behav 8(3):649–650, 2006 16531122

Bortz JJ: Medically unexplained symptoms in older adults, in Clinical Neurology of the Older Adult. Edited by Sirven JI, Malamut BL. Philadelphia, PA, Lippincott Williams & Wilkins, 2008, pp 561–573

Chabolla DR, Krahn LE, So EL, Rummans TA: Psychogenic nonepileptic seizures. Mayo Clin Proc 71(5):493–500, 1996 8628032

D'Alessio L, Giagante B, Oddo S, et al: Psychiatric disorders in patients with psychogenic nonepileptic seizures, with and without comorbid epilepsy. Seizure 15(5):333–339, 2006 16720097

Deen HG: Back and neck pain, in Clinical Neurology of the Older Adult. Edited by Sirven JI, Malamut BL. Philadelphia, PA, Lippincott Williams & Wilkins, 2008, pp 213–221

de Waal MWM, Arnold IA, Eekhof JAH, van Hemert AM: Somatoform disorders in general practice: prevalence, functional impairment and comorbidity with anxiety and depressive disorders. Br J Psychiatry 184(6):470–476, 2004 15172939

Egloff N, Cámara RJ, von Känel R, et al: Hypersensitivity and hyperalgesia in somatoform pain disorders. Gen Hosp Psychiatry 36(3):284–290, 2014 24650586

Haftgoli N, Favrat B, Verdon F, et al: Patients presenting with somatic complaints in general practice: depression, anxiety and somatoform disorders are frequent and associated with psychosocial stressors. BMC Fam Pract 11:67, 2010 20843358

Hasin D, Katz H: Somatoform and substance use disorders. Psychosom Med 69(9):870–875, 2007 18040097

Karp JF, Weiner DK: Persistent pain and older adults, in Principles and Practice of Geriatric Psychiatry, 2nd Edition. Edited by Agronin ME, Maletta G. Philadelphia, PA, Lippincott Williams & Wilkins 2011, pp 763–782

Krautwurst S, Gerlach AL, Gomille L, et al: Health anxiety—an indicator of higher interoceptive sensitivity? J Behav Ther Exp Psychiatry 45(2):303–309, 2014 24584036

Leveille SG, Ling S, Hochberg MC, et al: Widespread musculoskeletal pain and the progression of disability in older disabled women. Ann Intern Med 135(12):1038–1046, 2001 11747382

Mari F, Di Bonaventura C, Vanacore N, et al: Video-EEG study of psychogenic nonepileptic seizures: differential characteristics in patients with and without epilepsy. Epilepsia 47(Suppl 5):64–67, 2006 17239109

Otis JAD, McGeeney B: Managing pain in the elderly. Clin Geriatr 8:48–62, 2000

Sack M, Lahmann C, Jaeger B, Henningsen P: Trauma prevalence and somatoform symptoms: are there specific somatoform symptoms related to traumatic experiences? J Nerv Ment Dis 195(11):928–933, 2007 18000455

Sawyer P, Lillis JP, Bodner EV, Allman RM: Substantial daily pain among nursing home residents. J Am Med Dir Assoc 8(3):158–165, 2007 17349944

Scudds RJ, Ostbye T: Pain and pain-related interference with function in older Canadians: the Canadian Study of Health and Aging. Disabil Rehabil 23(15):654–664, 2001 11720115

Tomenson B, McBeth J, Chew-Graham CA, et al: Somatization and health anxiety as predictors of health care use. Psychosom Med 74(6):656–664, 2012 22753632

CHAPTER 14

Sexuality and Aging

14.1 According to major studies and recent surveys of sexual activity, which of the following accurately describes sexual behaviors in individuals ages 65 years and older?

A. A majority of older men and women continue to be sexually active.
B. The quality of the relationship is the most influential factor for both men and women.
C. Previous level of sexual activity has little influence on late-life sexual activity.
D. Older gay and lesbian individuals report low levels of satisfaction with their sex lives.

The correct response is option A: A majority of older men and women continue to be sexually active.

Several major studies over the past 25 years have shown that a majority of middle-aged and older individuals continue to be sexually active (option A). In general, sexual interest and activity in late life depend on the previous level of sexual activity (option C); the availability, health, and sexual interest of the partner; and the individual's overall physical health (Lindau et al. 2007; Schick et al. 2010). Physical health appears to be the most important factor for older men, whereas the quality of the relationship is most influential for older women (option B). A small but growing literature indicates that older gay and lesbian individuals continue to be sexually active and to feel high levels of satisfaction with both their lifestyle and their sex lives (Adelman 1990) (option D). **(pp. 389, 391)**

14.2 Which of the following accurately describes normal age-related changes in sexual function?

A. In older men, the resolution or refractory stage decreases.
B. Compared with women, sexual changes in aging men occur more gradually and are less predictable.
C. The effects of physiological changes in sexual function are rarely influenced by psychosocial factors.
D. Erections take longer to achieve but are easier to sustain.

The correct response is option B: Compared with women, sexual changes in aging men occur more gradually and are less predictable.

In both sexes, the effects of physiological changes in sexual function are mediated by a number of psychosocial factors. The more an individual knows about what constitutes normal age-associated changes in sexual function, the easier it may be for him or her to accept these changes (option C). Compared with women, the sexual changes in aging men occur more gradually with a less predictable time frame (Morley 2003; Westheimer and Lopater 2002) (option B). Older men require more physical stimulation to achieve erections, which tend to be less frequent, less durable, and less reliable (option D). In older men, the resolution or refractory stage is much longer, lasting hours to days instead of minutes to hours as in younger men (option A). **(p. 394)**

14.3 Which of the following best describes the more common sexual dysfunctions seen in late life?

A. Oral erectogenic agents are ineffective in men with psychogenic erectile dysfunction.
B. The physiological cause of female sexual interest/arousal disorder in older women is primarily due to reduced levels of free testosterone.
C. In older women, female orgasmic disorder is often permanent and unresponsive to treatment.
D. Premature (early) ejaculation is most common in younger men and almost always resolves with normal aging.

The correct response is option B: The physiological cause of female sexual interest/arousal disorder in older women is primarily due to reduced levels of free testosterone.

Oral erectogenic agents sildenafil, tadalafil, and vardenafil improve erectile function in men with both organic and psychogenic erectile dysfunction by serving as selective inhibitors of phosphodiesterase type 5 (option A). Premature ejaculation is the most common sexual dysfunction in younger men, reported in 20%–38% of various samples, and may remain relatively constant even in older ages (Laumann et al. 1999; Lindau et al. 2007; Porst et al. 2007; Westheimer and Lopater 2002) (option D). The critical physiological cause of low desire in women appears to be the menopause-associated reduction in levels of free testosterone (option B). In the treatment of female orgasmic disorder, individual sex therapy, testosterone supplementation, and sildenafil have been used with some success (option C). **(pp. 403–404)**

14.4 Which of the following medications is *least likely* to cause sexual dysfunction in late life?

A. Antidepressants (tricyclic antidepressants, selective serotonin reuptake inhibitors, monoamine oxidase inhibitors).
B. Antiandrogens (e.g., leuprolide, ketoconazole).

C. Mood stabilizers (e.g., lithium, valproic acid, carbamazepine)
D. Phosphodiesterase type 5 inhibitors (e.g., sildenafil, tadalafil)

The correct response is option D: Phosphodiesterase type 5 inhibitors (e.g., sildenafil, tadalafil).

Several medications can cause sexual dysfunction and can affect both men and women at any point in the sexual response cycle (Crenshaw and Goldberg 1996; Goodwin and Agronin 1997; Ludwig and Phillips 2014; Thomas 2003). Antidepressants (option A), antiandrogens (option B), and mood stabilizers (option C) are commonly associated with sexual dysfunction. The oral erectogenic agents sildenafil, tadalafil, and vardenafil, which serve as selective inhibitors of phosphodiesterase type 5 (option D), are used to treat sexual dysfunction. **(pp. 396–397, 404; Table 14–4, "Medications associated with sexual dysfunction in late life," p. 399)**

14.5   A geriatric psychiatry fellow is preparing to provide nursing home staff with education about how dementia affects sexuality. Which of the following is most consistent with current knowledge?

A. Sexual desire in individuals with dementia may remain strong and even increase.
B. The percentage of individuals with dementia who demonstrate sexual aggression or inappropriate sexual behaviors is high.
C. Sexual disinhibition and innocuous behaviors are easy for staff and caregivers to differentiate.
D. In nursing home settings, health care professionals are not required to inquire about ethical issues associated with sexuality and dementia.

The correct response is option A: Sexual desire in individuals with dementia may remain strong and even increase.

Dementia affects sexuality in several ways. Sexual desire may remain strong and even increase, especially if inhibitions are reduced by cognitive impairment (option A). Although the percentage of individuals with dementia who demonstrate sexually aggressive or inappropriate behaviors is relatively small, these conditions tend to generate a disproportionate amount of anxiety for caregivers and to require a greater amount of clinical attention from long-term-care staff (Joller et al. 2013) (option B). When assessing an individual who has allegedly demonstrated problematic behaviors, it is critical to identify the context of the behaviors. For example, public disrobing or touching of genitals in public may not be due to sexual urges but may instead reflect underlying confusion, delirium, motor restlessness, or stereotypy associated with dementia. However, caregivers and long-term-care staff sometimes misinterpret innocuous behaviors as evidence of sexual disinhibition (Hajjar and Kamel 2004b; Redinbaugh et al. 1997) (option C). Unfortunately, health care professionals often fail to inquire about ethical issues associated with sexuality and dementia, despite the frequency with which they affect couples (Agronin 2014; Robinson and Davis 2013) (option D). **(pp. 405–406)**

14.6 Which of the following is most accurate concerning sexually transmitted diseases (STDs) in people 65 years and older since 2008?

A. Rates of STDs (chlamydia, gonorrhea, syphilis) have significantly increased.
B. Extensive data on STDs have been collected in published surveys about late-life sexuality.
C. With respect to HIV and AIDS, the rates of individuals living with HIV infection have not changed appreciably.
D. Older individuals remain at risk for STDs but may neglect safe sex practices.

The correct response is option D: Older individuals remain at risk for STDs but may neglect safe sex practices.

According to surveillance data from the Centers for Disease Control and Prevention (2012), rates of STDs including chlamydia, gonorrhea, and syphilis in individuals ages 65 years and older were the lowest of any group and had not changed appreciably in the previous 5 years (option A). None of the published surveys about late-life sexuality asked respondents about STDs, even though older people are certainly at risk for contracting them (option B). With respect to HIV and AIDS, the largest increase in individuals living with HIV infection from 2008 to 2010 was among individuals older than 65 years, with a rate at the end of 2010 of 85.7 per 100,000 persons in the United States (option C). Older individuals remain at risk for STDs because they continue to be sexually active. Adding to this risk is the fact that many older people never received the sex education provided to today's younger population. Thus, they may neglect safe-sex practices due to lack of knowledge, the absence of pregnancy risk, and a false sense of safety from knowing that STDs are more prevalent in younger people (option D). **(p. 395)**

14.7 Which of the following is most accurate with regard to sexuality in long-term-care settings?

A. Many residents report the desire for sexual relationships is extinguished.
B. Common barriers to sexual activity in facilities include negative attitudes of staff.
C. Obtaining a sexual history during long-term-care facility intake is often irrelevant.
D. Couples wishing to be intimate must arrange for visits outside the care facility.

The correct response is option B: Common barriers to sexual activity in facilities include negative attitudes of staff.

Not surprisingly, the rate of sexual activity is low in most nursing homes (Hajjar and Kamel 2004a; Mulligan and Palguta 1991). For many residents, however, the desire for sexual relationships still exists (option A). Some of the common barriers to sexual activity among long-term-care residents include loss of interest, chronic illness, sexual dysfunction, and negative attitudes of staff (Hajjar and Kamel 2004a; Richardson and Lazur 1995; Wasow and Loeb 1979) (option B). Residents should be educated about sexuality in late life and about their sexual rights. One way to facilitate these educational goals for residents and staff in long-term-care settings is to develop and promote a policy on sexuality. To carry out such a policy, clinical staff in long-term-care facilities should ensure that a sexual history is obtained during intake and routine nursing, medical, and mental health evaluations (option C). These evaluations can also be used to assess residents' concerns and capacities with respect to sexual function and relationships. Long-term-care facilities must ensure adequate privacy for couples wishing to be intimate and must facilitate conjugal or home visits (option D). **(p. 392)**

14.8 A couple in their early 70s recently started dating. They come for a consultation regarding issues with fear of intimacy. Which of the following best describes current sex therapy treatment models in older adults?

A. Sex therapy is best done conjointly with sexual partners.
B. A psychodynamic model is often more successful than cognitive-behavioral techniques.
C. Sensate focus exercises should be avoided in older, anxious couples.
D. Cognitive distortions toward sexual activity in older adults are often fixed and treatment resistant.

The correct response is option A: Sex therapy is best done conjointly with sexual partners.

Sex therapy is always best done conjointly, where both partners participate because both are an integral part of the problem and solution (option A). Historically, a psychodynamic model was used in sex therapy to uncover underlying unconscious conflicts, but that approach is now viewed as less successful, and cognitive-behavioral techniques are used in current treatment models (Brotto and Luria 2014; Kaplan 1974, 1983; Westheimer and Lopater 2002) (option B). Behavioral techniques used during sex therapy begin with exercises called *sensate focus,* in which a couple practices physical relaxation techniques during nonpressured sensual touching. Sensate focus helps to reduce performance anxiety and restore the natural flow of the sexual response cycle (option C). Sex therapy involves both cognitive and behavioral techniques, with an overall goal of building an association between relaxed and sensual physical intimacy and sexual relations. The same principles can be applied across the life span, with several refinements in late life (option D). **(pp. 401–402)**

14.9 Which of the following antidepressants is associated with lower rates of sexual dysfunction?

A. Tricyclic antidepressants (TCAs).
B. Venlafaxine.
C. Bupropion.
D. Serotonin selective reuptake inhibitors (SSRIs).

The correct response is option C: Bupropion.

Many of the antidepressants used to treat mood or anxiety disorders can cause or exacerbate sexual dysfunction. Erectile disorder, delayed or inhibited orgasm, and/or a decrease in desire is experienced by 10%–60% of men taking SSRIs (option D), venlafaxine (option B), or TCAs (option A) (Montejo et al. 2001; Segraves 1998). Lower rates of sexual dysfunction have been associated with the antidepressants mirtazapine (25%), bupropion (5%–15%) (option C), and nefazodone (8%) (Kavoussi et al. 1997; Montejo et al. 2001; Reichenpfader et al. 2014). **(p. 397)**

14.10 Which of the following options most accurately describes antipsychotic medications and sexual function in older adults?

A. Higher rates of dysfunction occur with prolactin-sparing agents.
B. All antipsychotics can cause sexual dysfunction, usually in proportion to the dose.
C. Less potent agents with higher anticholinergic effects may cause less dysfunction.
D. Atypical antipsychotics are used to enhance libido and sexual arousal.

The correct response is option B: All antipsychotics can cause sexual dysfunction, usually in proportion to the dose.

All antipsychotic medications can cause sexual dysfunction, usually in proportion to the dose (option B); higher rates of dysfunction occur with prolactin-raising agents such as risperidone, haloperidol, olanzapine, and clozapine (40%–60%) than with prolactin-sparing agents such as quetiapine, aripiprazole, and ziprasidone (16%–27%) (Baggaley 2008; Serretti and Chiesa 2011) (option A). Like antidepressant and anxiolytic medications, antipsychotics can decrease libido, interfere with sexual arousal, and inhibit erections, ejaculation, and orgasm (Baggaley 2008) (option D). With regard to antipsychotic medications, more potent agents with fewer anticholinergic side effects and prolactin-sparing agents may cause less dysfunction (Baggaley 2008; Serretti and Chiesa 2011) (option C). **(pp. 398, 400)**

References

Adelman M: Stigma, gay lifestyles, and adjustment to aging: a study of later-life gay men and lesbians. J Homosex 20(3–4):7–32, 1990 2086652

Agronin ME: Sexuality and aging, in Principles and Practice of Sex Therapy, 5th Edition. Edited by Binik YM, Hall KSK. New York, Guilford, 2014, pp 525–539

Baggaley M: Sexual dysfunction in schizophrenia: focus on recent evidence. Hum Psychopharmacol 23(3):201–209, 2008 18338766

Brotto L, Luria M: Sexual interest/arousal disorder in woman, in Principles and Practice of Sex Therapy, 5th Edition. Edited by Binik YM, Hall KSK. New York, Guilford, 2014, pp 17–41

Centers for Disease Control and Prevention: Sexually Transmitted Disease Surveillance, 2012. Available at: http://www.cdc.gov/sTD/stats12/Surv2012.pdf. Accessed April 2014.

Crenshaw TL, Goldberg JP: Sexual Pharmacology: Drugs That Affect Sexual Function. New York, WW Norton, 1996

Goodwin AJ, Agronin ME: A Women's Guide to Overcoming Sexual Fear and Pain. Oakland, CA, New Harbinger, 1997

Hajjar RR, Kamel HK: Sexuality in the nursing home, part 1: attitudes and barriers to sexual expression. J Am Med Dir Assoc 5 (2 suppl):S42–S47, 2004a 14984610

Hajjar RR, Kamel HK: Sexuality in the nursing home, part 2: managing abnormal behavior—legal and ethical issues. J Am Med Dir Assoc 5 (2 suppl):S48–S52, 2004b 14984611

Joller P, Gupta N, Seitz DP, et al: Approach to inappropriate sexual behaviour in people with dementia. Can Fam Physician 59(3):255–260, 2013 23486794

Kaplan HS: The New Sex Therapy. New York, Brunner/Mazel, 1974

Kaplan HS: The Evaluation of Sexual Disorders: Psychological and Medical Aspects. New York, Brunner/Mazel, 1983

Kavoussi RJ, Segraves RT, Hughes AR, et al: Double-blind comparison of bupropion sustained release and sertraline in depressed outpatients. J Clin Psychiatry 58(12):532–537, 1997 9448656

Laumann EO, Paik A, Rosen RC: Sexual dysfunction in the United States: prevalence and predictors. JAMA 281(6):537–544, 1999 10022110

Lindau ST, Schumm LP, Laumann EO, et al: A study of sexuality and health among older adults in the United States. N Engl J Med 357(8):762–774, 2007 17715410

Ludwig W, Phillips M: Organic causes of erectile dysfunction in men under 40. Urol Int 92(1):1–6, 2014 24281298

Montejo AL, Llorca G, Izquierdo JA, et al: Incidence of sexual dysfunction associated with antidepressant agents: a prospective multicenter study of 1022 outpatients. J Clin Psychiatry 62 (suppl 3):10–21, 2001 11229449

Morley JE: Testosterone and behavior. Clin Geriatr Med 19(3):605–616, 2003

Mulligan T, Palguta RF Jr: Sexual interest, activity, and satisfaction among male nursing home residents. Arch Sex Behav 20(2):199–204, 1991 2064543

Porst H, Montorsi F, Rosen RC, et al: The Premature Ejaculation Prevalence and Attitudes (PEPA) survey: prevalence, comorbidities, and professional help-seeking. Eur Urol 51(3):816–823, 2007 16934919

Redinbaugh EM, Zeiss AM, Davies HD, et al: Sexual behavior in men with dementing illnesses. Clin Geriatr 5:45–50, 1997

Reichenpfader U, Gartlehner G, Morgan LC, et al: Sexual dysfunction associated with second-generation antidepressants in patients with major depressive disorder: results from a systematic review with network meta-analysis. Drug Saf 37(1):19–31, 2014 24338044

Richardson JP, Lazur A: Sexuality in the nursing home patient. Am Fam Physician 51(1):121–124, 1995 7810464

Robinson KM, Davis SJ: Influence of cognitive decline on sexuality in individuals with dementia and their caregivers. J Gerontol Nurs 39(11):30–36, 2013 24066786

Schick V, Herbenick D, Reece M, et al: Sexual behaviors, condom use, and sexual health of Americans over 50: implications for sexual health promotion for older adults. J Sex Med 7 (suppl 5):315–329, 2010 21029388

Segraves RT: Antidepressant-induced sexual dysfunction. J Clin Psychiatry 59 (suppl 4):48–54, 1998 9554321

Serretti A, Chiesa A: A meta-analysis of sexual dysfunction in psychiatric patients taking antipsychotics. Int Clin Psychopharmacol 26(3):130–140, 2011 21191308

Thomas DR: Medications and sexual function. Clin Geriatr Med 19(3):553–562, 2003 14567007

Wasow M, Loeb MB: Sexuality in nursing homes. J Am Geriatr Soc 27(2):73–79, 1979 762368

Westheimer RK, Lopater S: Human Sexuality: A Psychosocial Perspective. Philadelphia, PA, Lippincott Williams & Wilkins, 2002

CHAPTER 15

Bereavement

15.1 Which of the following events that can cause bereavement is the most common and traumatic in late life?

A. Death of spouse.
B. Death of an adult child.
C. Deterioration of one's health.
D. Divorce.

The correct response is option A: Death of spouse.

The terms *bereavement* and *grief reaction* have been used to refer to any number of losses. These losses include (but are not limited to) the death of a spouse, an adult child (option B), another family member, or a close personal friend; divorce (option D) (Cain 1988); anticipatory grief associated with caregiving for a severely impaired loved one (Bass et al. 1991); and a significant decline in one's own health (option C), attractiveness, capabilities, opportunities, and so forth (Kalish 1987). When used in its narrowest sense, however, bereavement refers to the reaction or process that results after the death of someone close. The death of a spouse (option A) is generally accepted as the most common and traumatic life event in late life (Jacobs and Ostfeld 1977). **(p. 415)**

15.2 How does the mortality rate compare for men and women in the first year after a spouse's death?

A. The rate is 2 times less for men than for women.
B. The rate is the same for men as for women.
C. The rate is 2 times greater for men than for women.
D. The rate is 12 times greater for men than for women.

The correct response is option D: The rate is 12 times greater for men than for women.

Although elderly women may live without a spouse longer than their male peers, they also have lower mortality rates. For example, in the University of Southern

California longitudinal study of spousal bereavement, the first year after bereavement saw a mortality rate of 12% in men but only about 1% in women (Gallagher-Thompson et al. 1993; Thompson et al. 1991) (option D; options A, B, and C are incorrect). **(p. 416)**

15.3 Which of the following is a significant differentiating factor between grieving and major depression?

A. Problems with sleep.
B. Poor appetite.
C. Feelings of global dejection or complete anhedonia.
D. Attention and concentration problems.

The correct response is option C: Feelings of global dejection or complete anhedonia.

Specific symptoms such as frequent crying, chronic sleep disturbance (option A), blue mood, poor appetite (option B), low energy, feelings of fatigue, loss of interest in daily living, and problems with attention and concentration (option D) are common in both grief and major depression. Even though these symptoms can also be indicative of depression, most grieving individuals do not develop major depression; the sadness that accompanies bereavement is specific to the loss of the loved person, rather than the more global dejection that characterizes major depression (option C). **(p. 416)**

15.4 Which of the following approaches to a loss is found in those individuals having the best psychological outcome from bereavement?

A. Focusing on the individual who died and his or her contributions.
B. Accepting the loss as a part of life.
C. Constructing a meaning in life from the loss.
D. Focusing on finding a balance between loss-oriented stressors and restoration-oriented stressors.

The correct response is option D: Focusing on finding a balance between loss-oriented stressors and restoration-oriented stressors.

Grieving is not only a process involving preoccupation with the deceased (option A), accepting the loss (option B), trying to make sense of what has happened, and so on; it also involves attempts to construct meaning from the loss (option C) and reduce the chaos associated with such traumatic events. As Stroebe and Schut (1999, 2010) address with their dual process model, the bereaved oscillate between dealing with loss-oriented stressors and restoration-oriented stressors. Limited empirical support for this model is emerging, with individuals reporting actively dealing with both loss-oriented stressors and restoration-oriented stressors showing the best psychological outcomes (Bennett et al. 2010) (option D). **(p. 418)**

15.5 Which of the following coping strategies is more likely to be used by resilient individuals?

A. Supportive counseling.
B. Religious or faith-based coping.
C. Physical exercise.
D. Medications to maximize sleep.

The correct response is option B: Religious or faith-based coping.

Individuals identified as resilient demonstrate consistently low levels of depression or negative affect across the postloss period. Resilient individuals did not differ from common or chronic grief groups in either relationship quality or interviewer ratings of interpersonal skill or warmth (Bonanno et al. 2004; Ott et al. 2007), but they were more likely than the other groups to use religious coping (Ott et al. 2007) (option B; options A, C, and D are incorrect). **(pp. 418–419)**

15.6 Which of the following statements best characterizes chronic or abnormal grief?

A. Individuals with chronic grief display both intrusive symptoms and signs of avoidance and failure to adapt more than a year after the loss.
B. Individuals with chronic grief display episodic symptoms of distress for up to a year after the loss.
C. Individuals with chronic grief display signs of avoidance and failure to adapt for only the first month after the loss.
D. Individuals with chronic grief display both intrusive symptoms and signs of avoidance and failure to adapt within the first 6 months after the loss.

The correct response is option A: Individuals with chronic grief display both intrusive symptoms and signs of avoidance and failure to adapt more than a year after the loss.

Chronic grief (also referred to as complicated bereavement, traumatic grief, or prolonged grief disorder) occurs in 10%–15% of individuals (Bonanno et al. 2002; Ott et al. 2007) and is characterized by unremitting distress that lasts for an extended period following a loss. For abnormal grief, Horowitz et al. (1997) emphasized the importance of both intrusive symptoms and signs of avoidance and failure to adapt. Evidence of these signs and symptoms must be present for 14 months after the loss (option A; options B, C, and D are incorrect). **(p. 419)**

15.7 Cultural differences exist among bereaved individuals in different parts of the world. What pattern best describes Chinese bereavement?

A. Emotional experiences.
B. Spiritual rituals.
C. Cognitive practices.
D. Behavioral rituals.

The correct response is option D: Behavioral rituals.

Diverse cultural norms further complicate the distinction between adaptive and abnormal grieving practices. In contrast to the Western focus on the emotional experience of the grieving person, the Chinese focus on the behavior of the bereaved and the importance of demonstrating proper respect and love for the deceased by carrying out mourning rituals in an appropriate manner (option D; options A, B, and C are incorrect). **(p. 420)**

15.8 Which of the following is true regarding gender differences in bereavement?

A. Widowers are at relatively higher risk of death than widows.
B. Bereavement has a greater impact on depression scores in women than in men.
C. Following the loss of a spouse, men experience more personal growth than women.
D. In the "dual process" model, men are more focused on psychological aspects of coping with the loss, whereas women are more focused on restoring their life pattern without the loved one.

The correct response is option A: Widowers are at relatively higher risk of death than widows.

Gender differences in bereavement are complex. Stroebe et al. (2001) concluded that "widowers are indeed at relatively higher risk [of death] than widows (option A), and, given that death is the most extreme consequence of bereavement, much weight may be attached to this finding" (p. 69). The differential psychological impact of bereavement on men and women also appears unbalanced. Several studies have found that bereavement has a greater impact on depression scores in men than in women (van Grootheest et al. 1999; Williams 2003) (option B), but it may be that the elevated depression scores for men indicate that men begin to experience greater depression before the loss of their wives and then this level of comorbid depression is maintained in bereavement (Lee and DeMaris 2007). Women have been found to have less life satisfaction than men following the loss of a spouse (Lichtenstein et al. 1996; Williams 2003), but they may also experience more personal growth after the loss (Carr 2004) (option C). Referring to their "dual process" model, Stroebe et al. (2001) hypothesized that women are more focused on psychological aspects of coping with the loss, whereas men are more focused on restoring their life pattern without the loved one (option D). However, societal and structural demands may prompt flexible coping in women who have followed more traditional gender roles (e.g., in addition to loss-focused coping, women must adjust to new financial and domestic circumstances), whereas less pressure exists for men to engage with their nonpreferred coping focus. **(pp. 421–422)**

15.9 Of the risk factors for complicated bereavement, which of the following is associated with poor coping with loss 2 years later?

A. Clinically significant depression within the first 2 weeks postloss.
B. Intense negative emotions at 2 months postloss, such as a desire to die and frequent crying.

C. Self-reported depression in the mild range.

D. Spouse died of violent causes.

The correct response is option B: Intense negative emotions at 2 months post-loss, such as a desire to die and frequent crying.

Clinically significant depression within the first 2 months postloss (option A) is a significant risk factor for poor outcome over time. Lund et al. (1993) found that intense negative emotions at 2 months postloss—such as a desire to die and frequent crying—were associated with poor coping 2 years later (option B). Wortman and Silver (1989) reviewed a number of studies indicating that depression confounds successful resolution of grief. Both preloss depression and depression early in bereavement may play a significant role in adjustment. In a prospective longitudinal study of the course of bereavement outcomes, it appears that a higher proportion of individuals with preloss depression remained depressed at 18 months postloss (43%) than of those without preloss depression (21%; Bonanno et al. 2002). In work investigating the relationship between depression and later bereavement outcome, Gilewski et al. (1991) found that individuals with self-reported depression in the moderate to severe range (option C) were at greatest risk for all other psychopathological symptoms, such as increased anxiety, hostility, and interpersonal sensitivity. This result occurred whether their spouses had committed suicide or died of natural causes (option D). **(p. 422)**

15.10 Which of the following psychological treatments for complicated grief has been found to be more effective than other form of therapies?

A. Cognitive-behavioral therapy.

B. Supportive therapy.

C. Interpersonal therapy.

D. Waitlist control conditions.

The correct response is option A: Cognitive-behavioral therapy.

A growing number of psychological interventions have been developed specifically to target symptoms of complicated grief. A meta-analysis found a medium effect size favoring these targeted interventions, especially interventions grounded in cognitive-behavioral therapy (option A), as more effective than other supportive therapies (option B), interpersonal therapy (option C), or waitlist control conditions (option D) (Wittouck et al. 2011). Cognitive and cognitive-behavioral therapies of various forms are effective in treating patients with complex bereavement reactions (Currier et al. 2010). One such strategy focuses on core constructs known to be disrupted during intense grief (Viney 1990). As these disrupted constructs are identified through self-monitoring and Socratic questioning during treatment sessions, the client learns methods of reconstructing shattered beliefs about the self, the present surroundings, and future events. A blend of cognitive and behavioral techniques (such as challenging dysfunctional thoughts and teaching specific behavioral skills for use in resolving interpersonal problems) has been applied successfully with individual patients (for an example, see Florsheim and Gallagher-Thompson 1990). **(p. 425)**

15.11 Which of the following reflects the use of pharmacological interventions in bereavement?

    A. Antidepressants should be prescribed to reduce symptoms of grief whether or not the person has symptoms of depression.
    B. The empirical literature is equivocal with regard to effectiveness of medication use in uncomplicated grief.
    C. Antidepressants, including tricyclic antidepressants (TCAs) and selective serotonin reuptake inhibitors (SSRIs), have not been found to be effective in reducing symptoms of grief that are also present in depression.
    D. World Health Organization (WHO) guidelines in management of stress and trauma-related disorders recommend the use of benzodiazepines in the management of bereavement.

The correct response is option B: The empirical literature is equivocal with regard to effectiveness of medication use in uncomplicated grief.

Using medication to treat uncomplicated grief (other than for specific symptoms such as insomnia) has been questioned. Many clinicians feel that medication, if used at all, should be minimal and brief. For example, Raphael et al. (2001) argued that if depression is not evident, then antidepressants should not be prescribed to reduce symptoms of grief (option A). The empirical literature is equivocal with regard to effectiveness of medication use in uncomplicated grief (option B). There is some indication that antidepressants, including TCAs and SSRIs, are effective for reducing symptoms that are also present in depression (option C). A small randomized controlled trial comparing benzodiazepine use to placebo noted no significant differences between groups in bereavement symptoms, although there was a trend for negative impact of benzodiazepine use on sleep initiation and bad dreams (Warner et al. 2001). Recently released WHO guidelines in management of stress and trauma-related disorders specifically recommend against the use of benzodiazepines in the management of bereavement (Tol et al. 2013) (option D). **(p. 427)**

15.12 Which of the following is one of the eight developmental levels in the Assimilation of Problematic Experiences Sequence model?

    A. Full immersion in the painful situation.
    B. Development of heightened awareness of the painful situation.
    C. Reduction of understanding/insight.
    D. Integration/mastery.

The correct response is option D: Integration/mastery.

To assist practitioners in assessing the efficacy of their bereavement treatment, Wilson (2011) developed the Assimilation of Problematic Experiences Sequence model, which describes the psychosocial changes exhibited by clients as they deal with a challenging experience such as grief. The complete assimilation sequence includes eight developmental levels, from 0 to 7, and describes an individual's progression from being warded off/dissociated from the experience (option A) to developing a vague awareness of the painful situation (option B), to gaining understanding/insight (option C), and eventually moving to problem solution and ultimately to integration/mastery (option D). **(p. 426)**

References

Bass DM, Bowman K, Noelker LS: The influence of caregiving and bereavement support on adjusting to an older relative's death. Gerontologist 31(1):32–42, 1991 2007473

Bennett KM, Gibbons K, Mackenzie-Smith S: Loss and restoration in later life: an examination of dual process model of coping with bereavement. Omega (Westport) 61(4):315–332, 2010 21058612

Bonanno GA, Wortman CB, Lehman DR, et al: Resilience to loss and chronic grief: a prospective study from preloss to 18-months postloss. J Pers Soc Psychol 83(5):1150–1164, 2002 12416919

Bonanno GA, Wortman CB, Nesse RM: Prospective patterns of resilience and maladjustment during widowhood. Psychol Aging 19(2):260–271, 2004 15222819

Cain BS: Divorce among elderly women: a growing social phenomenon. Soc Casework 69:563–568, 1988

Carr D: Gender, preloss marital dependence, and older adults' adjustment to widowhood. J Marriage Fam 66:220–235, 2004

Currier JM, Holland JM, Neimeyer RA: Do CBT-based interventions alleviate distress following bereavement? A review of the current evidence. Int J Cogn Ther 3:77–93, 2010

Florsheim M, Gallagher-Thompson D: Cognitive/behavioral treatment of atypical bereavement: a case study. Clin Gerontol 10:73–76, 1990

Gallagher-Thompson D, Futterman A, Farberow N: The impact of spousal bereavement on older widows and widowers, in Handbook of Bereavement. Edited by Stroebe MS, Stroebe W, Hansson R, et al. Cambridge, UK, Cambridge University Press, 1993, pp 227–239

Gilewski MJ, Farberow NL, Gallagher DE, Thompson LW: Interaction of depression and bereavement on mental health in the elderly. Psychol Aging 6(1):67–75, 1991 2029370

Horowitz MJ, Siegel B, Holen A, et al: Diagnostic criteria for complicated grief disorder. Am J Psychiatry 154(7):904–910, 1997 9210739

Kalish RA: Older people and grief. Generations 11:33–38, 1987

Jacobs S, Ostfeld A: An epidemiological review of the mortality of bereavement. Psychosom Med 39(5):344–357, 1977 333498

Lee GR, DeMaris A: Widowhood, gender, and depression: a longitudinal analysis. Res Aging 29:56–72, 2007

Lichtenstein P, Gatz M, Pedersen NL, et al: A co-twin–control study of response to widowhood. J Gerontol B Psychol Sci Soc Sci 51(5):279–289, 1996 8809004

Lund DA, Caserta M, Dimond M: The course of spousal bereavement in later life, in Handbook of Bereavement. Edited by Stroebe MS, Stroebe W, Hansson R. Cambridge, UK, Cambridge University Press, 1993, pp 240–254

Ott CH, Lueger RJ, Kelber ST, Prigerson HG: Spousal bereavement in older adults: common, resilient, and chronic grief with defining characteristics. J Nerv Ment Dis 195(4):332–341, 2007 17435484

Raphael B, Minkov C, Dobson M: Psychotherapeutic and pharmacological intervention for bereaved persons, in Handbook of Bereavement Research: Consequences, Coping, and Care. Edited by Stroebe MS, Hansson RO, Stroebe W, et al. Washington, DC, American Psychological Association, 2001, pp 587–612

Stroebe M, Schut H: The dual process model of coping with bereavement: rationale and description. Death Stud 23(3):197–224, 1999 10848151

Stroebe M, Schut H: The dual process model of coping with bereavement: a decade on. Omega (Westport) 61(4):273–289, 2010 21058610

Stroebe MS, Stroebe W, Schut H: Gender differences in adjustment to bereavement: an empirical and theoretical review. Rev Gen Psychol 5:62–83, 2001

Thompson LW, Gallagher-Thompson D, Futterman A, et al: The effects of late-life spousal bereavement over a 30-month interval. Psychol Aging 6(3):434–441, 1991 1930760

Tol WA, Barbui C, van Ommeren M: Management of acute stress, PTSD, and bereavement: WHO recommendations. JAMA 310(5):477–478, 2013 23925613

van Grootheest DS, Beekman ATF, Broese van Groenou MI, Deeg DJ: Sex differences in depression after widowhood. Do men suffer more? Soc Psychiatry Psychiatr Epidemiol 34(7):391–398, 1999 10477960

Viney L: The construing widow: dislocation and adaptation in bereavement. Psychother Patient 6:207–222, 1990

Warner J, Metcalfe C, King M: Evaluating the use of benzodiazepines following recent bereavement. Br J Psychiatry 178(1):36–41, 2001 11136208

Williams K: Has the future of marriage arrived? A contemporary examination of gender, marriage, and psychological well-being. J Health Soc Behav 44(4):470–487, 2003 15038144

Wilson J: The assimilation of problematic experiences sequence: an approach to evidence-based practice in bereavement counseling. J Soc Work End Life Palliat Care 7(4):350–362, 2011 22150179

Wittouck C, Van Autreve S, De Jaegere E, et al: The prevention and treatment of complicated grief: a meta-analysis. Clin Psychol Rev 31(1):69–78, 2011 21130937

Wortman CB, Silver RC: The myths of coping with loss. J Consult Clin Psychol 57(3):349–357, 1989 2661609

CHAPTER 16

Sleep and Circadian Rhythm Disorders

16.1 Which of the following correctly states the prevalence of sleep problems in geriatric patients?

A. Sleep complaints are rarely reported by seniors with Parkinson's disease.
B. More than half of all seniors who live at home report sleep difficulties.
C. Restless legs syndrome (RLS) is reported by less than 10% of patients older than 65 years.
D. Nocturia is reported by less than 50% of seniors as a cause of sleep difficulties.

The correct response is option B: More than half of all seniors who live at home report sleep difficulties.

More than half of noninstitutionalized individuals older than 65 years report chronic sleep difficulties (Foley et al. 1995; National Institutes of Health Consensus Development Conference Statement 1991; Prinz et al. 1990) (option B). Sleep disturbances affect quality of life, increase the risk of accidents and falls, and, perhaps most important, are among the leading reasons for long-term-care placement (Pollak and Perlick 1991; Pollak et al. 1990; Sanford 1975). Sleep complaints are noted in 60%–90% of individuals with Parkinson's disease (Trenkwalder 1998) (option A). RLS is present in up to 28% of patients older than 65 years (Clark 2001) (option C). It has been reported that nocturia is the most common explanation given by elderly individuals for difficulty in maintaining sleep; 63%–72% of elderly individuals cite nocturia as a reason for sleep maintenance problems (Middelkoop et al. 1996) (option D). **(pp. 435, 439, 441, 443)**

16.2 Which of the following is true regarding the changes in sleep with aging?

A. Decreased total sleep time, reduced sleep efficiency, and increased awakenings.
B. Increased total sleep time, increased sleep efficiency, and increased awakenings.
C. Decreased total sleep time, increased sleep efficiency, and reduced awakenings.
D. Increased total sleep time, reduced sleep efficiency, and reduced awakenings.

The correct response is option A: Decreased total sleep time, reduced sleep efficiency, and increased awakenings.

Perhaps the most striking change in sleep patterns in older adults is the frequent interruption of sleep by periods of wakefulness (Ohayon 2002). Older adults also have decreased total sleep time, reduced sleep efficiency, decreased slow-wave sleep and rapid eye movement (REM) sleep, and increased stage 1 and 2 sleep (option A; options B, C, and D are incorrect). **(p. 436)**

16.3   An 85-year-old man comes to your office with concerns that his family has noticed changes in his sleep pattern. His grandson complains that he goes to bed too early, and his daytime napping worries his daughter. The patient admits that he is more tired than he used to be and he goes to bed and wakes up earlier than in the past. Which statement most adequately addresses the concerns of this patient?

   A. The increased likelihood of napping is associated with aging, but the tendency to fall asleep and wake earlier is not.
   B. The tendency to fall asleep and wake earlier is associated with aging, but an increased likelihood of napping is not.
   C. Aging is not associated with the increased likelihood of napping or the tendency to fall asleep and wake earlier.
   D. Aging is associated with an increased likelihood of napping and a tendency to fall asleep and wake up earlier.

The correct response is option D: Aging is associated with an increased likelihood of napping and a tendency to fall asleep and wake up earlier.

The sleep-wake cycle appears to change significantly with age. The amplitudes of both the sleep-wake cycle and the 24-hour body temperature rhythm appear to decrease with aging (Bliwise 2000; Czeisler et al. 1999). Aging is also associated with a tendency to fall asleep and awaken earlier (Monk 2005). Additionally, compared with younger people, older adults are more likely to be sleepy and nap during the day (Buysse et al. 1992; Martin and Ancoli-Israel 2006) (option D; options A, B, and C are incorrect). **(p. 436)**

16.4   A divorced 78-year-old man comes to your office for an evaluation. He has a medical history significant for obesity, hypertension, coronary artery disease, and diabetes mellitus. The patient complains of excessive daytime sleepiness and foggy thinking. He falls asleep between 10 and 11 P.M. and wakes up between 6 and 7 A.M. What is the most appropriate next step?

   A. Obtain a subjective sleep log.
   B. Order a brain magnetic resonance imaging (MRI) scan.
   C. Start actigraphy.
   D. Get a polysomnogram.

The correct response is option D: Get a polysomnogram.

The patient is obese and reporting excessive daytime sleepiness and foggy thinking. Polysomnography (option D) is the primary laboratory test in sleep medicine. Although this patient's symptoms may warrant a brain MRI (option B), the patient's symptoms all point to possible sleep apnea, which is best diagnosed through polysomnography. Actigraphy is an objective assessment of activity throughout the day and night. A person who complains of an inability to fall asleep until 3 A.M. and difficulty in awakening before noon may need actigraphy (option C), but this is not the issue the patient describes. A subjective sleep log (option A) can be useful, particularly in the assessment of insomnia and circadian rhythm disturbances, neither of which the patient is reporting. **(p. 445)**

16.5   A 68-year-old woman comes to your office reporting sleep difficulties. She notes that when she is falling asleep her legs become very uncomfortable and she has to kick her legs back and forth to relieve the sensation. What is the best next step?

A. Start ropinerole or pramipexole.
B. Check glucose, complete blood count (CBC), and ferritin.
C. Start clonazepam or gabapentin.
D. Get a polysomnogram.

The correct response is option B: Check glucose, complete blood count (CBC), and ferritin.

RLS is often associated with periodic limb movement disorder (PLMD) and is often described as an uncomfortable feeling in the lower extremities that creates an irresistible urge to move. Symptoms are worse when the individual is at rest rather than active. In fact, patients experience improvement in symptoms with movement. Polysomnography (option D) is not needed for a diagnosis of RLS, which is made through history taking. In elderly patients, ferritin levels lower than 45 µg/L have a positive correlation with an increased risk of RLS. Also associated with PLMD and RLS are diabetes mellitus, pregnancy, iron deficiency anemia, and use of certain medications, including antidepressants and antipsychotics (Bliwise et al. 1985) (option B). Workup to exclude these conditions is typically carried out before initiating medication treatment (options A and C). **(p. 439)**

16.6   An 86-year-old patient with moderate Alzheimer's disease (AD) is brought to your office by his family. Concerns are voiced around the patient's going to bed at 7 P.M. and waking up around 2 A.M. The patient needs a significant amount of attention, and the family is having difficulties being up in the middle of the night. The family hopes to keep their loved one at home as long as possible. What would you recommend for managing the patient's sleep?

A. Begin evening bright light therapy.
B. Give evening melatonin.
C. Start a cholinesterase inhibitor.
D. Place the patient in a nursing facility.

The correct response is option A: Begin evening bright light therapy.

Individuals with AD have been found to experience an increased number of arousals and awakenings, to take more daytime naps, and to have a diminished amount of REM sleep and slow-wave sleep (Prinz et al. 1982). Patients may develop circadian rhythm disturbances leading to the decreased night-time sleep and increased daytime sleep (Bliwise 2004). Moreover, cholinesterase inhibitors (option C), the primary treatment for AD, can cause vivid dreaming and insomnia. Nocturnal sleep disruption is among the leading reasons that individuals with dementia become institutionalized (Pollak and Perlick 1991; Pollak et al. 1990; Sanford 1975) (option D), but placing the patient would not currently fit with the family's stated goal to "keep their loved one at home as long as possible." Many aspects of good sleep hygiene that are emphasized in the general population can help patients with dementia who have sleep disturbance. Morning light therapy and caregiver education may also be helpful (Bliwise 2000; McCurry et al. 2005). For patients who go to bed very early and awaken in the very early hours of the morning, exposure to light in the evening hours (option A) or exercise in the evening hours can help postpone bedtime and consequently time of awakening. A recent Cochrane review found no evidence that melatonin (option B) improved any major sleep outcomes in patients with AD (McCleery et al. 2014). **(pp. 440–441)**

16.7   What would you advise to a family practice colleague who has questions about managing the sleep complaints of depressed patients?

A. Treating depressed patients' insomnia will not affect their mood.
B. Improving their sleep will decrease their suicide risk.
C. You can expect an antidepressant to fix patients' insomnia.
D. If the depression has resolved, there is no need to treat insomnia.

The correct response is option B: Improving their sleep will decrease their suicide risk.

Depression is frequently associated with sleep disruption in individuals older than 60 years. Major depressive disorder is the condition in which there is the strongest evidence for a complex bidirectional relationship with sleep disturbance (Krystal 2006). Although insomnia has long been viewed as a secondary symptom of underlying depression, the results of a series of studies are inconsistent with this point of view (National Institutes of Health Consensus Conference 1984). The findings include evidence that those with insomnia have an increased future risk of major depressive disorder, that insomnia is an independent risk factor for suicide in depressed individuals (option B), that antidepressant treatment frequently does not result in resolution of insomnia (option C), and that this residual insomnia is associated with an increased risk of depression (Breslau et al. 1996; Fawcett et al. 1990; Livingston et al. 1993; Reynolds et al. 1997) (option D). The strongest evidence of the importance of depression is a study that examined the administration of the insomnia agent eszopiclone along with the antidepressant fluoxetine for initial therapy of depression (Fava et al. 2006; Krystal et al. 2007). Compared with subjects treated with fluoxetine and placebo, those receiving fluoxetine and eszopiclone not only slept significantly better but also experienced more rapid and greater improvement in nonsleep aspects of depression (option A). **(p. 440)**

16.8   A middle-aged man presents with his wife for consultation. He reports sleeping well, but his wife reports that he "fights" in his sleep and has accidentally injured her in the past. Which condition is he most likely to develop in the next 5 years?

A. Alzheimer's disease.
B. Frontotemporal dementia.
C. Vascular dementia.
D. Parkinson's disease.

The correct response is option D: Parkinson's disease.

A sleep problem seen in patients with Parkinson's disease is REM sleep behavior disorder (RBD), in which the patient acts out dreams because the paralysis that usually occurs during REM sleep is absent (Clarenbach 2000). Patients (typically men) with the idiopathic form of RBD are at increased risk of developing a parkinsonian disorder or dementia, usually linked to α-synuclein pathology, the risk being 20%–40% after an average of 5 years follow-up (Postuma et al. 2009; Schenck et al. 1996) (option D; options A, B, and C are incorrect). **(pp. 441–442)**

16.9   A 52-year-old man presents complaining of sleep difficulties. He notes that he wakes "countless" times a night to urinate and feels that he can never sleep more than an hour or two at a time. His home medications include hydrochlorothiazide, simvastatin, and finasteride. Which of the following recommendations is most appropriate at this time for this patient?

A. Restrict evening fluids.
B. Take diuretics in the afternoon.
C. Restrict alcohol intake to moderate evening consumption.
D. Lower finasteride dose.

The correct response is option A: Restrict evening fluids.

The most common causes of nocturia in men are conditions that increase in frequency with age: benign prostatic hypertrophy and sleep apnea. Nocturia can generally be treated effectively by addressing the underlying condition, so having the patient lower his finasteride dose (option D) is not recommended. Patients with nocturia should be advised to restrict fluids in the evening (option A), to avoid alcohol (option C), and to ensure that diuretics are dosed in the mornings (option B). **(pp. 443–444)**

16.10 A middle-aged woman with no significant medical conditions reports ongoing sleep difficulties since menopause. She notes that she used to wake in the middle of the night with hot flashes and now continues to wake regularly, but she doesn't know why. She would like a long-term solution to this issue. What would you recommend?

A. Hormone replacement therapy.
B. Low-dose venlafaxine.
C. Cognitive-behavioral therapy.
D. Zolpidem before bedtime.

The correct response is option C: Cognitive-behavioral therapy.

There appears to be clear evidence that many women experience sleep disruption in association with vasomotor symptoms that are caused by decreased levels of circulating estrogen and progesterone (Bliwise 2000; Krystal et al. 1998). Although hormone replacement therapy (option A), venlafaxine (option B), and zolpidem (option D) can be effective in improving sleep difficulties associated with vaso-motor symptoms, the patient is no longer complaining of hot flashes. Although menopausal sleep disturbance is poorly understood, it has been suggested that behavioral conditioning occurs. In recent years, the term *cognitive-behavioral therapy for insomnia* (CBT-I) has been used to refer to a specific combination of therapies for insomnia that include stimulus control, sleep restriction, and cognitive strategies to alter dysfunctional sleep-related beliefs. A meta-analytic comparison suggests that behavioral therapies compare favorably with hypnotic pharmacotherapies in terms of short-term treatment effects and, unlike hypnotics, have enduring benefits and few side effects (Smith et al. 2002) (option C). **(pp. 444, 447)**

16.11 A middle-aged woman with a history of degenerative joint disease and diabetes mellitus presents with sleep difficulties that started during perimenopause. She reports that when she gets hot flashes and night sweats, she awakens and cannot get back to sleep. She sleeps well when she is not experiencing vasomotor symptoms. What treatment would you recommend for her sleep complaints?

A. Hormone replacement therapy.
B. Low-dose venlafaxine.
C. Cognitive-behavioral therapy.
D. Zolpidem before bedtime.

The correct response is option A: Hormone replacement therapy.

Many women experience sleep disruption in association with vasomotor symptoms that are caused by decreased levels of circulating estrogen and progesterone (Bliwise 2000; Krystal et al. 1998). If an association between insomnia and menopausal changes appears to exist, a trial of hormone replacement therapy could be considered (option A). If hormone replacement therapy is contraindicated, the antidepressants venlafaxine (option B), paroxetine, and fluoxetine, as well as gabapentin, have shown some efficacy in the management t of vasomotor symptoms with good tolerability (North American Menopause Society 2004). If an insomnia complaint persists after amelioration of vasomotor symptoms, other treatments such as pharmacological management of insomnia (option D) or CBT-I (option C) should be considered. **(p. 444)**

16.12 A 71-year-old man comes to your office complaining of difficulties falling asleep, noting that he goes to bed at 10 P.M. but cannot fall asleep until 2 or 3 A.M. He often does not wake up until noon. What is the best step in evaluating this patient?

A. Order a polysomnogram.
B. Order a thorough urologic evaluation.
C. Monitor symptoms with a sleep log and actigraphy.
D. Administer the Multiple Sleep Latency Test.

The correct response is option C: Monitor symptoms with a sleep log and actigraphy.

Each of the methods of evaluating a patient with sleep difficulties may be useful, depending on the nature of the complaint. A person who complains of an inability to fall asleep until 3 A.M. and difficulty in awakening before noon may need actigraphy and a sleep log assessment (option C). Actigraphy is an objective assessment of activity throughout the day and night that is used to determine the amount of wakefulness during the sleep period. A subjective sleep log can be useful in evaluating complaints of insomnia and circadian rhythm disturbances (as this patient reports). A polysomnogram (option A) is most appropriate in an individual who complains of excessive daytime sleepiness and nighttime snoring because polysomnography is primarily used to evaluate for sleep apnea, PLMD, nocturnal seizures, and nocturnal medical or psychiatric events. The Multiple Sleep Latency Test (option D) evaluates daytime sleepiness, which the patient is not reporting. The first step in evaluating patients with sleep-related complaints is a comprehensive clinical evaluation, and sometimes the treatment plan may include further testing and consultation, but nothing in the patient's story suggests a significant urologic component to his sleep difficulties (option B). **(p. 445)**

16.13 An 83-year-old man with hypertension, presbycusis, degenerative joint disease, diabetes mellitus, and cataracts reports difficulty sleeping at night. What is the most likely cause of his insomnia?

A. Unplanned daytime napping.
B. Untreated major depression.
C. Unrecognized sleep apnea.
D. Undiagnosed midbrain lesion.

The correct response is option A: Unplanned daytime napping.

Many elderly individuals experience decrements in hearing, vision, and mobility. Changes in these vital functions can have a profound effect on sleep. Most frequently, this effect stems from a loss of activities in which the affected individual can engage; to pass the time, the person takes unplanned naps (option A) or tries to sleep more than he or she is physiologically able to. The result is fragmentation of sleep and loss of circadian rhythmicity. Affected individuals report spending many frustrating hours awake in bed at night. Major depressive disorder is frequently associated with sleep disruption and is seen in roughly 10%–15% of individuals older than age 65, but no depressive symptoms have been mentioned in this case (option B). It has been suggested that the frequency of obstructive sleep apnea increases with age, but the patient is not complaining of daytime sleepiness or snoring (option C). Hypersomnia has been associated with lesions of the cephalad portions of the ascending reticular activating system, which includes the midbrain and paramedian region of the thalamus, but the patient is experiencing hyposomnia, not hypersomnia (option D). **(pp. 437, 440, 443, 444–445)**

16.14 Which of the following describes stimulus control to treat insomnia?

A. Using the bed only for sleeping, not napping, and having a routine schedule.
B. Using a sleep log to determine how much time to spend in bed at night.
C. Using relaxation therapies that decrease sleep latency and manage night awakenings.
D. Addressing dysfunctional beliefs and encouraging increased daytime activity.

The correct response is option A: Using the bed only for sleeping, not napping, and having a routine schedule.

Stimulus control therapy, developed by Bootzin (1972), is particularly useful for older individuals who have fallen out of a normal sleep-wake routine and for those who compromise their nighttime sleep by excessive daytime napping. It addresses such problems by curtailing daytime napping and by enforcing a consistent sleep-wake schedule. In addition, this treatment enhances sleep-inducing qualities of the bedroom by eliminating sleep-incompatible behaviors in bed (option A). Nonpharmacological interventions that address dysfunctional beliefs about sleep and the sleep-disruptive habits they sustain are often useful for combating insomnia in older patients (option D), but this does not describe stimulus control. Relaxation therapies (option C) can potentially help patients fall asleep, but they are not stimulus control. Because older adults appear to have a reduced homeostatic sleep drive (Dijk et al. 1997) as well as a propensity to spend excessive time in bed (Carskadon et al. 1982), measures are often needed to reduce the amount of time older patients with insomnia routinely allot for nocturnal sleep. Such a reduction is the aim of sleep restriction therapy (Spielman et al. 1987; Wohlgemuth and Edinger 2000) (option B). **(pp. 445–447)**

16.15 Which agent has been found to improve sleep maintenance and decrease early morning awakenings for older adults?

A. Ramelteon.
B. Mirtazapine.

C. Doxepin.

D. Trazodone.

The correct response is option C: Doxepin.

Eszopiclone (2 mg at bedtime) and doxepin (3 mg at bedtime) have been demonstrated to improve the ability to stay asleep in older adults with insomnia (Krystal et al. 2010; McCall et al. 2006). The doxepin study, which lasted for 12 weeks, is particularly notable for its effect on sleep maintenance and early morning awakenings given that these are the primary sleep complaints of elderly people (option C). Trazodone (option D), mirtazapine (option B), and amitriptyline have not been studied in older adults with insomnia. Ramelteon (option A) has been found to sustain sleep onset efficacy (Mayer et al. 2009), not sleep maintenance efficacy. **(pp. 448–450)**

References

Bliwise DL: Normal aging, in Principles and Practice of Sleep Medicine, 3rd Edition. Edited by Kryger MH, Roth T, Dement WC. Philadelphia, PA, WB Saunders, 2000, pp 26–42

Bliwise DL: Sleep disorders in Alzheimer's disease and other dementias. Clin Cornerstoner 6 (suppl 1A):S16–S28, 2004 15259536

Bliwise DL, Petta D, Seidel W, et al: Periodic leg movements during sleep in the elderly. Arch Gerontol Geriatr 4(3):273–282, 1985 4074025

Bootzin RR: A stimulus control treatment for insomnia. Proceedings of the American Psychological Association 7:395–396, 1972

Breslau N, Roth T, Rosenthal P, Andreski P: Sleep disturbance and psychiatric disorders: a longitudinal epidemiological study of young adults. Biol Psychiatry 39(6):411–418, 1996 8679786

Buysse DJ, Browman KE, Monk TH: Napping and 24-hour sleep/wake patterns in healthy elderly and young adults. J Am Geriatr Soc 40(8):779–786, 1992 1634721

Carskadon MA, Brown ED, Dement WC: Sleep fragmentation in the elderly: relationship to daytime sleep tendency. Neurobiol Aging 3(4):321–327, 1982 7170049

Clarenbach P: Parkinson's disease and sleep. J Neurol 247 (suppl 4):IV20–IV23, 2000 1199812

Clark MM: Restless legs syndrome. J Am Board Fam Pract 14(5):368–374, 2001 11572542

Czeisler CA, Duffy JF, Shanahan TL, et al: Stability, precision, and near-24-hour period of the human circadian pacemaker. Science 284(5423):2177–2181, 1999 10381883

Dijk DJ, Duffy JF, Riel E, et al: Altered interaction of circadian and homeostatic aspects of sleep propensity results in awakening at an earlier circadian phase in older people. Sleep Res 26:710, 1997

Fava M, McCall WV, Krystal A, et al: Eszopiclone co-administered with fluoxetine in patients with insomnia coexisting with major depressive disorder. Biol Psychiatry 59(11):1052–1060, 2006 16581036

Fawcett J, Scheftner WA, Fogg L, et al: Time-related predictors of suicide in major affective disorder. Am J Psychiatry 147(9):1189–1194, 1990 2104515

Foley DJ, Monjan AA, Brown SL: Sleep complaints among elderly persons: an epidemiologic study of three communities. Sleep 18(6):425–432, 1995 7481413

Krystal AD: Sleep and psychiatric disorders: future directions. Psychiatr Clin North Am 29(4):1115–1130, abstract xi, 2006 17118285

Krystal AD, Edinger J, Wohlgemuth W, et al: Sleep in peri-menopausal and post-menopausal women. Sleep Med Rev 2(4):243–253, 1998 15310495

Krystal AD, Fava M, Rubens R, et al: Evaluation of eszopiclone discontinuation after cotherapy with fluoxetine for insomnia with coexisting depression. J Clin Sleep Med 3(1):48–55, 2007 17557453

Krystal AD, Durrence HH, Scharf M, et al: Efficacy and safety of doxepin 1 mg and 3 mg in a 12-week sleep laboratory and outpatient trial of elderly subjects with chronic primary insomnia. Sleep 33(11):1553–1561, 2010 21102997

Livingston G, Blizzard B, Mann A: Does sleep disturbance predict depression in elderly people: A study in inner London. Br J Gen Pract 43(376):445–448, 1993 8292414

Martin JL, Ancoli-Israel S: Napping in older adults. Sleep Med Clin 1:177–186, 2006

Mayer G, Wang-Weigand S, Roth-Schechter B, et al: Efficacy and safety of 6-month nightly ramelteon administration in adults with chronic primary insomnia. Sleep 32(3):351–360, 2009 19294955

McCall WV, Erman M, Krystal AD, et al: A polysomnography study of eszopiclone in elderly patients with insomnia. Curr Med Res Opin 22(9):1633–1642, 2006 16968566

McCleery J, Cohen DA, Sharpley AL, et al: Pharmacotherapies for sleep disturbances in Alzheimer's disease. Cochrane Review. Cochrane Database Syst Rev (3):CD009178, 2014 24659320

McCurry SM, Gibbons LE, Logsdon RG, et al: Nighttime insomnia treatment and education for Alzheimer's disease: a randomized, controlled trial. J Am Geriatr Soc 53(5):793–802, 2005 15877554

Middelkoop HA, Smilde-van den Doel DA, Neven AK, et al: Subjective sleep characteristics of 1,485 males and females aged 50–93: effects of sex and age, and factors related to self-evaluated quality of sleep. J Gerontol A Biol Sci Med Sci 51(3): M108–M115, 1996 8630703

Monk TH: Aging human circadian rhythms: conventional wisdom may not always be right. J Biol Rhythms 20(4):366–374, 2005 16077155

National Institutes of Health Consensus Conference: Drugs and insomnia: the use of medications to promote sleep. JAMA 251(18):2410–2414, 1984 6142971

National Institutes of Health Consensus Development Conference Statement: The treatment of sleep disorders of older people March 26–28, 1990. Sleep 14(2):169–177, 1991 1866532

North American Menopause Society: Treatment of menopause-associated vasomotor symptoms: position statement of the North American Menopause Society. Menopause 11(1):11–33, 2004 14716179

Ohayon MM: Epidemiology of insomnia: what we know and what we still need to learn. Sleep Med Rev 6(2):97–111, 2002 12531146

Pollak CP, Perlick D: Sleep problems and institutionalization of the elderly. J Geriatr Psychiatry Neurol 4(4):204–210, 1991 1789908

Pollak CP, Perlick D, Linsner JP, et al: Sleep problems in the community elderly as predictors of death and nursing home placement. J Community Health 15(2):123–135, 1990 2355110

Postuma RB, Gagnon JF, Vendette M, et al: Quantifying the risk of neurodegenerative disease in idiopathic REM sleep behavior disorder. Neurology 72(15):1296–1300, 2009 19109537

Prinz PN, Peskind ER, Vitaliano PP, et al: Changes in the sleep and waking EEGs of nondemented and demented elderly subjects. J Am Geriatr Soc 30(2):86–93, 1982 7199061

Prinz PN, Vitiello MV, Raskind MA, et al: Geriatrics: sleep disorders and aging. N Engl J Med 323(8):520–526, 1990 2198467

Reynolds CF III, Frank E, Houck PR, et al: Which elderly patients with remitted depression remain well with continued interpersonal psychotherapy after discontinuation of antidepressant medication? Am J Psychiatry 154(7):958–962, 1997 9210746

Sanford JRA: Tolerance of debility in elderly dependants by supporters at home: its significance for hospital practice. BMJ 3(5981):471–473, 1975 1156826

Schenck CH, Bundlie SR, Mahowald MW: Delayed emergence of a parkinsonian disorder in 38% of 29 older men initially diagnosed with idiopathic rapid eye movement sleep behaviour disorder. Neurology 46(2):388–393, 1996 8614500

Smith MT, Perlis ML, Park A, et al: Comparative meta-analysis of pharmacotherapy and behavior therapy for persistent insomnia. Am J Psychiatry 159(1):5–11, 2002 11772681

Spielman AJ, Saskin P, Thorpy MJ: Treatment of chronic insomnia by restriction of time in bed. Sleep 10(1):45–56, 1987 3563247

Trenkwalder C: Sleep dysfunction in Parkinson's disease. Clin Neurosci 5(2):107–114, 1998 23711168

Wohlgemuth WK, Edinger JD: Sleep restriction therapy, in Treatment of Late-Life Insomnia. Edited by Lichstein KL, Morin CM. Thousand Oaks, CA, Sage, 2000, pp 147–184

CHAPTER 17

Substance-Related and Addictive Disorders

17.1   What effect do the physiological changes associated with aging have on the pharmacokinetics of alcohol?

A. Decreased serum concentration and absorption and increased distribution.
B. Increased serum concentration and absorption and decreased distribution.
C. Increased serum concentration, absorption, and distribution.
D. Decreased serum concentration, absorption, and distribution.

The correct response is option C: Increased serum concentration, absorption, and distribution.

Lean body mass and total water volume decrease relative to total fat volume later in life. As a result, total body volume decreases, thereby increasing the serum concentration, absorption, and distribution of alcohol and drugs in the body (option C; options A, B, and D are incorrect). **(p. 461)**

17.2   According to national guidelines, which of the following represents the upper limit of recommended alcohol consumption for adults older than age 65 years?

A. 1 standard drink per day or 7 standard drinks per week.
B. 2 standard drinks per day or 14 standard drinks per week.
C. No more than 3 standard drinks per drinking occasion.
D. At least 1 standard drink per day for health benefits unless there is a medical comorbidity or past history of alcohol use disorder.

The correct response is option A: 1 standard drink per day or 7 standard drinks per week.

Taking age-related factors into account, guidelines for alcohol use are lower for older relative to younger adults. Recommendations set forth by the National Institute on Alcohol Abuse and Alcoholism (2005) and the Center for Substance Abuse Treatment (Blow 1998) on older adults state that adults age 65 years or older should consume no more than one standard drink per day or seven standard drinks per week (option A; option B is incorrect). Moreover, older adults should not consume more than two standard drinks on any one occasion (binge drinking) (option C). Although the literature suggests that low to moderate use of alcohol can lead to various health benefits among older adults, it is important to recognize that there is no evidence to support the notion that recommending that nondrinkers initiate drinking will translate into reduced health risks (option D). **(pp. 462, 469)**

17.3 An elderly individual who consumes 10 standard drinks per week and has no substance-related health, social, or emotional problems would be classified as which of the following?

A. Low-risk drinker.
B. Moderate drinker.
C. Social drinker.
D. At-risk drinker.

The correct response is option D: At-risk drinker.

Older adults who consume substances above recommended levels yet experience minimal or no substance-related health, social, or emotional problems are considered at-risk or excessive substance users. The recommended guidelines specify no more than seven standard drinks per week (option D). Those who drink within the recommended guidelines, do not exhibit any alcohol-related problems, and use caution when driving or when using contraindicated medications are classified as low-risk (option A), social (option C), or moderate (option B) drinkers. **(pp. 462, 464)**

17.4 Which of the following symptoms of substance use disorder is valid for young to middle-aged adults but may be of questionable validity in diagnosing the disorder in later life?

A. Unsuccessful attempts to cut down on use.
B. Cravings or a strong desire to use the substance.
C. Presence of withdrawal.
D. Failure to fulfill major role obligations at work or home.

The correct response is option D: Failure to fulfill major role obligations at work or home.

The criteria for substance use disorder are based mostly on research with young to middle-aged adults and have not been sufficiently validated among older populations; therefore, the symptoms and consequences set forth in DSM-5 may not be sensitive enough to capture disorder in later life. For example, some of the standard symptoms of substance use disorder listed in DSM-5, such as employment problems or interpersonal difficulties, may not be as readily applied to older individuals, given age-related factors such as retirement, widowhood, and resultant changes in occupational and social roles and network composition. As a result, the risks associated with this pattern of substance use may be underestimated (option D; options A, B, and C are incorrect). **(pp. 464–465)**

17.5   Which of the following substances is more likely to be misused by older women than older men?

A. Alcohol.
B. Marijuana.
C. Cocaine.
D. Psychoactive medications.

The correct response is option D: Psychoactive medications.

Older men are more likely to drink greater quantities of alcohol than older women and are more likely to have alcohol-related problems (Moore et al. 2005) (option A). Illicit drug use (options B and C) among older adults is rare, with a lifetime history of use of 2.88% for men and 0.66% for women (Anthony and Helzer 1991). Women, though less likely than men to use and abuse alcohol, are more likely than men to use and misuse psychoactive medications (Simoni-Wastila and Yang 2006) (option D), particularly if they are divorced or widowed, have lower socioeconomic status (e.g., education and income), or have been diagnosed with a mood disorder or anxiety (Closser and Blow 1993). **(pp. 467–469)**

17.6   Older adults who are moderate drinkers are at increased risk of developing which of the following?

A. Type 2 diabetes mellitus.
B. Hemorrhagic stroke.
C. Cardiovascular disease.
D. Physical limitations.

The correct response is option B: Hemorrhagic stroke.

Low-risk or moderate alcohol consumption is associated with a reduced risk of cardiovascular disease (option C), a lower incidence of type 2 diabetes mellitus (option A), and lower odds of reporting physical limitations (option D) when compared with abstinence or heavy use. However, even moderate alcohol use can lead to adverse health outcomes. For example, whereas moderate alcohol consumption decreases the risk of strokes caused by blocked blood vessels, it increases the risk of having a stroke caused by bleeding or hemorrhaging (option B). **(pp. 469, 470)**

17.7   Which of the following techniques is considered the gold standard for assessing the frequency and quantity of alcohol use by patients?

A. Prospective diary method.
B. Timeline followback (TLFB) method.

C. Assessing average drinking practices.

D. CAGE questionnaire.

The correct response is option A: Prospective diary method.

Techniques used to assess the quantity and frequency of alcohol and drug use fall into three categories: prospective monitoring and recording of alcohol and drug use, retrospective accounts of daily use of some defined period of time (i.e., TLFB), and questions regarding average consumption practices. The prospective monitoring (diary) method is considered to be the gold standard because it elicits the greatest number of reports of consumption and is highly associated with sales data for alcoholic beverages among younger adults (Lemmens et al. 1992; Tucker et al. 2007) (option A; options B and C are incorrect). The CAGE questionnaire (option D) is often used to screen for at-risk substance use or misuse as a complement to questions assessing the quantity and frequency of use; it does not, itself, assess either quantity or frequency. **(pp. 472, 473)**

17.8 Among individuals who participated in age-integrated residential treatment, older adults were as likely as middle-aged adults to do which of the following?

A. Contact a sponsor.

B. Self-identify as being a 12-step group member.

C. Engage in 12-step programs.

D. Call a fellow group member for help.

The correct response is option C: Engage in 12-step programs.

In their matched comparison of older versus younger and middle-aged adults who participated in age-integrated residential treatment, Lemke and Moos (2003) found that older patients engaged in 12-step programs as frequently as their younger and middle-aged counterparts when assessed at follow-up (option C). Results also indicated that more involvement in self-help groups posttreatment was associated with better treatment outcomes across all three age groups. However, older adults were less likely than middle-aged adults to self-identify as being a 12-step group member (option B) and were less likely than younger and middle-aged adults to report calling a fellow group member for help (option D). Additionally, older adults were significantly less likely to contact a sponsor (option A). **(p. 477)**

17.9 Which of the following medications has the most evidence to support its use in reducing heavy drinking and craving in older adults with alcohol use disorders?

A. Disulfiram.

B. Naltrexone.

C. Acamprosate.

D. Lorazepam.

The correct response is option B: Naltrexone.

Although disulfiram (option A) was originally the only medication approved for the treatment of alcohol dependence, it was seldom used in older patients because of the potential for adverse effects. Naltrexone (option B) has been shown to be effective among older adults. Meta-analytic work supports the notion that although acamprosate might be considered more effective in promoting and sustaining abstinence, naltrexone may be more effective in reducing heavy drinking and craving (Maisel et al. 2013). Unfortunately, no studies of the efficacy or safety of acamprosate (option C) among older patients have been conducted to date. Benzodiazepines such as lorazepam (option D) are associated with an increased risk of falls and fractures, impaired driving, disruptions in sleep cycles, and, among the frail elderly, excessive disability (Charlson et al. 2009; Madhusoodanan and Bogunovic 2004), and as such would not be appropriate in this population. **(pp. 470, 477–478)**

17.10 Which of the following symptoms, when present with other withdrawal symptoms, is an indicator of severe alcohol withdrawal?

A. Autonomic hyperactivity.
B. Tremor.
C. Nausea.
D. Hallucinations.

The correct response is option D: Hallucinations.

The classic set of symptoms associated with alcohol withdrawal includes autonomic hyperactivity (increased pulse rate, increased blood pressure, and increased temperature) (option A), restlessness, disturbed sleep, anxiety, nausea (option C), and tremor (option B). Severe withdrawal is marked by auditory, visual, or tactile hallucinations (option D); delirium; seizures; and coma. Autonomic hyperactivity, tremor, and nausea are symptoms of alcohol withdrawal, but they are not markers of severe withdrawal. **(p. 478)**

17.11 Which of the following changes in sleep patterns is associated with alcohol use?

A. Decrease in stage 4 sleep.
B. Increase in rapid eye movements (REM).
C. Increased sleep latency.
D. Decrease in stage 3 sleep.

The correct response is option A: Decrease in stage 4 sleep.

It is well established that alcohol causes changes in sleep patterns such as decreased sleep latency (option C), decreased stage 4 sleep (option A), and precipitation or aggravation of sleep apnea (National Institute on Alcohol Abuse and Alcoholism 1998; Wagman et al. 1977). Increase in REM episodes (option B) and decrease in stage 3 sleep (option D) are age-related (not alcohol-related) sleep changes. **(pp. 480–481)**

17.12 In the modified version of the CAGE questionnaire, problem drinking in older adults is indicated by a minimum of how many positive responses?

    A. One.
    B. Two.
    C. Three.
    D. Four.

The correct response is option A: One.

The CAGE questionnaire (Mayfield et al. 1974) is the most widely used alcohol screening test in clinical practice. A modified version of the CAGE questionnaire asks only about recent problems, and the threshold is often reduced to one positive response as an indicator of problems in older adults (option A; options B, C, and D are incorrect). This modified version of the CAGE has demonstrated high specificity for detecting alcohol abuse but relatively low sensitivity for alcohol use disorder (Buchsbaum et al. 1992; Moore et al. 2002). **(p. 473)**

17.13 In older adults, what is the minimum score on the Alcohol Use Disorders Identification Test (AUDIT-C) that indicates a positive screen and the need for further evaluation?

    A. 1.
    B. 3.
    C. 5.
    D. 10.

The correct response is option B: 3.

The AUDIT and its abbreviated version, the AUDIT-C, are simple screening measures that capture the frequency of drinking and bingeing in the past year (Bush et al. 1998; Dawson et al. 2005; Rubinsky et al. 2013). The AUDIT-C is scored on a scale of 0–12, with a score of 0 indicating no alcohol use during the preceding year. For older adults, a score of 3 or more reflects a positive screen and suggests the need for further evaluation (option B; options A, C, and D are incorrect). Generally, the higher the AUDIT-C score, the more likely it is that the individual's drinking is affecting his or her health and safety and is indicative of an alcohol use disorder (Bush et al. 1998; Rubinsky et al. 2013). **(p. 473)**

17.14 The majority of drugs of abuse will remain detectable in a urine drug screen for a minimum of how many days?

    A. 4.
    B. 7.

C. 10.

D. 14.

The correct response is option A: 4.

Urine drug screens are useful as both screening tools and confirmation of self-report when assessing prescription/over-the-counter medication and illicit drug abuse. The majority of drugs of abuse will remain detectable in a urine drug screen for 4 or more days (option A; options B, C, and D are incorrect), with some still detectable after several weeks. **(p. 475)**

17.15 What is the rate of heavy and binge drinking among adults older than 65 years?

A. 3%.

B. 10%.

C. 15%.

D. 25%.

The correct response is option B: 10%.

From the early 1990s until 2002, the prevalence of alcohol abuse or dependence has tripled to 3.1% among adults ages 65 years and older (Grant et al. 2004). Heavy and binge drinking among adults older than 65 years has increased, with recent reports citing rates near 10.2% (Substance Abuse and Mental Health Services Administration 2013) (option B; options A, C, and D are incorrect). **(p. 460)**

References

Anthony JC, Helzer JE: Syndromes of drug abuse and dependence, in Psychiatric Disorders in America: The Epidemiologic Catchment Area Study. Edited by Robins LN, Regier DA. New York, Free Press, 1991, pp 116–154

Blow FC: (Consensus Panel Chair): Substance Abuse Among Older Adults. Treatment Improvement Series Protocol (TIP) Series No. 26. Center for Substance Abuse Treatment. Rockville, MD, U.S. Department of Health and Human Services, 1998

Buchsbaum DG, Buchanan RG, Welsh J, et al: Screening for drinking disorders in the elderly using the CAGE questionnaire. J Am Geriatr Soc 40(7):662–665, 1992 1607581

Bush K, Kivlahan DR, McDonell MB, et al: The AUDIT alcohol consumption questions (AUDIT-C): an effective brief screening test for problem drinking. Ambulatory Care Quality Improvement Project (ACQUIP). Alcohol Use Disorders Identification Test. Arch Intern Med 158(16):1789–1795, 1998 9738608

Charlson F, Degenhardt L, McLaren J, et al: A systematic review of research examining benzodiazepine-related mortality. Pharmacoepidemiol Drug Saf 18(2):93–103, 2009 19125401

Closser MH, Blow FC: Recent advances in addictive disorders. Special populations. Women, ethnic minorities, and the elderly. Psychiatr Clin North Am 16(1):199–209, 1993 8456045

Dawson DA, Grant BF, Stinson FS, Zhou Y: Effectiveness of the derived Alcohol Use Disorders Identification Test (AUDIT-C) in screening for alcohol use disorders and risk drinking in the US general population. Alcohol Clin Exp Res 29(5):844–854, 2005 15897730

Grant BF, Dawson DA, Stinson FS, et al: The 12-month prevalence and trends in DSM-IV alcohol abuse and dependence: United States, 1991-1992 and 2001-2002. Drug Alcohol Depend 74(3):223–234, 2004 15194200

Lemke S, Moos RH: Outcomes at 1 and 5 years for older patients with alcohol use disorders. J Subst Abuse Treat 24(1):43–50, 2003 12646329

Lemmens P, Tan ES, Knibbe RA: Measuring quantity and frequency of drinking in a general population survey: a comparison of five indices. J Stud Alcohol 53(5):476–486, 1992 1405641

Madhusoodanan S, Bogunovic OJ: Safety of benzodiazepines in the geriatric population. Expert Opin Drug Saf 3(5):485–493, 2004 15335303

Maisel NC, Blodgett JC, Wilbourne PL, et al: Meta-analysis of naltrexone and acamprosate for treating alcohol use disorders: when are these medications most helpful? Addiction 108(2):275–293, 2013 23075288

Mayfield D, McLeod G, Hall P: The CAGE questionnaire: validation of a new alcoholism screening instrument. Am J Psychiatry 131(10):1121–1123, 1974 4416585

Moore AA, Beck JC, Babor TF, et al: Beyond alcoholism: identifying older, at-risk drinkers in primary care. J Stud Alcohol 63(3):316–324, 2002 12086132

Moore AA, Gould R, Reuben DB, et al: Longitudinal patterns and predictors of alcohol consumption in the United States. Am J Public Health 95(3):458–465, 2005 15727977

National Institute on Alcohol Abuse and Alcoholism: Alcohol and sleep. Alcohol Alert No. 41 (July). Bethesda, MD, U.S. Department of Health and Human Services, Public Health Services, National Institutes of Health, 1998

National Institute on Alcohol Abuse and Alcoholism: Module 10C: Older adults and alcohol problems. Bethesda, MD, U.S. Department of Health and Human Services, Public Health Services, National Institutes of Health, 2005

Rubinsky AD, Dawson DA, Williams EC, et al: AUDIT-C scores as a scaled marker of mean daily drinking, alcohol use disorder severity, and probability of alcohol dependence in a U.S. general population sample of drinkers. Alcohol Clin Exp Res 37(8):1380–1390, 2013 23906469

Simoni-Wastila L, Yang HK: Psychoactive drug abuse in older adults. Am J Geriatr Pharmacother 4(4):380–394, 2006 17296542

Substance Abuse and Mental Health Services Administration: Results from the 2012 National Survey on Drug Use and Health: Summary of National Findings, NSDUH Series H-46 (HHS Publ No SMA-13-4795). Rockville, MD, Substance Abuse and Mental Health Services Administration, 2013

Tucker JA, Foushee HR, Black BC, Roth DL: Agreement between prospective interactive voice response self-monitoring and structured retrospective reports of drinking and contextual variables during natural resolution attempts. J Stud Alcohol Drugs 68(4):538–542, 2007 17568958

Wagman AM, Allen RP, Upright D: Effects of alcohol consumption upon parameters of ultradian sleep rhythms in alcoholics. Adv Exp Med Biol 85A:601–616, 1977 920494

CHAPTER 18

Personality Disorders

18.1 Which of the following is true about personality disorders in the geriatric population?

A. Personality disorders are unlikely to have an effect on comorbid depressive disorders in elderly persons.
B. Because of the high prevalence of chronic medical disorders in this population, functional impairment leads to an increase in the prevalence of personality disorders.
C. Problems related to personality disorders are less frequently a focus in the patients of geriatric psychiatrists than their general psychiatrist colleagues.
D. The prevalence of cluster B personality disorders is higher in the elderly than in the young.

The correct response is option C: Problems related to personality disorders are less frequently a focus in the patients of geriatric psychiatrists than their general psychiatrist colleagues.

The prevalence of personality disorders in the general population of older persons (3%–13%) is lower by about half than in younger persons (Agronin and Maletta 2000; Schuster et al. 2013) (option B). It is not uncommon for geriatric psychiatrists to comment that problems related to personality disorders are less frequently a focus in their patients compared with the patients of their general psychiatry colleagues (option C). Prevalence studies tend to support this observation. In part, the lower prevalence of personality disorders in the elderly appears to be due to a decline in severity over the years, especially of Cluster B disorders (Hunt 2007; Tracie Shea et al. 2009; Tyrer and Seiverwright 1988) (option D). The presence of a personality disorder in the context of a depressive disorder complicates differential diagnosis and treatment planning (Lynch et al. 2007). For depressive disorders, the worst outcomes occur among patients with comorbid personality disorders (Abrams et al. 2001; Morse and Lynch 2004) (option A). This comorbidity is associated with a longer time to response and greater nonresponse to treatment. **(pp. 491, 493)**

18.2   Which of the following correctly identifies the relationship between the specified personality disorder and aspects of aging?

A. Elderly paranoid patients may improve from forced intimate contact associated with hospital stays and nursing facilities.
B. Narcissistic patients are particularly susceptible to losses associated with retirement and bereavement, which aggravate regulation of self-esteem.
C. Borderline patients continue to have problems with impulsivity and self-harm at high rates as they age, whereas their sense of self becomes more stable over time.
D. Antisocial personality disorder is as prevalent in the elderly as in younger adults.

The correct response is option B: Narcissistic patients are particularly susceptible to losses associated with retirement and bereavement, which aggregate regulation of self-esteem.

Forced intimate contact associated with hospitals and nursing facilities highlights paranoid personality disorder (option A). For patients with narcissistic personalities, increased losses, such as retirement and bereavement, aggravate regulation of self-esteem (option B). In persons with borderline personality disorder, problems related to sense of self, including phenomena such as splitting, intense and unstable interpersonal relationships, impaired affective regulation, and extreme difficulty with control and regulation of anger, often persist through the life cycle. Problems such as severe impulsivity, risky behavior, and self-mutilation tend to diminish with advancing age (Zanarini et al. 2007) (option C). Elderly individuals are more law abiding, and antisocial personality is less common in older prisoners (option D). **(p. 499; Table 18–1, "Personality disorders and related aspects of aging," p. 494)**

18.3   Using the five-factor model of personality, nonclinical samples of older persons are more likely to display which of the following traits in comparison with younger persons?

A. Extraversion.
B. Neuroticism.
C. Openness.
D. Conscientiousness.

The correct response is option D: Conscientiousness.

The most frequent model of personality traits is the five-factor model consisting of neuroticism, extraversion, openness, agreeableness, and conscientiousness (Digman 1990). In general, higher levels of neuroticism (having more anxiety, depression, and vulnerability to stress) are associated with poorer outcomes, whereas higher levels of extraversion (being more outgoing and sociable) and conscientiousness (being better organized and having more self-discipline and willpower) are associated with better outcomes. In nonclinical samples younger persons are somewhat higher on traits of extraversion (option A), neuroticism (option B), and openness (option C), whereas older persons are higher on agreeableness and conscientiousness (option D), with most of the change occurring in young adulthood rather than later life (Roberts et al. 2006). **(p. 495)**

18.4　An older patient with a personality disorder is likely to display fewer of which of the following diagnostic criteria?

A. Feelings of emptiness.
B. Impaired affect regulation.
C. Intense anger.
D. Breaking the law.

The correct response is option D: Breaking the law.

Older substance abusers show lower levels of crime and drug use compared with when they were younger (Hanlon et al. 1990), older homicide offenders are far less likely to have personality disorders than younger offenders are (Putkonen et al. 2010), and in general the elderly are more law abiding, with far fewer arrests (Harlow 1998). Therefore, it is not inconsistent for older patients with personality disorders to exhibit fewer "high-energy" diagnostic criteria (e.g., law-breaking, identity disturbance, promiscuity) (option D). In contrast, a 10-year follow-up study of 362 patients with personality disorders diagnosed at an inpatient admission showed that symptoms related to impulsivity (such as self-mutilation and suicide attempts) resolved relatively quickly, whereas mood symptoms such as anger (option C), loneliness, and emptiness (option A) were more stable. In persons with borderline personality disorder, phenomena such as splitting, intense and unstable interpersonal relationships, impaired affective regulation (option B), and extreme difficulty with control and regulation of anger often persist throughout the life cycle. **(pp. 493, 496, 499)**

18.5　Which of the following best represents Erikson's stage theory of late development?

A. Older adults develop more mature defense mechanisms than do younger adults.
B. The development of mature defenses has been found to be independent of education and social privilege.
C. Cluster B personality disorders become less severe as people age.
D. The major goal of adjustment to old age is to look back across the lifespan in order to find meaning.

The correct response is option D: The major goal of adjustment to old age is to look back across the lifespan in order to find meaning.

Erikson's stage theory of late-life development (Erikson et al. 1986) proposed that the major developmental task of older age is to look back and seek meaning across the lifespan, rather than looking forward as in previous developmental modes that are now in decline. The goal of this task, as discussed by Erikson, is to maintain more integrity than despair about one's life (option D). Options A, B, and C are not propositions of Erikson's theory. **(p. 496)**

18.6   A well-adjusted elderly person might be expected to make frequent use of which one of these defense mechanisms?

   A. Anticipation.
   B. Projection.
   C. Splitting.
   D. Problem-focused coping.

The correct response is option A: Anticipation.

Defenses are involuntary mental mechanisms for regulating the realities that persons are powerless to change. Vaillant (2012) and others (Haan 1977) have described a hierarchy of defenses from immature and maladaptive to mature and adaptive. Mature defenses include humor, altruism, sublimation, anticipation (option A), and suppression. Mature and adaptive defenses synthesize and attenuate conflicts rather than distorting or denying them. In a "Defensive Functioning Scale" for defense mechanisms (Vaillant 1994), defense mechanisms were categorized into seven levels ranging from high adaptive (e.g., altruism) to defensive dysregulation (e.g., delusional projection) (option B). Problem-focused coping (option D) is not a specific defense mechanism per se but a set of coping strategies used when a situation can be changed, in contrast to emotion-focused coping, which is used when a situation cannot be changed. To cope effectively with stress, individuals must learn to recognize the difference between situations that can and cannot be changed and then must match the right coping skill with the right situation. **(pp. 495–497)**

18.7   Patients with frontal lobe syndromes are more likely to show preservation in which of the following domains?

   A. Executive function, including planning.
   B. Obeying rules of interpersonal social behavior.
   C. Memory.
   D. Verbal reasoning.

The correct response is option C: Memory.

Syndromes based on frontal lobe pathology that result in loss of normal executive function present some of the most difficult diagnostic challenges, especially if the onset of symptoms is subtle, the rate of progression is slow, and the main attributes of the premorbid personality are obscure. Individuals with frontal or frontotemporal lobe disease may show good preservation of memory function (option C). They are, however, prone to trouble with "mechanistic planning, verbal reasoning, or problem solving" (options A and D) and "obeying rules of interpersonal social behaviour (option B), the experience of reward and punishment, and the interpretation of complex emotions" (Grafman and Litvan 1999, p. 1921; Passant et al. 2005). **(p. 499)**

18.8   Which symptom if it appears independently should raise suspicion for organic brain pathology when onset is late in life?

   A. Obsessive-compulsive traits.
   B. Irritability.
   C. Fatigue.
   D. Suicidal ideation.

The correct response is option A: Obsessive-compulsive traits.

Late-onset obsessive-compulsive symptoms or traits (option A) are particularly likely to have a basis in brain disease. Geriatric psychiatrists are familiar with the phenomenon that acquired brain disease in later life appears to strengthen undesirable personality traits that were present, although less intense and conspicuous, in earlier adult life. However, if signs and symptoms of personality disorder were not present before the onset of a neurocognitive illness or brain injury, it is rational to assume that such illnesses play a causative role in the personality change. Irritability and fatigue are common features of multiple psychiatric illnesses, including mood and anxiety disorders. For example, associated features of generalized anxiety disorder are muscle tension, restlessness (or feeling keyed up or on edge), sleep difficulties, concentration problems (often thought by older adults to be memory problems), fatigue (option C), and irritability (option B). Suicidal ideation is a common symptom in a major depressive episode, which can be made when the individual exhibits one or both of two core symptoms—depressed mood and lack of interest or pleasure—as well as four or more of the following symptoms, for at least 2 weeks: significant weight loss, insomnia or hypersomnia, psychomotor agitation or retardation, fatigue or loss of energy, feelings of worthlessness or excessive or inappropriate guilt, diminished ability to concentrate or make decisions, and recurrent thoughts of death or suicidal ideation (option D) (American Psychiatric Association 2013). First-onset episodes of major depression after age 60 years (referred to as late onset) are common, making up about one-half of all episodes in older adults. **(pp. 258, 346, 499, 500)**

18.9   Which of the following is a core feature of any successful psychotherapy for geriatric patients?

   A. Global revision of maladaptive aspects of personality.
   B. Empathic and respectful listening.
   C. Cognitive restructuring.
   D. Behavioral analysis.

The correct response is option B: Empathic and respectful listening.

The principal features of successful psychotherapy for geriatric patients are a structure with consistency, availability, empathic and respectful listening (option B), flexibility, and open-mindedness on the part of the psychotherapist. These features are probably more important than a particular theoretical orientation (Clarkin et al. 2007). Psychotherapy of any type, either by itself or in combination with pharmacotherapy, with a goal of a global revision of maladaptive aspects of personality in later life (option A), is unlikely to succeed. Individualized treatment targeting specific symptoms that discomfort, threaten, or endanger patients or their family or caregivers is far more realistic and more likely to realize success. Helping patients recognize and alter erroneous or distorted thinking (options C and D) is also important and possible, as in cognitive-behavioral therapy and its variant Dialectical-Behavioral Therapy (Lynch et al. 2007), but these are not core features of psychotherapy for geriatric patients. **(pp. 500, 501)**

18.10   Which of the following is a component of a good pharmacological treatment plan to target symptoms of personality disorder?

A. Use of repeatable self-report assessments.
B. Use of selective serotonin reuptake inhibitors (SSRIs) as first-line treatment.
C. Development of a plan for continued long-term use of the medication.
D. Use of antipsychotics as first-line treatment.

The correct response is option A: Use of repeatable self-report assessments.

Pharmacological treatment should be a systematic trial guided by three principles. First, a medication should be selected for an identified target symptom area (e.g., affect, impulsivity, aggression, anxiety). Second, such trials should include a repeatable assessment strategy (e.g., global rating, self-report, or caregiver report targeted to the symptom area) (option A). Third, trials should have a specified duration at the end of which a decision is made whether or not to continue the medication (option C). SSRIs (option B) and other newer antidepressant drugs, anticonvulsants, and atypical antipsychotic drugs (option D), used alone or in combinations, may be useful in systematic trials for specified symptoms. **(p. 501)**

References

Abrams RC, Alexopoulos GS, Spielman LA, et al: Personality disorder symptoms predict declines in global functioning and quality of life in elderly depressed patients. Am J Geriatr Psychiatry 9(1):67–71, 2001 11156754

Agronin ME, Maletta G: Personality disorders in late life. Understanding and overcoming the gap in research. Am J Geriatr Psychiatry 8(1):4–18, 2000 10648290

American Psychiatric Association: Diagnostic and Statistical Manual of Mental Disorders, 5th Edition. Arlington, VA, American Psychiatric Association, 2013

Clarkin JF, Levy KN, Lenzenweger MF, Kernberg OF: Evaluating three treatments for borderline personality disorder: a multiwave study. Am J Psychiatry 164(6):922–928, 2007 17541052

Digman JM: Personality structure: emergence of the five-factor model. Annu Rev Psychol 41:417–440, 1990

Erikson EH, Erikson JM, Kivnick HQ: Vital Involvement in Old Age. New York, WW Norton, 1986

Grafman J, Litvan I: Importance of deficits in executive functions. Lancet 354(9194):1921–1923, 1999 10622291

Haan NA: Coping and Defending. San Francisco, CA, Jossey-Bass, 1977

Hanlon TE, Nurco DN, Kinlock TW, Duszynski KR: Trends in criminal activity and drug use over an addiction career. Am J Drug Alcohol Abuse 16(3-4):223–238, 1990 2288322

Harlow CW: Special Report: Profile of Jail Inmates 1996 (Publ No NCJ 164620). Washington, DC, U.S. Department of Justice, 1998

Hunt M: Borderline personality disorder across the lifespan. J Women Aging 19(1–2):173–191, 2007 17588886

Lynch TR, Cheavens JS, Cukrowicz KC, et al: Treatment of older adults with co-morbid personality disorder and depression: a dialectical behavior therapy approach. Int J Geriatr Psychiatry 22(2):131–143, 2007 17096462

Morse JQ, Lynch TR: A preliminary investigation of self-reported personality disorders in late life: prevalence, predictors of depressive severity, and clinical correlates. Aging Ment Health 8(4):307–315, 2004 15370047

Passant U, Elfgren C, Englund E, Gustafson L: Psychiatric symptoms and their psychosocial consequences in frontotemporal dementia. Alzheimer Dis Assoc Disord 19(Suppl 1):S15–S18, 2005 16317252

Putkonen H, Weizmann-Henelius G, Repo-Tiihonen E, et al: Homicide, psychopathy, and aging—a nationwide register-based case-comparison study of homicide offenders aged 60 years or older. J Forensic Sci 55(6):1552–1556, 2010 20629908

Roberts BW, Walton KE, Viechtbauer W: Patterns of mean-level change in personality traits across the life course: a meta-analysis of longitudinal studies. Psychol Bull 132(1):1–25, 2006 16435954

Schuster JP, Hoertel N, Le Strat Y, et al: Personality disorders in older adults: findings from the National Epidemiologic Survey on Alcohol and Related Conditions. Am J Geriatr Psychiatry 21(8):757–768, 2013 23567365

Tracie Shea M, Edelen MO, Pinto A, et al: Improvement in borderline personality disorder in relationship to age. Acta Psychiatr Scand 119(2):143–148, 2009 18851719

Tyrer P, Seiverwright H: Studies of outcome, in Personality Disorders: Diagnosis, Management and Course. Edited by Tyrer P. London, Wright, 1988, pp 119–136

Vaillant GE: Ego mechanisms of defense and personality psychopathology. J Adnorm Psychol 103(1):44–50, 1994 8040479

Vaillant GE: Triumphs of Experience: The Men of the Harvard Grant Study. Cambridge, MA, London, 2012

Zanarini MC, Frankenburg FR, Reich DB, et al: The subsyndromal phenomenology of borderline personality disorder: a 10-year follow-up study. Am J Psychiatry 164(6):929–935, 2007 17541053

CHAPTER 19

Agitation in Older Adults

19.1 You are asked to see a 75-year-old man with a known diagnosis of Alzheimer's disease. The patient has lived in a nursing facility for many years, and staff note that the patient is agitated, intermittently confused, and combative over the course of the night. Nursing notes indicate that this is new behavior for the patient, and staff have never known him to be violent in the past. Which of the following is the most likely underlying diagnosis?

A. Delirium due to a general medical etiology.
B. Change in the patient's routine.
C. Gradual progression of Alzheimer's disease.
D. Change in staffing and in patient's caregiver.

The correct response is option A: Delirium due to a general medical etiology.

A careful psychiatric evaluation and history are key components of the initial approach to the individual who is presenting with agitation. It is important to determine whether the onset of agitation is acute, subacute, or chronic. A sudden onset of disruptive behavior typically suggests a medical etiology (option A), whereas a slower, insidious onset of agitation may be a distress response to a change in caregiver (option D), routine (option B), or environment in a patient who is losing capacity to express him- or herself. Agitation may also be seen without obvious precipitants in the course of gradual progression of neurocognitive disorder (option C). **(p. 508)**

19.2 What is the preferred approach to management of agitation in neurocognitive disorders?

A. Pharmacological approach.
B. Nonpharmacological approach.
C. Relocating the patient to a new, unfamiliar setting.
D. Ignoring agitation because it usually occurs without a distinct reason.

The correct response is option B: Nonpharmacological approach.

Disruptive behaviors do not occur in a vacuum (option D). Agitation has a person-specific situational context and meaning that may often, but not always, be understood. In neurocognitive disorders, the preferred approach to management of agitation is nonpharmacological (option B), with pharmacological approaches (option A) used as second-line. Agitated individuals with dementia generally respond well to calm, dignified, familiar settings (option C) with predictable routines. **(pp. 509–510)**

19.3   Which of the following strategies to reduce agitation in older adults should be considered as a first-line approach?

A. Immediately calling social services to investigate the home or nursing facility.
B. Prescribing a high-dose antipsychotic.
C. Assessing patient preferences.
D. Increasing the patient's physical activity throughout the day.

The correct response is option C: Assessing patient preferences.

Nonpharmacological strategies to reduce agitation begin with assessment of retained abilities, patient preferences (option C), and available family and staff resources. If an agitated patient is paranoid, part of the task of the clinician is to determine whether the patient's mistrustful and suspicious demeanor may be warranted. If after such exploration the clinician is not convinced that the accusations are wholly explained by a delusion, a social services agency or department should be requested to investigate further (option A). In neurocognitive disorders, the preferred approach to management is nonpharmacological, with pharmacological approaches used as second-line (option B). Other nonpharmacological strategies include allowing adequate rest or passive observation between stimulating activities (option D). **(pp. 508–509, 511)**

19.4   What is the best approach when trying to communicate with an agitated person with dementia?

A. Do not repeat yourself because it will further agitate the person.
B. Speak loudly if the person is hard of hearing.
C. Make eye contact.
D. Do not ask any questions if you are unsure of the person's meaning because that may agitate him or her further.

The correct response is option C: Make eye contact.

The following are suggestions for trying to communicate with an agitated person with dementia: Make eye contact (option C). Using a clear adult tone, call the person by a preferred or recognizable name. Words are not as important as a calm tone (option B). Repeat your words exactly, if necessary (option A). If you are unsure of the person's meaning, ask questions (option D). **(p. 512)**

19.5   Which of the following is a true statement regarding agitation in frail elderly patients?

   A. Agitation occurs only in the context of delirium.
   B. Agitation most commonly occurs in the context of delirium superimposed on dementia.
   C. Agitation often occurs without a cause.
   D. Agitation is never a feature of depression.

The correct response is option B: Agitation most commonly occurs in the context of delirium superimposed on dementia.

Agitation most commonly occurs in the context of delirium or dementia, and often these conditions coexist in frail elderly patients (option B). Disruptive behaviors do not occur in a vacuum (option C). Agitation in older adults is associated with a variety of diagnoses (option A), including mood disorders, psychotic disorders, neurocognitive disorders, and substance use disorders. Agitation can also be a feature of late-life depression (option D), and although treatment of the underlying depression should also treat the agitation, the full effect of antidepressant medications may not be apparent for several weeks. **(pp. 507, 509, 513)**

19.6   When are benzodiazepines the appropriate treatment for agitation in older adults?

   A. Only in the context of suspected delirium.
   B. When agitation is the result of hypoxia in patients with chronic obstructive pulmonary disease.
   C. In late-life depression.
   D. In cases of alcohol withdrawal.

The correct response is option D: In cases of alcohol withdrawal.

Benzodiazepines should generally be avoided in an agitated patient because of their high potential for worsening delirium as well as potentially disinhibiting the patient further (options A, B, and C); however, they may be appropriately used in cases of alcohol or benzodiazepine withdrawal (option D). More recently, benzodiazepines have also been linked to adverse respiratory outcomes in older patients with chronic obstructive pulmonary disease (Vozoris et al. 2014) (option B). In older patients, detrimental effects of benzodiazepines and benzodiazepine receptor agonists frequently outweigh any short-term symptomatic relief that they may provide and they should be avoided (American Geriatrics Society 2012 Beers Criteria Update Expert Panel 2012). Benzodiazepines may be used as a temporary adjunctive treatment for anxiety- or depression-related sleep disturbance when the primary pharmacotherapy is an antidepressant (option C). **(pp. 513, 556–557)**

19.7   Management of agitation in the context of delirium should be focused on which of the following interventions?

A. Administration of anticholinergic medications.
B. Ensuring proper use of physical restraints.
C. Identification and treatment of the underlying causes.
D. Administration of psychoactive medication.

The correct response is option C: Identification and treatment of the underlying causes.

In patients with diminished cognitive reserve, even small anticholinergic effects can substantially impair cognition (Mulsant et al. 2003; Nebes et al. 2005) (option A). The use of physical restraints should be minimized due to their role in prolonging delirium, worsening agitation, and increasing complications such as strangulation (Inouye et al. 2007) (option B). Strategies that increase the patient's mobility, self-care, and independence should be promoted. Management of delirium is focused on primary prevention, identifying and treating the underlying causes (option C), minimizing psychoactive medications, reorientation, safe and early mobilization, and normalization of the sleep-wake cycle (Inouye et al. 2006). Medications with known psychoactive effects should be discontinued or minimized whenever possible (option D). **(pp. 166, 169, 513, 558)**

19.8   You are called to see a 75-year-old man with Alzheimer's disease who has been verbally abusive and physically violent with hospital staff over the course of the day. He is refusing to take medication orally. The team plans to give the patient intravenous (IV) haloperidol. Which of the following is true regarding IV haloperidol?

A. IV haloperidol is known to cause hypotension.
B. IV haloperidol is associated with significant sedation.
C. IV haloperidol is best used in patients with parkinsonism.
D. IV haloperidol is associated with prolongation of the QT interval.

The correct response is option D: IV haloperidol is associated with prolongation of the QT interval.

Although haloperidol typically does not cause hypotension (option A) or significant sedation (option B), it may cause extrapyramidal symptoms at higher doses and should be avoided in patients with parkinsonism (option C). Intravenous haloperidol is associated with prolongation of the QT interval (option D). **(p. 514)**

19.9   You are asked to evaluate a 75-year-old man with cirrhosis who has been confused and agitated with staff in his nursing facility over the course of the night. Medical workup is significant for electrocardiogram with QTc interval of 515 ms and an elevated ammonia level. What treatment should you consider in this case?

A. IV haloperidol.
B. IV lorazepam.

C. Lactulose.
D. Oral clonazepam.

The correct response is option C: Lactulose.

Delirium secondary to hepatic encephalopathy has its own treatment pathway and relies primarily on the administration of either lactulose (option C) or nonabsorbable antibiotics (rifaximin). Intravenous haloperidol is associated with prolongation of the QT interval (option A). Benzodiazepines (options B and D) should generally be avoided in an agitated patient because of their high potential for worsening delirium as well as potentially disinhibiting the patient further; however, they may be appropriately used in cases of alcohol or benzodiazepine withdrawal. **(pp. 513–514)**

19.10 When evaluating a patient with Alzheimer's disease with acute onset of agitation, what is the first step in the evaluation?

A. Identifying potential precipitants associated with acute onset of agitation.
B. Prescribing opiates because the patient is likely in pain.
C. Prescribing antipsychotics to manage agitation.
D. Prescribing benzodiazepines to ensure sedation.

The correct response is option A: Identifying potential precipitants associated with acute onset of agitation.

As with all behavioral problems, the first step in treatment is to identify potential precipitants (option A). In neurocognitive disorders, the preferred approach to management is nonpharmacological, with pharmacological approaches used as second-line (options B, C, and D). **(pp. 509, 515)**

19.11 Older adults who are receiving carbamazepine for management of agitation should be monitored for which of the following abnormalities?

A. Hypernatremia.
B. Leukocytosis.
C. Hyponatremia.
D. Eosinophilia.

The correct response is option C: Hyponatremia.

Patients receiving carbamazepine should be monitored for hyponatremia (option C; option A is incorrect), agranulocytosis (options B and D), and the possibility of drug interactions because of hepatic cytochrome P450 enzyme induction by carbamazepine. **(p. 516)**

19.12 A 70-year-old woman with Alzheimer's disease living in a nursing home has been intermittently agitated, yelling and cursing at staff over the course of the week. The patient has also been noted to be tearful, lamenting over the infrequency of her family's visits. The consulting psychiatrist's differential diagnosis includes late-life depression. Which of the following medications has been shown to be effective for treating agitation in depressed patients with dementia?

A. Carbamazepine.
B. Citalopram.
C. Trazodone.
D. Valproic acid.

The correct response is option B: Citalopram.

Citalopram (option B) has been shown to be efficacious in double-blind placebo-controlled trials for treating agitation in dementia (Pollock et al. 2002; Porsteinsson et al. 2014). Carbamazepine (option A) and valproic acid (option D) have been studied in placebo-controlled trials for agitation in dementia (not depression). A placebo-controlled study of trazodone (option C), haloperidol, and behavior management techniques did not find a difference between placebo and any of the treatment groups (Teri et al. 2000). In a very small study, trazodone was found to be efficacious for treating agitation in patients with frontotemporal dementia (Lebert et al. 2004). **(pp. 516–517)**

19.13 A family brings their 65-year-old grandmother to the emergency department for evaluation of ongoing agitation in the context of pronounced visual hallucinations over the course of the past 6 months. The family has also noted memory difficulties during this time, and most recently, the patient has been walking very slowly with a slight resting tremor involving her arms. Medical workup is unrevealing, and the consulting psychiatrist suspects a neurocognitive disorder. Which of the following medications can the physician consider for management of agitation in this patient?

A. Rivastigmine.
B. Haloperidol.
C. Quetiapine.
D. Lorazepam.

The correct response is option A: Rivastigmine.

Dementia with Lewy bodies is characterized by early fluctuations in cognition and attention, recurrent and persistent visual hallucinations, and extrapyramidal motor symptoms. Perhaps the strongest evidence for use of cholinesterase inhibitors to target agitation was in patients with Lewy body dementia. McKeith et al. (2000) demonstrated that rivastigmine 12 mg/day (option A) was superior to placebo in addressing behavioral symptoms in patients with Lewy body dementia. This finding is particularly exciting given the neuroleptic sensitivity of patients with Lewy body pathology (options B and C). Benzodiazepines (option D) should generally be avoided in an agitated patient because of their high potential for worsening delirium as well as potentially disinhibiting the patient further; however, they may be appropriately used in cases of alcohol or benzodiazepine withdrawal. **(pp. 142, 513, 517)**

19.14 Which of the following classes of medications used to treat agitation in older adults has a black box warning regarding increased mortality rates issued by the U.S. Food and Drug Administration (FDA) in 2008?

A. Antidepressants.
B. Mood stabilizers.
C. Benzodiazepines.
D. Antipsychotics.

The correct response is option D: Antipsychotics.

In 2004, the FDA conducted a meta-analysis of 17 placebo-controlled trials of atypical antipsychotics and found an increased risk of all-cause mortality of 4.5% in the drug group versus 2.6% in the placebo group over a mean trial duration of 10 weeks; as a result, all atypical antipsychotics received a black box warning for use in patients with dementia. The FDA expanded the black box warning to include typical antipsychotics in 2008 (option D; options A, B, and C are incorrect). **(p. 515)**

19.15 A family brings their 70-year-old grandmother with no prior psychiatric history to the emergency department for evaluation of approximately 1 year of verbal agitation that has worsened over the past 2 months. After a thorough medical and psychiatric evaluation, the evaluating physician determines that the patient likely has Alzheimer's dementia and is considering treatment for agitation. Which of the following is important for the physician to consider when deciding on treatment?

A. Pharmacological approaches are always preferred for treatment of agitation in older adults.
B. Antipsychotics are the safest treatments available for agitation.
C. Antipsychotics should be prescribed in high doses when used in agitation in older adults.
D. Antipsychotics should be used at the lowest possible dosages for the shortest possible duration.

The correct response is option D: Antipsychotics should be used at the lowest possible dosages for the shortest possible duration.

Nonpharmacological approaches are the preferred treatment for agitation in older adults (option A). When the patient does not respond to nonpharmacological approaches or if symptoms are severe, pharmacological approaches may be warranted. If pharmacological means are used, ongoing risk-benefit analyses should guide treatment; the lowest possible dosages should be used for the shortest possible times (option D; option C is incorrect). In 2004, all atypical antipsychotics received a black box warning for use in patients with dementia. The FDA expanded its warning to include atypical antipsychotics in 2008 (option B). **(pp. 515, 519)**

References

American Geriatrics Society 2012 Beers Criteria Update Expert Panel: American Geriatrics Society updated Beers Criteria for potentially inappropriate medication use in older adults. J Am Geriatr Soc 60(4):616–631, 2012 23376048

Inouye SK, Baker DI, Fugal P, et al: Dissemination of the hospital elder life program: implementation, adaptation, and successes. J Am Geriatr Soc 54(10):1492–1499, 2006 17038065

Inouye SK, Zhang Y, Jones RN, et al: Risk factors for delirium at discharge: development and validation of a predictive model. Arch Intern Med 167(13):1406–1413, 2007 17620535

Lebert F, Stekke W, Hasenbroekx C, Pasquier F: Frontotemporal dementia: a randomised, controlled trial with trazodone. Dement Geriatr Cogn Disord 17(4):355–359, 2004 15178953

McKeith I, Del Ser T, Spano P, et al: Efficacy of rivastigmine in dementia with Lewy bodies: a randomised, double-blind, placebo-controlled international study. Lancet 356(9247):2031–2036, 2000 11145488

Mulsant BH, Pollock BG, Kirshner M, et al: Serum anticholinergic activity in a community-based sample of older adults: relationship with cognitive performance. Arch Gen Psychiatry 60(2):198–203, 2003 12578438

Nebes RD, Pollock BG, Meltzer CC, et al: Serum anticholinergic activity, white matter hyperintensities, and cognitive performance. Neurology 65:1487–1489, 2005 16275844

Pollock BG, Mulsant BH, Rosen J, et al: Comparison of citalopram, perphenazine, and placebo for the acute treatment of psychosis and behavioral disturbances in hospitalized, demented patients. Am J Psychiatry 159(3):460–465, 2002 11870012

Porsteinsson AP, Drye LT, Pollock BG, et al; CitAD Research Group: Effect of citalopram on agitation in Alzheimer disease: the CitAD randomized clinical trial. JAMA 311(7):682–691, 2014 24549548

Teri L, Logsdon RG, Peskind E, et al; Alzheimer's Disease Cooperative Study: Treatment of agitation in AD: a randomized, placebo-controlled clinical trial. Neurology 55(9):1271–1278, 2000 11087767

Vozoris NT, Fischer HD, Wang X, et al: Benzodiazepine drug use and adverse respiratory outcomes among older adults with COPD. Eur Respir J 44(2):332–340, 2014 24743966

CHAPTER 20

Psychopharmacology

20.1 Which of the following describes the efficacy data regarding treatment of depression in the elderly?

A. Antidepressants have not demonstrated efficacy for any disorder in this population.

B. No class of antidepressants is considered first-line treatment.

C. Antidepressants have not demonstrated efficacy in the treatment of depression in elderly patients with dementia.

D. Antidepressants work for depressive disorders but not for anxiety disorders.

The correct response is option C: Antidepressants have not demonstrated efficacy in the treatment of depression in elderly patients with dementia.

Six selective serotonin reuptake inhibitors (SSRIs) are available in the United States: citalopram, escitalopram, fluoxetine, fluvoxamine, paroxetine, and sertraline. They are approved by the U.S. Food and Drug Administration (FDA) for the treatment of major depressive disorder (all except fluvoxamine) and several anxiety disorders. In older adults, SSRIs remain first-line antidepressants (Sonnenberg et al. 2008) (option B) because of their broad spectrum of action, high efficacy (Mukai and Tampi 2009; Pinquart et al. 2006; Tedeschini et al. 2011), ease of use, good tolerability, and relative safety (Mulsant et al. 2014) (options A and D). More than 40 randomized controlled trials (RCTs) of SSRIs involving more than 6,000 geriatric patients with depression have been published. Some open studies and small single-site controlled trials also supported the use of SSRIs for the treatment of depression associated with Alzheimer's dementia (Katona et al. 1998; Lyketsos et al. 2003; Nyth and Gottfries 1990; Nyth et al. 1992; Olafsson et al. 1992; Petracca et al. 2001; Taragano et al. 1997). However, a larger multicenter trial failed to confirm these results; in this study, sertraline was not more efficacious and was less well tolerated than placebo for the treatment of depression in Alzheimer's disease (Rosenberg et al. 2010; Weintraub et al. 2010) (option C). Another multicenter study also showed no differences in the efficacy of sertraline, mirtazapine, or placebo in treating depression in patients with Alzheimer's disease, but the tolerability of either drug was worse than placebo (Banerjee et al. 2011). **(pp. 528, 529, 532)**

20.2   Which physiological change in the elderly results in an increase in the elimination half-life of lipid-soluble drugs?

A. Decreases in concentration of plasma albumin.
B. Decreases in hepatic blood flow.
C. Decreases in intestinal blood flow.
D. Decreases in lean body mass.

The correct response is option D: Decreases in lean body mass.

As seen in Table 20–1, decreased concentration of plasma albumin (option A) results in increased or decreased free concentration of drugs in plasma. Decreased hepatic blood flow (option B) results in decreased hepatic clearance and higher serum concentrations of drugs. Decreased intestinal blood flow (option C) results in decreased rate of drug absorption. Decreased lean body mass alters the distribution of lipid-soluble drugs and increases the elimination half-life (option D). **(Table 20–1, "Physiological changes in elderly persons associated with altered pharmacokinetics," p. 529)**

20.3   Which of the following antidepressants has linear plasma concentrations across the entire dosing range?

A. Sertraline.
B. Fluoxetine.
C. Paroxetine.
D. Fluvoxamine.

The correct response is option A: Sertraline.

As seen in Table 20–3, the proportionality of dosage to plasma concentration for sertraline (option A) is linear across the therapeutic range. Fluoxetine (option B), paroxetine (option C), and fluvoxamine (option D) do not have linear dosage to plasma concentration across the entire therapeutic range. **(Table 20–3, "Pharmacokinetic properties of second-generation antidepressants," p. 533)**

20.4   Which of the following medications has the highest potential to cause clinically significant drug-drug interactions secondary to the pharmacokinetic effects on hepatic metabolism?

A. Sertraline.
B. Fluoxetine.
C. Escitalopram.
D. Venlafaxine.

The correct response is option B: Fluoxetine.

As seen in Table 20–4, fluoxetine (option B) has the highest probability of inhibition of hepatic CYP2C9, 2C19, 2D6, and 3A4 enzymes. Sertraline (option A), escitalopram (option C), and venlafaxine (option D) have a low potential for causing clinically significant drug-drug interactions. **(Table 20–4, "Second-generation antidepressants' inhibition of cytochrome P450 (CYP) and potential for causing or being involved in significant drug-drug interactions," p. 535)**

20.5   Which of the following considerations limits the use of medications such as desipramine and nortriptyline in elderly patients?

A. High propensity to cause orthostasis and falls.
B. Effects on cardiac conduction.
C. Inability to use serum levels to monitor dosing.
D. Untreatable impact of bowel function.

The correct response is option: B: Effects on cardiac conduction.

The secondary amines desipramine and nortriptyline are preferred in older patients (Mulsant et al. 2014). They have a lower propensity to cause orthostasis and falls (option A), in addition to having linear pharmacokinetics and more modest anticholinergic effects (Chew et al. 2008). Their relatively narrow therapeutic index (i.e., the plasma level range separating efficacy and toxicity) necessitates monitoring of plasma levels and electrocardiograms in older patients. A single dose is given at bedtime; 5–7 days after initiation of desipramine at 50 mg or nortriptyline at 25 mg, plasma levels should be measured and dosages adjusted linearly, with targeted plasma levels of 200–400 ng/mL for desipramine and 50–150 ng/mL for nortriptyline (option C). These narrow ranges ensure efficacy while decreasing risks of cardiac toxicity and other side effects. Like the tertiary-amine tricyclic antidepressants (TCAs), desipramine and nortriptyline are type 1 antiarrhythmics: they have quinidine-like effects on cardiac conduction and should not be used in patients who have or are at risk for cardiac conduction defects (Roose et al. 1991) (option B). Most anticholinergic side effects of desipramine or nortriptyline (e.g., dry mouth, constipation) resolve with time or usually can be mitigated with symptomatic treatment (Rosen et al. 1993) (option D). TCAs have been associated with cognitive worsening compared with placebo (Reifler et al. 1989) and with less cognitive improvement than occurs with sertraline (Bondareff et al. 2000; Doraiswamy et al. 2003) or other SSRIs. **(pp. 543–544)**

20.6   In which of the following conditions should discontinuation of antipsychotics be considered for elderly patients?

A. Schizophrenia.
B. Major depressive disorder with psychosis.
C. Bipolar disorder.
D. Dementia with psychosis.

The correct response is option D: Dementia with psychosis.

In older adults, as in other age groups, atypical antipsychotics are now being prescribed as first-line drugs for the treatment of psychotic symptoms of any etiology. Studies support the efficacy of these agents in the treatment of late-life schizophrenia and late-onset psychoses (Scott et al. 2011; Suzuki et al. 2011) and in the treatment of behavioral and psychological symptoms of dementia (Maher and Theodore 2012; Maher et al. 2011). However, use of these agents in patients with dementia is being questioned (Ballard and Corbett 2010; Mulsant 2014; Salzman et al. 2008). Their long-term use is justified when they are used to treat schizophrenia (option A), bipolar disorder (option C), and possibly major depressive disorder with psychotic features (option B); discontinuation should be attempted in stable patients with other disorders. Although antipsychotics can be discontinued safely in most older patients with dementia (option D), their discontinuation can be associated with poor outcomes, in particular in older patients who had presented with more severe agitation or psychosis (Declercq et al. 2013). **(pp. 545–546)**

20.7   Which of the following is correct regarding the use of antipsychotics in the treatment of behavioral and psychological symptoms of dementia?

A. Second-generation antipsychotics have been shown to be significantly more likely to cause mortality compared with first-generation antipsychotics.
B. There is a tenfold increase in the rate of death in older patients treated with atypical antipsychotics compared with placebo.
C. Antipsychotics should be prescribed only to patients who have failed to respond to nonpharmacological interventions or alternative medications.
D. There is a substantially higher rate of falls in patients receiving second-generation antipsychotics compared with first-generation antipsychotics.

The correct response is option C: Antipsychotics should be prescribed only to patients who have failed to respond to nonpharmacological interventions or alternative medications.

In 2005, two highly publicized reports and an FDA warning indicated a nearly twofold increase in the rate of deaths in older patients with behavioral and psychological symptoms of dementia treated with atypical antipsychotics when compared with placebo (Kuehn 2005; Schneider et al. 2005) (option B). These reports have led to a reexamination of the safety of both conventional and atypical antipsychotics in older patients. Over the past decade, a series of studies have emphasized their association with mortality (Ballard et al. 2009; Langballe et al. 2014; Ray et al. 2009; Wang et al. 2005), stroke (Gill et al. 2005; Herrmann et al. 2004), severe hyperglycemia in patients with diabetes (Lipscombe et al. 2009), fractures (Liperoti et al. 2007), and venous thromboembolism (Kleijer et al. 2010). The relative safety of atypical compared with conventional antipsychotics remains unclear: atypical antipsychotics appear to be associated with lower mortality than typical antipsychotics (Langballe et al. 2014; Schneider et al. 2005) (option A) and they may cause fewer falls (Hien et al. 2005; Landi et al. 2005) (option D) and fewer extrapyramidal symptoms (Lee et al. 2004; Meagher et al. 2013; Rochon et al. 2005; van Iersel et al.

2005); however, they may cause more cerebrovascular events (Percudani et al. 2005), venous thromboembolism (Liperoti et al. 2005), and pancreatitis (Koller et al. 2003). Given the increased recognition of the risks associated with the use of antipsychotics in older patients, clinicians need to consider their potential risks and benefits for each individual patient (Gauthier et al. 2010; Rabins and Lyketsos 2005). Antipsychotics should be prescribed only to patients who have failed to respond to nonpharmacological interventions or alternative medications (Ballard and Corbett 2010; Mulsant 2014; Sink et al. 2005) (option C). **(pp. 545–546)**

20.8 Which of the following antipsychotic medications is considered to be the first-line treatment for agitation in elderly patients with dementia and distressing psychosis or agitation?

A. Olanzapine.
B. Quetiapine.
C. Risperidone.
D. Paliperidone.

The correct response is option C: Risperidone.

Of the atypical antipsychotics currently available in the United States, risperidone has the most published geriatric data for a variety of conditions (Schneider et al. 2005, 2006a; Sink et al. 2005; Suzuki et al. 2011). The efficacy and tolerability of risperidone in the treatment of behavioral and psychological symptoms of dementia have been reported in several randomized placebo-controlled trials (e.g., Brodaty et al. 2003; De Deyn et al. 1999, 2005b; Katz et al. 1999; Schneider et al. 2006a, Schneider et al. 2006b; Sink et al. 2005); in randomized comparisons with haloperidol (Chan et al. 2001; De Deyn et al. 1999; Suh et al. 2004), promazine and olanzapine (Gareri et al. 2004), and olanzapine (Fontaine et al. 2003; Mulsant et al. 2004); and in many uncontrolled studies or large case series. The efficacy of risperidone in the treatment of agitation or psychosis is further supported by a placebo-controlled trial showing that patients with Alzheimer's disease whose agitation or psychosis had responded acutely to risperidone experienced an increased risk of relapse when they were switched to placebo after 4 months (hazard ratio 1:9) or 8 months (hazard ratio 4:9) compared with those who remained on risperidone (Devanand et al. 2012). Taken together, these data support risperidone as a first choice among antipsychotics for the treatment of patients with dementia and distressing psychosis or severe agitation (option C; options A, B, and D are incorrect). **(p. 546)**

20.9 Which of the following issues in an elderly patient would limit the use of paliperidone?

A. There are no data on its use in the elderly.
B. The patient has reduced hepatic function.
C. The patient is receiving a potent CYP2D6 inhibitor.
D. The patient has end-stage renal disease.

The correct response is option D: The patient has end-stage renal disease.

Paliperidone is the active 9-hydroxy metabolite of risperidone, and therefore some of its pharmacological action, efficacy, and side effects are similar to those of risperidone. Its once-daily extended-release formulation takes 24 hours to reach a maximum concentration, and its clearance is not affected by hepatic impairment (option B) or CYP2D6 metabolism (option C) but is affected by renal function (option D). Its efficacy and tolerability in the treatment of older patients with psychosis is supported by data from 125 subjects ages 65 years and older who participated in three 6-week registration trials that led to the medication's approval by the FDA for the treatment of schizophrenia (e.g., Davidson et al. 2007; Kane et al. 2007) (option A). Otherwise, limited available data support the efficacy and safety of paliperidone in the treatment of older patients with schizophrenia (Madhusoodanan and Zaveri 2010): in a 6-week randomized placebo-controlled trial followed by a 24-week open-label extension, 114 patients ages 65 years and older (mean age of 70) received paliperidone 3–12 mg/day or placebo. Discontinuation due to adverse events and weight gain were similar in the two groups. **(pp. 547–548)**

20.10 Which of the following antipsychotic medications is often used as a first-line treatment in older patients with Parkinson's disease because of its low propensity to cause extrapyramidal symptoms?

A. Haloperidol.
B. Risperidone.
C. Quetiapine.
D. Olanzapine.

The correct response is option C: Quetiapine.

Because of its low propensity to cause extrapyramidal symptoms, quetiapine is often used as a first-line antipsychotic in older patients with Parkinson's disease (option C; options A, B, and D are incorrect), dementia with Lewy bodies, or tardive dyskinesia (Fernandez et al. 2002; Poewe 2005); however, quetiapine was not found to be efficacious in these patients in two double-blind trials (Kurlan et al. 2007; Rabey et al. 2007). **(p. 550)**

20.11 Aripiprazole treatment for older individuals with dementia is limited by which of the following concerns?

A. Orthostatic hypotension.
B. Lack of efficacy.
C. Akathisia.
D. Anticholinergic effects.

The correct response is option C: Akathisia.

Aripiprazole has partial dopamine type 2 (D_2) receptor agonist properties (i.e., in high dopaminergic states it acts as an antagonist, and in low dopaminergic states it acts as an agonist). This may explain why it is unlikely to cause extrapyramidal side effects or prolactin elevation (associated with osteoporosis), even at high D_2 receptor occupancy (Mamo et al. 2007). It has only moderate affinity to the adrenergic α_1 receptor and histamine H_1 receptor and negligible affinity to the muscarinic receptor (Chew et al. 2006). As a result, orthostatic hypotension (option A) and antihistaminergic and anticholinergic adverse effects (option D) are less likely to occur than with other atypical agents. However, akathisia (option C) may be a common side effect in older patients (Coley et al. 2009; Sheffrin et al. 2009). Several randomized placebo-controlled trials of aripiprazole in older patients with behavioral and psychological symptoms of dementia have been published (De Deyn et al. 2005a; Mintzer et al. 2007; Streim et al. 2008). Recent expert opinions (De Deyn et al. 2013; Herrmann et al. 2013) are congruent with a meta-analysis of these trials that concluded that "efficacy on rating scales was observed by meta-analysis for aripiprazole" (Schneider et al. 2006a, p. 191) and with a 2011 review published by the U.S. Agency for Healthcare Research and Quality that reached a similar conclusion (Maher and Theodore 2012; Maher et al. 2011) (option B). **(p. 551)**

20.12 Which of the following is a limitation to the use of lithium in older patients with bipolar disorder?

A. Lack of efficacy in suicidality.
B. Definitive evidence of adverse renal effects.
C. Changes in pharmacokinetics.
D. Need to reach very high serum lithium levels in order to achieve therapeutic effects.

The correct response is option C: Changes in pharmacokinetics.

Available data from open and controlled trials suggest that lithium is efficacious in the acute treatment and prophylaxis of mania in older patients (D'Souza et al. 2011; Sajatovic et al. 2005; Shulman 2010); however, age-related reductions in renal clearance and decreased total body water significantly affect the pharmacokinetics of lithium in older patients, increasing the risk of toxicity (D'Souza et al. 2011) (option C). Medical comorbidities common in late life—such as impaired renal function, hyponatremia, dehydration, and heart failure—further exacerbate the risk of toxicity (D'Souza et al. 2011; Sajatovic et al. 2006, 2013). Thiazide diuretics, angiotensin-converting enzyme inhibitors, and nonsteroidal anti-inflammatory drugs may precipitate toxicity by further diminishing the renal clearance of lithium. Lithium toxicity can produce persistent central nervous system impairment or be fatal: it is a medical emergency that requires careful correction of fluid and electrolyte imbalances and that may require administration of mannitol (or even hemodialysis) to increase lithium excretion. Older patients require lower lithium dosages than do younger patients to produce similar serum lithium levels, and their lithium levels, electrolytes, and thyroid-stimulating hormone should be monitored regularly (D'Souza et al. 2011; Rej et al. 2014a). Also, older persons are more sensitive to neurological side effects of lithium and experience them at lower lithium levels. Treatment in older patients may require lithium levels to be kept as low as 0.4–0.8 mEq/L (option D). In addition, despite the absence of definite evidence, concerns about the association between long-term use of lithium and renal disease and the possible causal role of lithium in this association remain (Rej et al. 2014b) (option B). Despite its potential toxicity, lithium remains an important drug in the treatment of bipolar disorder and treatment-resistant depression in late life because of its potential effect on suicidality (Müller-Oerlinghausen and Lewitzka 2010) (option A) and its potential neuroprotective properties (Foland et al. 2008; Germaná et al. 2010; Hajek et al. 2012a, 2012b; Macritchie et al. 2010). **(pp. 553–554)**

20.13 Which of the following is a true statement regarding the use of bupropion for treatment of geriatric depression?

A. There is no evidence base to support the safety or efficacy of bupropion in geriatric depression.
B. Expert consensus favors the use of bupropion as a first-line agent in older depressed patients.
C. Bupropion has been reported to be safe and effective in older patients who were partial responders to SSRIs or venlafaxine.
D. Bupropion can be helpful for patients who complain of nausea, diarrhea, unbearable fatigue, or sexual dysfunction during SSRI treatment.

The correct response is option D: Bupropion can be helpful for patients who complain of nausea, diarrhea, unbearable fatigue, or sexual dysfunction during SSRI treatment.

Published data supporting the safety and efficacy of bupropion in geriatric depression are limited to small controlled trials and one small open study (Steffens et al. 2001) (option A). Expert consensus favors the use of bupropion—alone or as an augmentation agent—in older depressed patients whose symptoms have not responded to SSRIs or who cannot tolerate them (Alexopoulos et al. 2001; Buchanan et al. 2006; Mulsant et al. 2001, 2014) (option B). In particular, bupropion can be helpful for patients who complain of nausea, diarrhea, unbearable fatigue, or sexual dysfunction during SSRI treatment (Nieuwstraten and Dolovich 2001; Thase et al. 2005) (option D). Although augmentation with bupropion has been reported to be helpful in patients who were partial responders to SSRIs or venlafaxine (Bodkin et al. 1997; Spier 1998), the safety of this combination has not been established (Joo et al. 2002) (option C). **(pp. 540–541)**

20.14 Which of the following was a finding in the Sequenced Treatment Alternatives to Relieve Depression (STAR*D) study regarding geriatric depression?

A. STAR*D established the safety of combination treatment with mirtazapine and venlafaxine XR in older patients with geriatric depression.
B. The STAR*D trial found that a combination of mirtazapine and venlafaxine XR was less effective than the monoamine oxidase inhibitor (MAOI) tranylcypromine for treatment-resistant depression.

C. Only a few STAR*D participants were elderly.

D. Data from the STAR*D trial suggest that a combination of mirtazapine and venlafaxine is safe but ineffective for treatment-resistant depression.

The correct response is option C: Only a few STAR*D participants were elderly.

The STAR*D study found that a combination of mirtazapine and venlafaxine XR had modest efficacy in patients with treatment-resistant depression (option D), comparable to the efficacy of the MAOI tranylcypromine (Rush et al. 2006) (option B); however, only a few STAR*D participants were elderly (option C), and the safety of this combination has not been established in older patients (options A and D). **(pp. 541–542)**

20.15 Which of the following is a true statement regarding the use of trazodone in geriatric patients?

A. Trazodone has no role in the treatment of agitation or aggression in patients with dementia.

B. Trazodone is more efficacious than placebo in the treatment of sleep disturbances of patients with Alzheimer's disease.

C. Adverse effects of trazodone are not dose-dependent.

D. At doses typically used to treat insomnia, trazodone may cause dry mouth, orthostatic hypotension, and QT prolongation.

The correct response is option B: Trazodone is more efficacious than placebo in the treatment of sleep disturbances of patients with Alzheimer's disease.

Trazodone is indicated for the treatment of major depressive disorder, but it is now almost exclusively used off-label as a hypnotic or sedative agent (Bossini et al. 2012) due to its sedative effect associated with antagonism of the 5-HT_{2A} receptor and, to a lesser extent, the 5-HT_{2B}, 5HT_{1A}, and α_1 receptors. To minimize adverse effects, doses should be kept low (e.g., 50–150 mg at bedtime) when trazodone is used as a hypnotic agent (option C). At doses typically used to treat depression (300–600 mg/day), trazodone antagonism of α_1-adrenergic receptors may cause dry mouth, orthostatic hypotension (with syncope), QT prolongation or arrhythmias, and priapism (which is rare in older adults) (option D). Some evidence going back to the early 1990s indicates that trazodone at low to moderate doses (50–300 mg/day) has an efficacy comparable to that of haloperidol in the treatment of agitation or aggression in patients with dementia (Henry et al. 2011; Houlihan et al. 1994; Sultzer et al. 1997; Teri et al. 2000) (option A). In a unique small ($N=30$) RCT, trazodone (50 mg given at 10 P.M.) was well tolerated, and it was more efficacious than placebo in the treatment of sleep disturbances of patients with Alzheimer's disease (Camargos et al. 2014) (option B). **(p. 542)**

20.16 Which of the following is the most evidence-based indication for use of psycho-stimulants in geriatric patients?

A. Treatment of depression in medically burdened elders.
B. Adjunctive treatment for negative symptoms of schizophrenia.
C. Treatment of apathy and fatigue in patients taking SSRIs.
D. Treatment augmentation for depressed patients taking SSRIs.

The correct response is option A: Treatment of depression in medically bur-dened elders.

Even though some clinicians prescribe psychostimulants for the treatment of late-life mood disorders, this practice has minimal empirical support. A few small dou-ble-blind trials suggested that methylphenidate is generally well tolerated and modestly efficacious for medically burdened depressed elders (Satel and Nelson 1989; Wallace et al. 1995) (option A). A small study suggested that methylpheni-date can be used in older depressed patients to augment SSRIs, which inhibit do-pamine release and may contribute to apathy and fatigue (Lavretsky et al. 2006) (option D). The wakefulness-promoting agent modafinil and its R-enantiomer ar-modafinil appear to induce a calm alertness through nondopaminergic mecha-nisms. These agents have been used to target apathy and fatigue in patients taking SSRIs (Dunlop et al. 2007; Fava et al. 2007; Goss et al. 2013) (option C) and as adjunctive treatment for negative symptoms of schizophrenia (Lindenmayer et al. 2013) (option B), but there are almost no published geriatric data for these drugs (Darwish et al. 2011; Varanese et al. 2013). **(pp. 544–545)**

20.17 Which of the following statements correctly reflects drug-drug interactions among the mood stabilizers?

A. Valproate decreases lamotrigine concentration.
B. Carbamazepine doubles lamotrigine concentrations.
C. Oxcarbazepine is more likely to be involved in drug interactions than carba-mazepine.
D. Carbamazepine can lower its own concentration.

The correct response is option D: Carbamazepine can lower its own concentra-tion.

Because valproate *increases* lamotrigine concentration (option A), the initial and target doses need to be halved in patients who are receiving divalproex and the titration of lamotrigine needs to be slowed down. Conversely, carbamazepine ap-proximately halves lamotrigine concentrations (option B), and the initial la-motrigine dose needs to be doubled in patients receiving carbamazepine. Carbamazepine is primarily eliminated by CYP3A4, and its clearance is reduced with aging. Its interactions with other drugs are protean: carbamazepine concen-trations are increased to potential toxicity by CYP3A4 inhibitors such as macro-lide antibiotics, antifungals, and some antidepressants. CYP3A4 inducers—such as phenobarbital, phenytoin, and carbamazepine itself—lower the concentration of carbamazepine (option D) and the concentrations of many drugs metabolized by this isoenzyme, including lamotrigine, valproate, some antidepressants, and antipsychotics (Fenn et al. 2006). Oxcarbazepine, the 10-keto analogue of carbamazepine, is a less potent CYP3A4 inducer and less likely to be involved in drug interactions (option C). **(p. 555)**

References

Alexopoulos GS, Katz IR, Reynolds CF III, et al: Pharmacotherapy of depression in older patients: a summary of the expert consensus guidelines. J Psychiatr Pract 7(6):361–376, 2001 15990550

Ballard C, Corbett A: Management of neuropsychiatric symptoms in people with dementia. CNS Drugs 24(9):729–739, 2010 20806986

Ballard C, Hanney ML, Theodoulou M, et al; DART-AD investigators: The dementia antipsychotic withdrawal trial (DART-AD): long-term follow-up of a randomised placebo-controlled trial. Lancet Neurol 8(2):151–157, 2009 19138567

Banerjee S, Hellier J, Dewey M, et al: Sertraline or mirtazapine for depression in dementia (HTA-SADD): a randomised, multicentre, double-blind, placebo-controlled trial. Lancet 378(9789):403–411, 2011 21764118 2011

Bodkin JA, Lasser RA, Wines JD Jr, et al: Combining serotonin reuptake inhibitors and bupropion in partial responders to antidepressant monotherapy. J Clin Psychiatry 58(4):137–145, 1997 9164423

Bondareff W, Alpert M, Friedhoff AJ, et al: Comparison of sertraline and nortriptyline in the treatment of major depressive disorder in late life. Am J Psychiatry 157(5):729–736, 2000 10784465

Bossini L, Casolaro I, Koukouna D, et al: Off-label uses of trazodone: a review. Expert Opin Pharmacother 13(12):1707–1717, 2012 22712761

Brodaty H, Ames D, Snowdon J, et al: A randomized placebo-controlled trial of risperidone for the treatment of aggression, agitation, and psychosis of dementia. J Clin Psychiatry 64(2):134–143, 2003 12633121

Buchanan D, Tourigny-Rivard MF, Cappeliez P, et al: National Guidelines for seniors' mental health: the assessment and treatment of depression. Can J Geriatr 9(suppl 2):S52–S58, 2006

Camargos EF, Louzada LL, Quintas JL, et al: Trazodone improves sleep parameters in Alzheimer disease patients: a randomized, double-blind, and placebo-controlled study. Am J Geriatr Psychiatry 22(12):1565–1574, 2014 24495406

Chan WC, Lam LC, Choy CN, et al: A double-blind randomised comparison of risperidone and haloperidol in the treatment of behavioural and psychological symptoms in Chinese dementia patients. Int J Geriatr Psychiatry 16(12):1156–1162, 2001 11748775

Chew ML, Mulsant BH, Pollock BG, et al: A model of anticholinergic activity of atypical antipsychotic medications. Schizophr Res 88(1-3):63–72, 2006 16928430

Chew ML, Mulsant BH, Pollock BG, et al: Anticholinergic activity of 107 medications commonly used by older adults. J Am Geriatr Soc 56(7):1333–1341, 2008 18510583

Coley KC, Scipio TM, Ruby C, et al: Aripiprazole prescribing patterns and side effects in elderly psychiatric inpatients. J Psychiatr Pract 15(2):150–153, 2009 19339850

Darwish M, Kirby M, Hellriegel ET, et al: Systemic exposure to armodafinil and its tolerability in healthy elderly versus young men: an open-label, multiple-dose, parallel-group study. Drugs Aging 28(2):139–150, 2011 21275439

Davidson M, Emsley R, Kramer M, et al: Efficacy, safety and early response of paliperidone extended-release tablets (paliperidone ER): results of a 6-week, randomized, placebo-controlled study. Schizophr Res 93(1–3):117–130, 2007 17466492

Declercq T, Petrovic M, Azermai M, et al: Withdrawal versus continuation of chronic antipsychotic drugs for behavioural and psychological symptoms in older people with dementia. Cochrane Database Syst Rev 3(3):CD007726, 2013 23543555

De Deyn PP, Rabheru K, Rasmussen A, et al: A randomized trial of risperidone, placebo, and haloperidol for behavioral symptoms of dementia. Neurology 53(5):946–955, 1999 10496251

De Deyn P, Jeste DV, Swanink R, et al: Aripiprazole for the treatment of psychosis in patients with Alzheimer's disease: a randomized, placebo-controlled study. J Clin Psychopharmacol 25(5):463–467, 2005a 16160622

De Deyn PP, Katz IR, Brodaty H, et al: Management of agitation, aggression, and psychosis associated with dementia: a pooled analysis including three randomized, placebo-controlled double-blind trials in nursing home residents treated with risperidone. Clin Neurol Neurosurg 107(6):497–508, 2005b 15922506

De Deyn PP, Drenth AF, Kremer BP, et al: Aripiprazole in the treatment of Alzheimer's disease. Expert Opin Pharmacother 14(4):459–474, 2013 23350964

Devanand DP, Mintzer J, Schultz SK, et al: Relapse risk after discontinuation of risperidone in Alzheimer's disease. N Engl J Med 367(16):1497–1507, 2012 23075176

Doraiswamy PM, Krishnan KR, Oxman T, et al: Does antidepressant therapy improve cognition in elderly depressed patients? J Gerontol A Biol Sci Med Sci 58(12):M1137–M1144, 2003 14684712

D'Souza R, Rajji TK, Mulsant BH, Pollock BG: Use of lithium in the treatment of bipolar disorder in late-life. Curr Psychiatry Rep 13(6):488–492, 2011 21847537

Dunlop BW, Crits-Christoph P, Evans DL, et al: Coadministration of modafinil and a selective serotonin reuptake inhibitor from the initiation of treatment of major depressive disorder with fatigue and sleepiness: a double-blind, placebo-controlled study. J Clin Psychopharmacol 27(6):614–619, 2007 18004129

Fava M, Thase ME, DeBattista C, et al: Modafinil augmentation of selective serotonin reuptake inhibitor therapy in MDD partial responders with persistent fatigue and sleepiness. Ann Clin Psychiatry 19(3):153–159, 2007 17729016

Fenn HH, Sommer BR, Ketter TA, Alldredge B: Safety and tolerability of mood-stabilising anticonvulsants in the elderly. Expert Opin Drug Saf 5(3):401–416, 2006 16610969

Fernandez HH, Trieschmann ME, Burke MA, Friedman JH: Quetiapine for psychosis in Parkinson's disease versus dementia with Lewy bodies. J Clin Psychiatry 63(6):513–515, 2002 12088163

Foland LC, Altshuler LL, Sugar CA, et al: Increased volume of the amygdala and hippocampus in bipolar patients treated with lithium. Neuroreport 19(2):221–224, 2008 18185112

Fontaine CS, Hynan LS, Koch K, et al: A double-blind comparison of olanzapine versus risperidone in the acute treatment of dementia-related behavioral disturbances in extended care facilities. J Clin Psychiatry 64(6):726–730, 2003 12823090

Gareri P, Cotroneo A, Lacava R, et al: Comparison of the efficacy of new and conventional antipsychotic drugs in the treatment of behavioral and psychological symptoms of dementia (BPSD). Arch Gerontol Geriatr Suppl 9(9):207–215, 2004 15207416

Gauthier S, Cummings J, Ballard C, et al: Management of behavioral problems in Alzheimer's disease. Int Psychogeriatr 22(3):346–372, 2010 20096151

Germaná C, Kempton MJ, Sarnicola A, et al: The effects of lithium and anticonvulsants on brain structure in bipolar disorder. Acta Psychiatr Scand 122(6):481–487, 2010 20560901

Gill SS, Rochon PA, Herrmann N, et al: Atypical antipsychotic drugs and risk of ischaemic stroke: population based retrospective cohort study. BMJ 330(7489):445, 2005 15668211

Goss AJ, Kaser M, Costafreda SG, et al: Modafinil augmentation therapy in unipolar and bipolar depression: a systematic review and meta-analysis of randomized controlled trials. J Clin Psychiatry 74(11):1101–1107, 2013 24330897

Hajek T, Cullis J, Novak T, et al: Hippocampal volumes in bipolar disorders: opposing effects of illness burden and lithium treatment. Bipolar Disord 14(3):261–270, 2012a 22548899

Hajek T, Kopecek M, Höschl C, Alda M: Smaller hippocampal volumes in patients with bipolar disorder are masked by exposure to lithium: a meta-analysis. J Psychiatry Neurosci 37(5):333–343, 2012b 22498078

Henry G, Williamson D, Tampi RR: Efficacy and tolerability of antidepressants in the treatment of behavioral and psychological symptoms of dementia, a literature review of evidence. Am J Alzheimers Dis Other Demen 26(3):169–183, 2011 21429956

Herrmann N, Mamdani M, Lanctôt KL: Atypical antipsychotics and risk of cerebrovascular accidents. Am J Psychiatry 161(6):1113–1115, 2004 15169702

Herrmann N, Lanctôt KL, Hogan DB: Pharmacological recommendations for the symptomatic treatment of dementia: the Canadian Consensus Conference on the Diagnosis and Treatment of Dementia 2012. Alzheimers Res Ther 5(Suppl 1):S5, 2013 24565367

Hien TT, Cumming RG, Cameron ID, et al: Atypical antipsychotic medications and risk of falls in residents of aged care facilities. J Am Geriatr Soc 53(8):1290–1295, 2005 16078953

Houlihan DJ, Mulsant BH, Sweet RA, et al: A naturalistic study of trazodone in the treatment of behavioral complications of dementia. Am J Geriatr Psychiatry 2(1):78–85, 1994 21629010

Joo JH, Lenze EJ, Mulsant BH, et al: Risk factors for falls during treatment of late-life depression. J Clin Psychiatry 63(10):936–941, 2002 12416604

Kane J, Canas F, Kramer M, et al: Treatment of schizophrenia with paliperidone extended-release tablets: a 6-week placebo-controlled trial. Schizophr Res 90(1–3):147–161, 2007 17092691

Katona CLE, Hunter BN, Bray J: A double-blind comparison of the efficacy and safety of paroxetine and imipramine in the treatment of depression with dementia. Int J Geriatr Psychiatry 13(2):100–108, 1998 9526179

Katz IR, Jeste DV, Mintzer JE, et al; Risperidone Study Group: Comparison of risperidone and placebo for psychosis and behavioral disturbances associated with dementia: a randomized, double-blind trial. J Clin Psychiatry 60(2):107–115, 1999 10084637

Kleijer BC, Heerdink ER, Egberts TC, et al: Antipsychotic drug use and the risk of venous thromboembolism in elderly patients. J Clin Psychopharmacol 30(5):526–530, 2010 20814323

Koller EA, Cross JT, Doraiswamy PM, Malozowski SN: Pancreatitis associated with atypical antipsychotics: from the Food and Drug Administration's MedWatch surveillance system and published reports. Pharmacotherapy 23(9):1123–1130, 2003 14524644

Kuehn BM: FDA warns antipsychotic drugs may be risky for elderly. JAMA 293(20):2462, 2005 15914734

Kurlan R, Cummings J, Raman R, Thal L; Alzheimer's Disease Cooperative Study Group: Quetiapine for agitation or psychosis in patients with dementia and parkinsonism. Neurology 68(17):1356–1363, 2007 17452579

Landi F, Onder G, Cesari M, et al; Silver Network Home Care Study Group: Psychotropic medications and risk for falls among community-dwelling frail older people: an observational study. J Gerontol A Biol Sci Med Sci 60(5):622–626, 2005 15972615

Langballe EM, Engdahl B, Nordeng H, et al: Short- and long-term mortality risk associated with the use of antipsychotics among 26,940 dementia outpatients: a population-based study. Am J Geriatr Psychiatry 22(4):321–331, 2014 24016844

Lavretsky H, Park S, Siddarth P, et al: Methylphenidate-enhanced antidepressant response to citalopram in the elderly: a double-blind, placebo-controlled pilot trial. Am J Geriatr Psychiatry 14(2):181–185, 2006 16473984

Lee PE, Gill SS, Freedman M, et al: Atypical antipsychotic drugs in the treatment of behavioural and psychological symptoms of dementia: systematic review. BMJ 329(7457):75, 2004 15194601

Lindenmayer JP, Nasrallah H, Pucci M, et al: A systematic review of psychostimulant treatment of negative symptoms of schizophrenia: challenges and therapeutic opportunities. Schizophr Res 147(2–3):241–252, 2013 23619055

Liperoti R, Pedone C, Lapane KL, et al: Venous thromboembolism among elderly patients treated with atypical and conventional antipsychotic agents. Arch Intern Med 165(22):2677–2682, 2005 16344428

Liperoti R, Onder G, Lapane KL, et al: Conventional or atypical antipsychotics and the risk of femur fracture among elderly patients: results of a case-control study. J Clin Psychiatry 68(6):929–934, 2007 17592919

Lipscombe LL, Lévesque L, Gruneir A, et al: Antipsychotic drugs and hyperglycemia in older patients with diabetes. Arch Intern Med 169(14):1282–1289, 2009 19636029

Lyketsos CG, DelCampo L, Steinberg M, et al: Treating depression in Alzheimer disease: efficacy and safety of sertraline therapy, and the benefits of depression reduction: the DIADS. Arch Gen Psychiatry 60(7):737–746, 2003 12860778

Macritchie KA, Lloyd AJ, Bastin ME, et al: White matter microstructural abnormalities in euthymic bipolar disorder. Br J Psychiatry 196(1):52–58, 2010 20044661

Madhusoodanan S, Zaveri D: Paliperidone use in the elderly. Curr Drug Saf 5(2):149–152, 2010 20406162

Maher AR, Theodore G: Summary of the comparative effectiveness review on off-label use of atypical antipsychotics. J Manag Care Pharm 18(5)(Suppl B):S1–S20, 2012 22784311

Maher AR, Maglione M, Bagley S, et al: Efficacy and comparative effectiveness of atypical antipsychotic medications for off-label uses in adults: a systematic review and meta-analysis. JAMA 306(12):1359–1369, 2011 21954480

Mamo D, Graff A, Mizrahi R, et al: Differential effects of aripiprazole on D(2), 5-HT(2), and 5-HT(1A) receptor occupancy in patients with schizophrenia: a triple tracer PET study. Am J Psychiatry 164(9):1411–1417, 2007 17728427

Meagher DJ, McLoughlin L, Leonard M, et al: What do we really know about the treatment of delirium with antipsychotics? Ten key issues for delirium pharmacotherapy. Am J Geriatr Psychiatry 21(12):1223–1238, 2013 23567421

Mintzer JE, Tune LE, Breder CD, et al: Aripiprazole for the treatment of psychoses in institutionalized patients with Alzheimer dementia: a multicenter, randomized, double-blind, placebo-controlled assessment of three fixed doses. Am J Geriatr Psychiatry 15(11):918–931, 2007 17974864

Mukai Y, Tampi RR: Treatment of depression in the elderly: a review of the recent literature on the efficacy of single- versus dual-action antidepressants. Clin Ther 31(5):945–961, 2009 19539096

Müller-Oerlinghausen B, Lewitzka U: Lithium reduces pathological aggression and suicidality: a mini-review. Neuropsychobiology 62(1):43–49, 2010 20453534

Mulsant BH: Challenges of the treatment of neuropsychiatric symptoms associated with dementia. Am J Geriatr Psychiatry 22(4):317–320, 2014 24635993

Mulsant BH, Alexopoulos GS, Reynolds CF 3rd, et al; PROSPECT Study Group: Pharmacological treatment of depression in older primary care patients: the PROSPECT algorithm. Int J Geriatr Psychiatry 16(6):585–592, 2001 11424167

Mulsant BH, Gharabawi GM, Bossie CA, et al: Correlates of anticholinergic activity in patients with dementia and psychosis treated with risperidone or olanzapine. J Clin Psychiatry 65(12):1708–1714, 2004 15641877

Mulsant BH, Blumberger DM, Ismail Z, et al: A systematic approach to pharmacotherapy for geriatric major depression. Clin Geriatr Med 30(3):517–534, 2014 25037293

Nieuwstraten CE, Dolovich LR: Bupropion versus selective serotonin-reuptake inhibitors for treatment of depression. Ann Pharmacother 35(12):1608–1613, 2001 11793630

Nyth AL, Gottfries CG: The clinical efficacy of citalopram in treatment of emotional disturbances in dementia disorders. A Nordic multicentre study. Br J Psychiatry 157:894–901, 1990 1705151

Nyth AL, Gottfries CG, Lyby K, et al: A controlled multicenter clinical study of citalopram and placebo in elderly depressed patients with and without concomitant dementia. Acta Psychiatr Scand 86(2):138–145, 1992 1529737

Olafsson K, Jørgensen S, Jensen HV, et al: Fluvoxamine in the treatment of demented elderly patients: a double-blind, placebo-controlled study. Acta Psychiatr Scand 85(6):453–456, 1992 1642129

Percudani M, Barbui C, Fortino I, et al: Second-generation antipsychotics and risk of cerebrovascular accidents in the elderly. J Clin Psychopharmacol 25(5):468–470, 2005 16160623

Petracca GM, Chemerinski E, Starkstein SE: A double-blind, placebo-controlled study of fluoxetine in depressed patients with Alzheimer's disease. Int Psychogeriatr 13(2):233–240, 2001 11495397

Pinquart M, Duberstein PR, Lyness JM: Treatments for later-life depressive conditions: a meta-analytic comparison of pharmacotherapy and psychotherapy. Am J Psychiatry 163(9):1493–1501, 2006 16946172

Poewe W: Treatment of dementia with Lewy bodies and Parkinson's disease dementia. Mov Disord 20(Suppl 12):S77–S82, 2005 16092095

Rabey JM, Prokhorov T, Miniovitz A, et al: Effect of quetiapine in psychotic Parkinson's disease patients: a double-blind labeled study of 3 months' duration. Mov Disord 22(3):313–318, 2007 17034006

Rabins PV, Lyketsos CG: Antipsychotic drugs in dementia: what should be made of the risks? JAMA 294(15):1963–1965, 2005 16234504

Ray WA, Chung CP, Murray KT, et al: Atypical antipsychotic drugs and the risk of sudden cardiac death. N Engl J Med 360(3):225–235, 2009 19144938

Reifler BV, Teri L, Raskind M, et al: Double-blind trial of imipramine in Alzheimer's disease patients with and without depression. Am J Psychiatry 146(1):45–49, 1989 2643356

Rej S, Beaulieu S, Segal M, et al: Lithium dosing and serum concentrations across the age spectrum: from early adulthood to the tenth decade of life. Drugs Aging 31(12):911–916, 2014a 25331906

Rej S, Shulman K, Herrmann N, et al: Prevalence and correlates of renal disease in older lithium users: a population-based study. Am J Geriatr Psychiatry 22(11):1075–1082, 2014b 24566239

Rochon PA, Stukel TA, Sykora K, et al: Atypical antipsychotics and parkinsonism. Arch Intern Med 165(16):1882–1888, 2005 16157833

Roose SP, Dalack GW, Glassman AH, et al: Cardiovascular effects of bupropion in depressed patients with heart disease. Am J Psychiatry 148(4):512–516, 1991 1900980

Rosen J, Sweet R, Pollock BG, et al: Nortriptyline in the hospitalized elderly: tolerance and side effect reduction. Psychopharmacol Bull 29(2):327–331, 1993 8290682

Rosenberg PB, Drye LT, Martin BK, et al; DIADS-2 Research Group: Sertraline for the treatment of depression in Alzheimer disease. Am J Geriatr Psychiatry 18(2):136–145, 2010 20087081

Rush AJ, Trivedi MH, Wisniewski SR, et al: Acute and longer-term outcomes in depressed outpatients requiring one or several treatment steps: a STAR*D report. Am J Psychiatry 163(11):1905–1917, 2006 17074942

Sajatovic M, Gyulai L, Calabrese JR, et al: Maintenance treatment outcomes in older patients with bipolar I disorder. Am J Geriatr Psychiatry 13(4):305–311, 2005 15845756

Sajatovic M, Blow FC, Ignacio RV: Psychiatric comorbidity in older adults with bipolar disorder. Int J Geriatr Psychiatry 21(6):582–587, 2006 16783798

Sajatovic M, Forester BP, Gildengers A, Mulsant BH: Aging changes and medical complexity in late-life bipolar disorder: emerging research findings that may help advance care. Neuropsychiatry (London) 3(6):621–633, 2013 24999372

Salzman C, Jeste DV, Meyer RE, et al: Elderly patients with dementia-related symptoms of severe agitation and aggression: consensus statement on treatment options, clinical trials methodology, and policy. J Clin Psychiatry 69(6):889–898, 2008 18494535

Satel SL, Nelson JC: Stimulants in the treatment of depression: a critical overview. J Clin Psychiatry 50(7):241–249, 1989 2567730

Schneider LS, Dagerman KS, Insel P: Risk of death with atypical antipsychotic drug treatment for dementia: meta-analysis of randomized placebo-controlled trials. JAMA 294(15):1934–1943, 2005 16234500

Schneider LS, Dagerman K, Insel PS: Efficacy and adverse effects of atypical antipsychotics for dementia: meta-analysis of randomized, placebo-controlled trials. Am J Geriatr Psychiatry 14(3):191–210, 2006a 16505124

Schneider LS, Tariot PN, Dagerman KS, et al; CATIE-AD Study Group: Effectiveness of atypical antipsychotic drugs in patients with Alzheimer's disease. N Engl J Med 355(15):1525–1538, 2006b 17035647

Scott J, Greenwald BS, Kramer E, Shuwall M: Atypical (second generation) antipsychotic treatment response in very late-onset schizophrenia-like psychosis. Int Psychogeriatr 23(5):742–748, 2011 21118614

Sheffrin M, Driscoll HC, Lenze EJ, et al: Pilot study of augmentation with aripiprazole for incomplete response in late-life depression: getting to remission. J Clin Psychiatry 70(2):208–213, 2009 19210951

Shulman KI: Lithium for older adults with bipolar disorder: Should it still be considered a first-line agent? Drugs Aging 27(8):607–615, 2010 20658789

Sink KM, Holden KF, Yaffe K: Pharmacological treatment of neuropsychiatric symptoms of dementia: a review of the evidence. JAMA 293(5):596–608, 2005 15687315

Sonnenberg CM, Deeg DJ, Comijs HC, et al: Trends in antidepressant use in the older population: results from the LASA-study over a period of 10 years. J Affect Disord 111(2–3):299–305, 2008 18442857

Spier SA: Use of bupropion with SRIs and venlafaxine. Depress Anxiety 7(2):73–75, 1998 9614595

Steffens DC, Doraiswamy PM, McQuoid DR: Bupropion SR in the naturalistic treatment of elderly patients with major depression. Int J Geriatr Psychiatry 16(9):862–865, 2001 11571765

Streim JE, Porsteinsson AP, Breder CD, et al: A randomized, double-blind, placebo-controlled study of aripiprazole for the treatment of psychosis in nursing home patients with Alzheimer disease. Am J Geriatr Psychiatry 16(7):537–550, 2008 18591574

Suh GH, Son HG, Ju YS, et al: A randomized, double-blind, crossover comparison of risperidone and haloperidol in Korean dementia patients with behavioral disturbances. Am J Geriatr Psychiatry 12(5):509–516, 2004 15353389

Sultzer DL, Gray KF, Gunay I, et al: A double-blind comparison of trazodone and haloperidol for treatment of agitation in patients with dementia. Am J Geriatr Psychiatry 5(1):60–69, 1997 9169246

Suzuki T, Remington G, Uchida H, et al: Management of schizophrenia in late life with antipsychotic medications: a qualitative review. Drugs Aging 28(12):961–980, 2011 22117095

Taragano FE, Lyketsos CG, Mangone CA, et al: A double-blind, randomized, fixed-dose trial of fluoxetine vs. amitriptyline in the treatment of major depression complicating Alzheimer's disease. Psychosomatics 38(3):246–252, 1997 9136253

Tedeschini E, Levkovitz Y, Iovieno N, et al: Efficacy of antidepressants for late-life depression: a meta-analysis and meta-regression of placebo-controlled randomized trials. J Clin Psychiatry 72(12):1660–1668, 2011 22244025

Teri L, Logsdon RG, Peskind E, et al; Alzheimer's Disease Cooperative Study: Treatment of agitation in AD: a randomized, placebo-controlled clinical trial. Neurology 55(9):1271–1278, 2000 11087767

Thase ME, Haight BR, Richard N, et al: Remission rates following antidepressant therapy with bupropion or selective serotonin reuptake inhibitors: a meta-analysis of original data from 7 randomized controlled trials. J Clin Psychiatry 66(8):974–981, 2005 16086611

van Iersel MB, Zuidema SU, Koopmans RT, et al: Antipsychotics for behavioural and psychological problems in elderly people with dementia: a systematic review of adverse events. Drugs Aging 22(10):845–858, 2005 16245958

Varanese S, Perfetti B, Gilbert-Wolf R, et al: Modafinil and armodafinil improve attention and global mental status in Lewy bodies disorders: preliminary evidence. Int J Geriatr Psychiatry 28(10):1095–1097, 2013 24038163

Wallace AE, Kofoed LL, West AN: Double-blind, placebo-controlled trial of methylphenidate in older, depressed, medically ill patients. Am J Psychiatry 152(6):929–931, 1995 7755127

Wang PS, Schneeweiss S, Avorn J, et al: Risk of death in elderly users of conventional vs. atypical antipsychotic medications. N Engl J Med 353(22):2335–2341, 2005 16319382

Weintraub D, Rosenberg PB, Drye LT, et al; DIADS-2 Research Group: Sertraline for the treatment of depression in Alzheimer disease: week-24 outcomes. Am J Geriatr Psychiatry 18(4):332–340, 2010 20220589

CHAPTER 21

Electroconvulsive Therapy and Other Forms of Brain Stimulation

21.1   Which of the following is a true statement regarding the effectiveness of electro-convulsive therapy (ECT) in the treatment of psychiatric disorders?

   A. ECT is effective in the treatment of melancholic depression, nonmelancholic depression, and unipolar depression but is *not* effective in the treatment of bipolar depression.
   B. In the treatment of acute mania, lithium is superior to ECT.
   C. There is an abundance of evidence showing that ECT effectively treats rapid-cycling bipolar disorder.
   D. Case series suggest that patients with schizoaffective disorder have a more robust response to ECT treatment than do those with schizophrenia.

The correct response is option D: Case series suggest that patients with schizoaffective disorder have a more robust response to ECT treatment than do those with schizophrenia.

The most common diagnostic indication for ECT is major depression (American Psychiatric Association 2001). Regarding subtypes of depression, ECT appears to be effective in treating both melancholic and severe nonmelancholic depression (Sackeim and Rush 1995), as well as bipolar and unipolar major depression (Weiner and Krystal 2001) (option A). Although ECT is used more frequently for major depression than for other illnesses and the vast majority of ECT research studies have focused on this condition, evidence suggests that ECT has efficacy in treating a number of other mental disorders. In the treatment of bipolar disorder, including mania, mixed states, and depressive episodes, ECT has been reported to achieve a response rate as high as 80%, to have efficacy equal to that of lithium, and to have a significant advantage over lithium in patients who have not responded to lithium or antipsychotic medication (Dierckx et al. 2012; Versiani et al. 2011) (option B). No systematic studies exist to indicate the utility of ECT in

291

individuals with rapid-cycling bipolar disorder (option C). Another disorder for which ECT has efficacy is schizophrenia. The presence of affective symptoms appears to increase the likelihood of response to ECT in individuals with schizophrenia (Pompili et al. 2013). Case reports and case series suggest that individuals with schizoaffective disorder may respond better to ECT than do patients with schizophrenia (American Psychiatric Association 2001) (option D). **(pp. 590–591)**

21.2   You recommend ECT for a 73-year-old woman with treatment-refractory depression. She has concerns about this modality because of stories she heard about "shock treatment" in the past. Which of the following would be an accurate statement about ECT treatment for someone in her age group?

A. ECT is more effective in young individuals than in elderly individuals.
B. ECT is at least as effective in elderly individuals as it is in middle-aged individuals.
C. ECT prevents recurrence of neuropsychiatric disorders.
D. ECT has a higher mortality rate than treatment with tricyclic antidepressants.

The correct response is option B: ECT is at least as effective in elderly individuals as it is in middle-aged individuals.

Several prospective studies suggest that ECT is a highly effective acute treatment for major depression in elderly individuals (Kamat et al. 2003; Kerner and Prudic 2014; O'Connor et al. 2001; Riva-Posse et al. 2013; Tew et al. 1999; van der Wurff et al. 2003; Wesson et al. 1997). There is consensus among the larger studies that elderly patients show at least equivalent improvement to middle-aged patients (option B) and greater improvement than those who are younger (option A). Although ECT is a highly effective treatment for a number of neuropsychiatric conditions, it is not a cure in the sense that it does not ensure that future episodes will not occur (Weiner and Krystal 2001; Weiner et al. 2000) (option C). The relatively low mortality rate of ECT appears to be comparable to the rate associated with minor surgery and has been considered to be less than that associated with pharmacotherapy with tricyclic antidepressants (Sackeim 1998) (option D). **(pp. 591–592, 593–594)**

21.3   Which of the following is a factor at the time of treatment that can worsen the cognitive side effects of ECT?

A. Using bifrontal instead of bitemporal electrode placement.
B. Stopping lithium while undergoing treatment.
C. The presence of basal ganglia disease.
D. The presence of pseudodementia.

The correct response is option C: The presence of basal ganglia disease.

The most important side effect with ECT is cognitive dysfunction, which remains a key factor limiting the use of this treatment modality (American Psychiatric Association 2001). Anterograde amnesia typically resolves within a few weeks after the treatment course, whereas retrograde amnesia tends to resolve more slowly (Weiner et al. 1986). Despite objective evidence that memory performance transiently decreases after ECT, some patients indicate that their memory function improves, likely a result of the lifting of depressive symptoms (American Psychiatric Association 2001; Weiner et al. 1986). This finding appears to be present in older adults as well as in younger individuals, particularly in individuals in whom the severity of depression-related cognitive deficits presents as a pseudodementia (Bosboom and Deijen 2006) (option D). A number of research studies have identified factors that can affect objective memory side effects of ECT (American Psychiatric Association 2001). Compared with unilateral placement of stimulus electrodes, bilateral placement has repeatedly been shown to increase the risk of amnesia, including in elderly populations (O'Connor et al. 2010; Stoppe et al. 2006). Studies suggest that both efficacy and cognitive effects of bifrontal ECT may be less than with bitemporal ECT and perhaps slightly greater than with unilateral ECT (option A). Some patients—including those taking lithium and medications with anticholinergic properties, as well as those having preexisting cerebral disease—appear to be at increased risk of cognitive side effects (American Psychiatric Association 2001) (option B). Individuals with diseases affecting the basal ganglia and subcortical white matter may be at particular risk (Figiel et al. 1990) (option C). **(pp. 594, 604)**

21.4   What is the only absolute contraindication to the use of ECT?

A. Unstable angina.
B. Unstable bone fractures.
C. Hyperkalemia.
D. There are no absolute contraindications.

The correct response is option D: There are no absolute contraindications.

Elderly patients referred for ECT frequently have preexisting medical illnesses (Christopher 2003; Weiner and Krystal 2001). Although some illnesses appear to increase the risks of ECT (Zielinski et al. 1993), no illness should be considered an absolute contraindication, given that risk is relative rather than absolute (Weiner and Krystal 2001; Weiner et al. 2000) (option D). The decision about whether to pursue a course of ECT should always involve a careful weighing of the risks and benefits of carrying out ECT versus those of not using it. Various medical problems, including central nervous system disorders, cardiovascular disorders, endocrinological disorders, metabolic disorders, hematological disorders, pulmonary disorders, gastrointestinal disorders, genitourinary disorders, and musculoskeletal disorders, as well as the specific issue of adverse effects of ECT in older adults should be taken into account. Fluctuations in pulse and blood pressure that occur during ECT treatments may be associated with cardiovascular complications (Weiner et al. 2000). Cardiovascular complications from ECT rarely occur in patients without preexisting cardiovascular risk factors (Takada et al.

2005; Weiner et al. 2000). The risk is increased in patients with recent myocardial infarction, uncompensated congestive heart failure, severe valvular disease, unstable aneurysm, unstable angina (option A) or active cardiac ischemia, uncontrolled hypertension, high-grade atrioventricular block, symptomatic ventricular arrhythmia, and supraventricular arrhythmia with uncontrolled ventricular rate (American Psychiatric Association 2001; Applegate 1997). The metabolic problems that are of primary concern are hyperkalemia (option C) and hypokalemia, both of which may lead to cardiac arrhythmias. The former is of particular concern because of the transient rise in serum potassium caused by succinylcholine and the muscle activity that may occur during the induced seizures (Christopher 2003; Weiner et al. 2000). Musculoskeletal conditions, such as osteoporosis, unstable fractures (option B), and loose or damaged teeth, are common in older adults and carry an increased risk of complications with ECT. **(pp. 594–599)**

21.5   Why is an anticholinergic medication, such as glycopyrrolate or atropine, administered before anesthesia during ECT treatment?

A. To prevent seizure-related tachycardia and hypertension.
B. To counteract the increased sympathetic effects of agents such as dexmedetomidine.
C. To counter the anticonvulsant properties of certain anesthetics.
D. To minimize the risk of stimulus-related asystole.

The correct response is option D: To minimize the risk of stimulus-related asystole.

ECT is a procedure involving general anesthesia. Airway management, the administration of medications necessary for anesthesia, and the handling of medical emergencies during and immediately following the ECT procedure are the responsibility of the anesthesia provider (American Psychiatric Association 2001). General anesthesia is usually provided by intravenous methohexital. Because seizure threshold (the amount of electricity necessary to induce a seizure) appears to increase with age, and stimulus output of ECT devices is limited by the U.S. Food and Drug Administration (FDA), difficulties in seizure induction can be experienced with older adults, particularly late in an index ECT course. In such situations, mexohexital dosage can be slightly diminished by concurrent usage of a short-acting sedative narcotic such as remifentanil (option C), or the anesthetic itself can be switched to one with less anticonvulsant properties (e.g., etomidate or ketamine). An anticholinergic medication, such as glycopyrrolate or atropine, may be administered before anesthesia to minimize the risk of stimulus-related asystole (option D) and the occurrence of postictal oral secretions. However, most practitioners use such agents selectively because they potentiate seizure-related tachycardia (option A). When seizure-related hypertension and tachycardia are severe or when prophylaxis is indicated on the basis of preexisting cardiovascular disease, β-blocking medications (e.g., labetalol) are often used to minimize these effects. Anticholinergic medications are not used to counteract agents such as dexmedetomidine. In fact, dexmedetomidine is interesting in that if it is administered preictally, it will blunt the sympathetically mediated rise in heart rate and blood pressure during the induced seizure (Aydogan et al. 2013) (option B). **(p. 602–603)**

21.6   What must an anesthesiologist consider when administering medications and monitoring an older adult during ECT treatment?

A. Because of altered metabolism or tolerance, older adults often need higher doses of medications than younger patients.
B. Time to effect may be longer in elderly patients.
C. Individuals with osteoporosis should be given less succinylcholine.
D. Haloperidol should be avoided in the treatment of postictal delirium or agitation.

The correct response is option B: Time to effect may be longer in elderly patients.

With older adults, it is important to recognize that lower doses of medications may be indicated because of altered metabolism or tolerance (option A). In addition, time to effect may be longer in older adults (option B). On the other hand, under some circumstances, higher doses may be necessary (e.g., more relaxant agent may be needed for an individual with osteoporosis) (option C). When necessary, postictal agitation or delirium can be managed with the use of intravenous midazolam (1 mg), haloperidol (2–5 mg) (option D), or the α_2 agonist dexmedetomidine (10–40 mcg), as well as by providing reassurance and maintaining a quiet, low-light environment for the postictal recovery process. **(pp. 602–603)**

21.7   Which type of stimulus electrode placement during ECT is associated with the least number of cognitive side effects?

A. Unilateral nondominant.
B. Bitemporal.
C. Bifrontal.
D. Cognitive side effects have been found to be equivalent among the three major types of stimulus electrode placement.

The correct response is option A: Unilateral nondominant.

There are three major types of stimulus electrode placement: bitemporal, bifrontal, and unilateral nondominant (the right side for the great majority of individuals). Bitemporal ECT involves placement of both stimulus electrodes over the frontotemporal regions, with the center of each electrode approximately 1 inch above the midpoint of a line transecting the external canthus of the eye and the tragus of the ear. Bifrontal electrode placement involves locating the center of the stimulus electrodes approximately 5 cm superior to each external canthus. The preferred type of unilateral nondominant placement involves location of one electrode over the right frontotemporal area (as described for bitemporal ECT) and the other over the right centroparietal area, just to the right of the vertex of the scalp, a point defined by the intersection of lines between the inion and nasion and between the tragi of both ears. ECT-associated amnesia is greater with bitemporal ECT (options B and D) than unilateral nondominant ECT (options A and D). With bifrontal electrode placement, the newest of the three techniques (Bailine et al. 2000), data are mixed, with some studies suggesting that cognitive effects of bifrontal ECT may be less than with bitemporal ECT and perhaps slightly greater than with unilateral ECT (options C and D). **(pp. 603–604)**

21.8   Which of the following statements is true regarding seizures induced during ECT?

A. It is easier to determine the quality of a seizure in geriatric patients.
B. ECT-induced seizures are identical to complex partial seizures in terms of electroencephalogram (EEG) findings.
C. The higher seizure threshold in older adults increases the risk of their being unable to receive a stimulus of sufficient intensity during ECT.
D. In unilateral ECT, there is no difference in therapeutic effect between a barely suprathreshold seizure and a moderately suprathreshold of the same duration.

The correct response is option C: The higher seizure threshold in older adults increases the risk of their being unable to receive a stimulus of sufficient intensity during ECT.

ECT-induced seizures are identical to spontaneous grand mal seizures except that with ECT the motor response is attenuated pharmacologically (option B). The EEG recording during ECT (ictal electroencephalogram) manifests the typical EEG features of a grand mal seizure, with irregular polyspike activity marking the tonic portion of the seizure and repetitive polyspike and slow-wave discharges during the clonic component. Compelling evidence indicates that not all seizures are equally potent from a therapeutic perspective. With unilateral ECT, barely suprathreshold seizures—despite having identical durations as seizures from more moderately suprathreshold stimuli—are only minimally therapeutic (Sackeim et al. 1993) (option D). Regardless of stimulus waveform, seizure quality determinations can be more difficult with elderly patients (option A), possibly because of the effects of age-related neuronal loss on the intensity of ictal hypersynchrony. Seizure threshold is a function of age, with substantially higher thresholds being present in older adults. This higher threshold leaves older adults at greater risk for being unable to receive a stimulus of sufficient intensity, because the maximum output of ECT devices used in the United States is limited by FDA regulations (Krystal et al. 2000) (option C). The risk that the threshold will exceed the maximum available stimulus intensity is greatest late in the treatment course, because seizure threshold rises to a varying extent with the number of treatments. **(p. 605)**

21.9   What is the most commonly recommended frequency and duration of ECT treatments in the United States?

A. Two times per week, between 4 and 8 treatments.
B. Two times per week, between 8 and 16 treatments.

C. Three times per week, between 3 and 9 treatments.

D. Three times per week, between 6 and 12 treatments.

The correct response is option D: Three times per week, between 6 and 12 treatments.

In the United States, ECT is typically administered three times a week, with an index course usually lasting between 6 and 12 treatments, although more or fewer are sometimes necessary (option D; options A, B, and C are incorrect). The frequency of ECT may be reduced to twice a week or even once a week if amnesia or confusion becomes a major problem (American Psychiatric Association 2001), something that is not infrequently indicated with elderly patients. The decision about when to end the index ECT course depends on treatment outcome. In general, the index ECT course is considered complete when a therapeutic plateau has occurred—that is, when the patient has reached a maximum level of response. **(pp. 605–606)**

21.10 Which of the following is a true statement regarding pharmacotherapy after an initial treatment of ECT?

A. Studies of maintenance pharmacotherapy after ECT treatment for major depression suggest that antidepressants should be augmented with a mood stabilizer.

B. A randomized trial showed that maintenance ECT is superior to maintenance pharmacological treatment with nortriptyline and lithium.

C. Initial ECT treatment typically eliminates preexisting resistance to antidepressants used prior to the initiation of ECT treatment.

D. Several studies of maintenance pharmacotherapy after ECT treatment for mania or schizophrenia suggest avoiding aggressive treatment with medications from different classes.

The correct response is option A: Studies of maintenance pharmacotherapy after ECT treatment for major depression suggest that antidepressants should be augmented with a mood stabilizer.

Pharmacological maintenance treatment is usually attempted after the initial index ECT course unless the patient indicates a strong preference for maintenance ECT. With major depression, evidence suggests that a combination of antidepressant and mood stabilizer may be more effective in maintaining remission than an antidepressant drug alone (Sackeim et al. 2001) (option A). Unfortunately, medication resistance during the index episode may diminish the likelihood of a sustained prophylactic effect (Sackeim et al. 1990) (option C). Maintenance pharmacotherapy following ECT treatment of mania or schizophrenia has not been well studied. In the absence of applicable data, an aggressive regimen of different drug classes should be considered (option D). After a flurry of largely positive case-series reports (Rabheru and Persad 1997), a randomized trial of maintenance ECT versus pharmacotherapy in patients treated for major depression was carried out, with results indicating that the efficacy of maintenance ECT over a 6-month period was comparable to that obtained by combination pharmacotherapy with both lithium and nortriptyline (Kellner et al. 2006) (option B). **(p. 606)**

21.11 Which of the following is a true statement regarding the use of repetitive transcranial magnetic stimulation (rTMS) in geriatric patients?

A. Elderly patients have shown a higher incidence of cognitive side effects.
B. The difficult side effects of rTMS cause more than a third of patients to discontinue treatment before completion.
C. Cortical atrophy in geriatric patients limits magnetic stimulation of deep brain structures.
D. rTMS is not associated with increased potential for seizure induction.

The correct response is option C: Cortical atrophy in geriatric patients limits magnetic stimulation of deep brain structures.

TMS involves the noninvasive use of rapidly alternating magnetic fields to stimulate areas of the brain related to mood regulation. One of the limitations of rTMS in geriatric patients is its restricted ability to stimulate deeper structures that have been affected by cortical atrophy (option C). TMS has demonstrated a strong safety record accompanied by minimal side effects, which is important in the treatment of elderly subjects. Studies have consistently shown that TMS is relatively well tolerated by patients, with only 4.5% of patients terminating early due to side effects (O'Reardon et al. 2007) (option B). Also important for geriatric patients is the fact that no significant adverse cognitive side effects were noted in these trials (option A). A more serious risk is posed by the increased potential for seizure induction (option D); to date there have been 13 documented cases of seizure related to TMS. Of note, many of these instances involved neurologically compromised patients or treatment parameters that fell outside the recommended standards (Wani et al. 2013). **(pp. 607–608)**

21.12 Which of the following is a reason why transcranial direct current stimulation (tDCS) may be a promising treatment for the geriatric population?

A. Multiple tDCS studies in the geriatric population have shown efficacy in the treatment of major depression.
B. Like rTMS, tDCS has shown specific benefits in the treatment of depression with psychosis and severe suicidal ideation.
C. tDCS provides a noninvasive method of stimulating neuronal excitation in cortical tissue, which is relatively well tolerated by patients.
D. tDCS is not associated with any adverse effects related to its administration.

The correct response is option C: tDCS provides a noninvasive method of stimulating neuronal excitation in cortical tissue, which is generally well tolerated by patients.

tDCS is a noninvasive brain stimulation therapy that has grown from its initial development as a research technique to encompass clinical application as well. It uses weak levels of direct current (usually ranging from 1 to 2.5 mA) to stimulate cortical neuronal activity. Administration involves placing two electrodes at targeted cortical areas (dorsolateral prefrontal cortex) on the patient's head, such that the electric current passing between them flows through the underlying cortical tissue, inducing neuronal excitation. tDCS is attractive as a brain stimulation treatment due to its demonstrated minimal risk of serious adverse events (option C). Minor adverse events commonly reported by patients include burning, tingling, and itching sensations at the site of stimulation during treatment (option D). rTMS trials typically exclude subjects with psychotic or severe suicidal ideation, but there is no corresponding evidence for tDCS in these populations (option B). Because it is in the early phases of development, tDCS has not yet been tested specifically in the geriatric population (option A). **(pp. 608–609)**

21.13 Direct stimulation of which of the following targets has been approved by the FDA as an invasive treatment for refractory major depression?

A. Vagus nerve.
B. Nucleus accumbens.
C. Ventral striatum.
D. Brodmann area 25.

The correct response is option A: Vagus nerve.

Vagus nerve stimulation (VNS) was the first FDA-approved invasive treatment to be developed for depression (option A). The vagus nerve is thought to affect depression through its relationship with areas of the brain associated with mood regulation (Wani et al. 2013). The use of neuroimaging technology has produced documentation that the VNS alters activity in mood-related cortical regions of the brain in research carried out on depressed patients (Daban et al. 2008). Deep brain stimulation (DBS) is an investigational approach to treating severe depression that continues to be evaluated, although the FDA approved use of DBS for Parkinson's disease in 2002. DBS involves surgical implantation of electrodes in a targeted area of the brain (e.g., Brodmann area 25) (option D). Other regions of the brain have also been targeted in patients with treatment-resistant depression, including the ventral striatum (option C) and the nucleus accumbens (option A) (Schlaepfer et al. 2008, 2014). **(pp. 609–610)**

21.14 Which of the following is an accurate statement regarding deep brain stimulation (DBS) in the treatment of chronic refractory depression?

A. DBS has not been shown to increase the risk of seizures.
B. DBS has not been shown to negatively affect cognitive functioning.
C. DBS targets various deep brain structures but does not target cortical areas.
D. DBS has not been effective for treating depression in patients with Parkinson's disease.

The correct response is option B: DBS has not been shown to negatively affect cognitive functioning.

DBS is an investigational approach to treating severe depression that continues to be evaluated, although the FDA approved use of DBS for Parkinson's disease in 2002. Many patients being treated for Parkinson's disease with DBS implants reported concomitant improvement in mood symptoms (Kuehn 2007), and this finding generated interest in DBS as an approach to treating severe depression (option D). Today, due to the invasive nature of the treatment, DBS is reserved for patients with severe treatment-resistant depression. DBS involves surgical implantation of electrodes in a targeted area of the brain (e.g., Brodmann area 25). These electrodes are attached to a neurostimulator that is implanted in the patient's chest wall, and electrical impulses are generated on a constant basis. Other regions of the brain have also been targeted in patients with treatment-resistant depression, including the ventral striatum and the nucleus accumbens (Schlaepfer et al. 2008, 2014). In spite of the invasive nature of DBS, an important strength is that it has not been shown to affect cognitive functioning (Mayberg et al. 2005) (option B). Still, there are risks associated with the surgical procedure, including infection, bleeding in the brain, and seizures (option A). Additionally, irritability, headaches, and pain at the generator site have been reported (Lozano et al. 2008). Further research is attempting to identify other cortical regions (option C) for stimulation and establish techniques and procedures that minimize such side effects (Schlaepfer et al. 2014). **(pp. 609–610)**

References

American Psychiatric Association: The Practice of Electroconvulsive Therapy: Recommendations for Treatment, Training, and Privileging. Washington, DC, American Psychiatric Press, 2001

Applegate RJ: Diagnosis and management of ischemic heart disease in the patient scheduled to undergo electroconvulsive therapy. Convuls Ther 13(3):128–144, 1997 9342129

Aydogan MS, Yücel A, Begec Z, et al: The hemodynamic effects of dexmedetomidine and esmolol in electroconvulsive therapy: a retrospective comparison. J ECT 29(4):308–311, 2013 23774056

Bailine SH, Rifkin A, Kayne E, et al: Comparison of bifrontal and bitemporal ECT for major depression. Am J Psychiatry 157(1):121–123, 2000 10618025

Bosboom PR, Deijen JB: Age-related cognitive effects of ECT and ECT-induced mood improvement in depressive patients. Depress Anxiety 23(2):93–101, 2006 16400627

Christopher EJ: Electroconvulsive therapy in the medically ill. Curr Psychiatry Rep 5(3):225–230, 2003 12773277

Daban C, Martinez-Aran A, Cruz N, Vieta E: Safety and efficacy of vagus nerve stimulation in treatment-resistant depression. A systematic review. J Affect Disord 110(1–2):1–15, 2008 18374988

Dierckx B, Heijnen WT, van den Broek WW, Birkenhäger TK: Efficacy of electroconvulsive therapy in bipolar versus unipolar major depression: a meta-analysis. Bipolar Disord 14(2):146–150, 2012 22420590

Figiel GS, Coffey CE, Djang WT, et al: Brain magnetic resonance imaging findings in ECT-induced delirium. J Neuropsychiatry Clin Neurosci 2(1):53–58, 1990 2136061

Kamat SM, Lefevre PJ, Grossberg GT: Electroconvulsive therapy in the elderly. Clin Geriatr Med 19(4):825–839, 2003 15024814

Kellner CH, Knapp RG, Petrides G, et al: Continuation electroconvulsive therapy vs pharmaco-therapy for relapse prevention in major depression: a multisite study from the Consortium for Research in Electroconvulsive Therapy (CORE). Arch Gen Psychiatry 63(12):1337–1344, 2006 17146008

Kerner N, Prudic J: Current electroconvulsive therapy practice and research in the geriatric population. Neuropsychiatry (London) 4(1):33–54, 2014 24778709

Krystal AD, Dean MD, Weiner RD, et al: ECT stimulus intensity: are present ECT devices too limited? Am J Psychiatry 157(6):963–967, 2000 10831477

Kuehn BM: Scientists probe deep brain stimulation: some promise for brain injury, psychiatric illness. JAMA 298(19):2249–2251, 2007 18029821

Lozano AM, Mayberg HS, Giacobbe P, et al: Subcallosal cingulate gyrus deep brain stimulation for treatment-resistant depression. Biol Psychiatry 64(6):461–467, 2008 18639234

Mayberg HS, Lozano AM, Voon V, et al: Deep brain stimulation for treatment-resistant depression. Neuron 45(5):651–660, 2005 15748841

O'Connor DW, Gardner B, Eppingstall B, Tofler D: Cognition in elderly patients receiving unilateral and bilateral electroconvulsive therapy: a prospective, naturalistic comparison. J Affect Disord 124(3):235–240, 2010 20053457

O'Connor MK, Knapp R, Husain M, et al: The influence of age on the response of major depression to electroconvulsive therapy: a C.O.R.E. Report. Am J Geriatr Psychiatry 9(4):382–390, 2001 11739064

O'Reardon JP, Solvason HB, Janicak PG, et al: Efficacy and safety of transcranial magnetic stimulation in the acute treatment of major depression: a multisite randomized controlled trial. Biol Psychiatry 62(11):1208–1216, 2007 17573044

Pompili M, Lester D, Dominici G, et al: Indications for electroconvulsive treatment in schizophrenia: a systematic review. Schizophr Res 146(1–3):1–9, 2013 23499244

Rabheru K, Persad E: A review of continuation and maintenance electroconvulsive therapy. Can J Psychiatry 42(5):476–484, 1997 9220110

Riva-Posse P, Hermida AP, McDonald WM: The role of electroconvulsive and neuromodulation therapies in the treatment of geriatric depression. Psychiatr Clin North Am 36(4):607–630, 2013 24229660

Sackeim HA: The use of electroconvulsive therapy in late-life depression, in Clinical Geriatric Psychopharmacology, 3rd Edition. Edited by Salzman C. Baltimore, MD, Williams & Wilkins, 1998, pp 262–309

Sackeim HA, Rush AJ: Melancholia and response to ECT. Am J Psychiatry 152(8):1242–1243, 1995 7625490

Sackeim HA, Prudic J, Devanand DP, et al: The impact of medication resistance and continuation pharmacotherapy on relapse following response to electroconvulsive therapy in major depression. J Clin Psychopharmacol 10(2):96–104, 1990 2341598

Sackeim HA, Prudic J, Devanand DP, et al: Effects of stimulus intensity and electrode placement on the efficacy and cognitive effects of electroconvulsive therapy. N Engl J Med 328(12):839–846, 1993 8441428

Sackeim HA, Haskett RF, Mulsant BH, et al: Continuation pharmacotherapy in the prevention of relapse following electroconvulsive therapy: a randomized controlled trial. JAMA 285(10):1299–1307, 2001 11255384

Schlaepfer TE, Cohen MX, Frick C, et al: Deep brain stimulation to reward circuitry alleviates anhedonia in refractory major depression. Neuropsychopharmacology 33(2):368–377, 2008 17429407

Schlaepfer TE, Bewernick BH, Kayser S, et al: Deep brain stimulation of the human reward system for major depression—rationale, outcomes and outlook. Neuropsychopharmacology 39(6):1303–1314, 2014 24513970

Stoppe A, Louzã M, Rosa M, et al: Fixed high-dose electroconvulsive therapy in the elderly with depression: a double-blind, randomized comparison of efficacy and tolerability between unilateral and bilateral electrode placement. J ECT 22(2):92–99, 2006 16801822

Takada JY, Solimene MC, da Luz PL, et al: Assessment of the cardiovascular effects of electroconvulsive therapy in individuals older than 50 years. Braz J Med Biol Res 38(9):1349–1357, 2005 16138218

Tew JD Jr, Mulsant BH, Haskett RF, et al: Acute efficacy of ECT in the treatment of major depression in the old-old. Am J Psychiatry 156(12):1865–1870, 1999 10588398

van der Wurff FB, Stek ML, Hoogendijk WJ, Beekman AT: The efficacy and safety of ECT in depressed older adults: a literature review. Int J Geriatr Psychiatry 18(10):894–904, 2003 14533122

Versiani M, Cheniaux E, Landeira-Fernandez J: Efficacy and safety of electroconvulsive therapy in the treatment of bipolar disorder: a systematic review. J ECT 27(2):153–164, 2011 20562714

Wani A, Trevino K, Marnell P, Husain MM: Advances in brain stimulation for depression. Ann Clin Psychiatry 25(3):217–224, 2013 23926577

Weiner RD, Krystal AD: Electroconvulsive therapy, in Treatments of Psychiatric Disorders, 3rd Edition. Edited by Gabbard GO, Rush AJ. Washington, DC, American Psychiatric Press, 2001, pp 1267–1293

Weiner RD, Rogers HJ, Davidson JR, Squire LR: Effects of stimulus parameters on cognitive side effects. Ann N Y Acad Sci 462:315–325, 1986 3458412

Weiner RD, Coffey CE, Krystal AD: Electroconvulsive therapy in the medical and neurologic patient, in Psychiatric Care of the Medical Patient, 2nd Edition. Edited by Stoudemire A, Fogel BS, Greenberg D. New York, Oxford University Press, 2000, pp 419–428

Wesson ML, Wilkinson AM, Anderson DN, Cracken CM: Does age predict the long-term outcome of depression treated with ECT? (a prospective study of the long-term outcome of ECT-treated depression with respect to age). Int J Geriatr Psychiatry 12(1):45–51, 1997 9050423

Zielinski RJ, Roose SP, Devanand DP, et al: Cardiovascular complications of ECT in depressed patients with cardiac disease. Am J Psychiatry 150(6):904–909, 1993 8494067

CHAPTER 22

Nutrition and Physical Activity

22.1 An 84-year-old woman with diabetes is brought in by her family for concerns of weight loss, weakness, and confusion. Which of the following dietary factors is least likely contributing to her current symptoms?

A. Negative energy balance from chronic inadequate food intake.
B. Decreased fluid intake due to the diminished thirst response.
C. A 20-year history of drinking 3 ounces of red wine nightly with dinner.
D. Poor glycemic control due to noncompliance with diabetic dietary restrictions.

The correct response is option D: A 20-year history of drinking 3 ounces of red wine nightly with dinner.

Although the effects of nutritional deficits might be transitory, the symptoms can be disabling and are likely to obscure any other underlying mechanisms of impairment. Chronic inadequate food intake is a concern and can lead to weakness, fatigue, and other vague symptoms due to negative energy balance (option A). Dehydration is an important contributor to delirium and confusion in older adults, who are known to have a diminished thirst response compared with younger adults (Luckey and Parsa 2003) (option B). Lack of compliance with therapeutic dietary restrictions and instructions can also contribute to poor mental status. Poor glycemic control can contribute to poor cognitive outcomes in the long term (Ravona-Springer et al. 2012; West et al. 2014) (option D). Although moderate alcohol intake in older adults (no more than one daily drink for women and two daily drinks for men) may preserve cognitive function, people with alcoholism often consume inadequate amounts of vitamins and minerals and may have an insufficient intake of protein (option C). Chronic alcohol misuse can lead to severe vitamin depletion and the development of Wernicke-Korsakoff syndrome in susceptible individuals (Thomson 2000). **(pp. 619, 620, 627)**

22.2　Which of the following aspects of the diet is associated with a reduced risk of cognitive decline, stroke, and depression?

A.　High intake of monounsaturated fats.
B.　High intake of saturated fats.
C.　Low intake of polyunsaturated fats.
D.　Consumption of a Western-style diet.

The correct response is option A: High intake of monounsaturated fats.

Adherence to the Mediterranean diet, characterized by high intake of monounsaturated and polyunsaturated omega-3 fats (option A; option C is incorrect), moderate ethanol consumption, and low intake of saturated fats (option B), has been associated with a reduced risk for cognitive decline (Scarmeas et al. 2006). In contrast, a Western-style diet (option D), characterized by high intake of high-fat (saturated) dairy products as well as meats, potatoes, and processed foods, is associated with greater cognitive decline (Parrott et al. 2013). **(p. 620)**

22.3　Which of the following is true regarding nutritional status and cognitive function?

A.　Reduced dietary folate intake is not associated with the development of dementia.
B.　Excessive vitamin B_{12} intake has been associated with dementia.
C.　Vitamin D plays a role in cognitive function.
D.　High plasma antioxidant levels are associated with cognitive impairment.

The correct response is option C: Vitamin D plays a role in cognitive function.

The most commonly studied vitamins are folate and vitamin B_{12}, the deficiencies of which have been linked with symptoms of dementia in older adults (Clarke 2007) (option A). Two longitudinal studies of adults older than age 65 years who were dementia free at baseline looked at predictors of incident dementia over 2–6 years. Intakes of folate at baseline (assessed by a food frequency questionnaire) and serum folate levels were associated with a decreased risk of dementia, including Alzheimer's disease, independent of other risk factors. Regarding vitamin B_{12}, the varied findings may indicate that only deficient states promote dementia (option B). A study by Przybelski and Binkley (2007) suggested that vitamin D has a role in cognitive function (option C). Other studies have linked low plasma antioxidant levels with cognitive impairment and brain white matter hyperintense lesions (option D). **(p. 621)**

22.4　Which of the following outcomes is *not* associated with adherence to a Mediterranean diet?

A.　Lower rates of vascular diseases.
B.　Increased risk of depression.
C.　Decreased risk of stroke.
D.　Decreased risk of cognitive impairment.

The correct response is option B: Increased risk of depression.

Preventive dietary factors for vascular diseases include monounsaturated fat, polyunsaturated fats (including omega-3 fatty acids), fiber, folate, ethanol (in moderation), fish, fruits, and vegetables, which are the primary components of a Mediterranean diet as well as other healthy diets (Almeida et al. 2009; Roberts et al. 2003) (option A). A meta-analysis examined the role of the Mediterranean diet in preventing mental and cognitive disorders (Psaltopoulou et al. 2013). Higher adherence to a Mediterranean diet was found to reduce risk not only for depression but also for stroke and cognitive impairment (option B; options C and D are incorrect). **(pp. 622, 623–624)**

22.5 What is the mechanism by which moderate alcohol intake helps in the preservation of cognitive function?

A. It increases generation of thromboxane A_2.
B. It increases white matter lesions.
C. It increases prostacyclin concentrations.
D. It increases platelet function.

The correct response is option C: It increases prostacyclin concentrations.

There is a considerable amount of evidence linking modest to moderate alcohol intake (no more than one daily drink for women and two daily drinks for men) with benefits related to preservation of cognitive function. Moderate alcohol intake has been found to reduce brain infarcts and white matter lesions (option B) and to reduce vascular risk by increasing prostacyclin concentrations (option C), reducing generation of thromboxane A_2 (option A), inhibiting platelet function (option D), and increasing high-density lipoprotein cholesterol levels (Frisardi et al. 2010; Panza et al. 2012). **(p. 620)**

22.6 Which of the following is true regarding physical activity and cognition?

A. Physical activity has been associated with decreased white matter integrity.
B. Physical activity has been associated with higher Mini-Mental State Examination scores.
C. Aerobic exercise has been associated with improved cognitive speed but not auditory and visual attention.
D. Physical activity does not affect brain volume.

The correct response is option B: Physical activity has been associated with higher Mini-Mental State Examination scores.

Physical activity has been associated with numerous cognitive benefits, including delayed onset of dementia (Larson et al. 2006), higher Mini-Mental State Examination scores (Almeida et al. 2006) (option B), and increased brain volumes (Colcombe et al. 2006) (option D). Also encouraging are reports linking greater aerobic fitness with white matter integrity in certain regions of the brain (Marks et al. 2007) (option A). A Cochrane review on the impact of aerobic exercise on cognition in adults ages 55 years and older found positive association on cognitive speed and auditory and visual attention (Angevaren et al. 2008) (option C). **(p. 624)**

22.7   Which statement is accurate regarding physical activity in healthy older adults?

A. Low to moderate physical activity is associated with a reduced risk of cognitive decline in older adults compared with sedentary individuals.
B. Vigorous, but not moderate, activity is associated prospectively with fewer depressive symptoms.
C. Living in a less walkable neighborhood is not associated with depressive symptoms.
D. Physical activity does not influence quality of life.

The correct response is option A: Low to moderate physical activity is associated with a reduced risk of cognitive decline in older adults compared with sedentary individuals.

In a meta-analysis of 15 prospective studies of healthy older adults, low to moderate physical activity was associated with a 35% reduced risk of cognitive decline compared with sedentary individuals (option A). Mental health is also associated with physical activity. Hamer et al. (2014) followed older adults for 8 years and found that those who were significantly less likely to report depressive symptoms participated either in moderate activity or in vigorous activity (option B); however, only those who participated in vigorous activity had reduced risk for cognitive impairment. Reported mental well-being is higher in older adults with good mobility status (Lampinen et al. 2006). Older adults who were regular participants in physical activity of at least moderate intensity for greater than 1 hour per week had higher health-related quality of life than those who were less active (option D). In contrast, older men living in neighborhoods where walkability was lower were more likely to be depressed than those living in environments that were more supportive of physical activity (Berke et al. 2007) (option C). **(p. 624)**

22.8   Which of the following is accurate regarding nutritional screening methods?

A. The Subjective Global Assessment (SGA) detects nutritional deficiencies in patients who are overweight at baseline.
B. The patient's body weight is the most important clinical measure of undernutrition.
C. The Mini Nutritional Assessment (MNA) is superior to other instruments in detecting nutritional deficiencies in patients who are overweight at baseline.
D. Serum albumin should be checked frequently in protein repletion.

The correct response is option B: The patient's body weight is the most important clinical measure of undernutrition.

The MNA is a validated tool that incorporates several domains, including functional status, lifestyle, diet, self-perception of health, and anthropometric indices (Donini et al. 2003). The SGA assesses nutritional status based on the patient's history and physical examination and is used to derive a clinical grade of that status (Detsky et al. 1994; Sacks et al. 2000). However, neither of these indices addresses the potential that being overweight could be masking the existence of micronutrient deficiencies (options A and C). The single most important clinical measure of undernutrition in older adults is that of current body weight and any recent changes (option B). Albumin is unlikely to be responsive to protein repletion in a timely manner (Omran and Morley 2000). Therefore, serum albumin (option D) is not recommended as a sole marker of nutritional status (Sullivan et al. 2002). **(p. 630)**

22.9   What is the recommendation regarding physical activity for older adults?

A. At least 150 minutes per week of moderate-intensity aerobic exercise is recommended.
B. When older adults are physically unable to complete 150 minutes of moderate-intensity physical activity, they should not be physically active.
C. To promote and maintain health, older adults should be physically active once a week.
D. Vigorous-intensity physical activity is not recommended for older adults.

The correct response is option A: At least 150 minutes per week of moderate-intensity aerobic exercise is recommended.

Older adults should do at least 150 minutes of moderate-intensity (option A) or 75 minutes of vigorous-intensity (option D) physical activity per week, with aerobic activity lasting longer than 10 minutes. Moderate-intensity aerobic activity is best described as producing noticeable increases in heart rate and breathing and reaching a level of 5 or 6 on a 10-point scale, where sitting is 0 and maximal effort is a 10. Vigorous-intensity aerobic activity is a level 7 or 8 on a 10-point scale. To promote and maintain health, older adults should be physically active throughout the entire week (option C). When older adults are physically unable to complete 150 minutes of moderate-intensity physical activity, they should be as physically active as their condition permits (option B). **(p. 637)**

22.10 Which of the following is a true statement regarding the nutritional status of older adults?

A. Serum albumin increases slightly with age.
B. Dietary intake is affected when older adults eat in social settings versus eating alone.
C. Risk of compromised nutritional status is reduced by residing in an assisted living facility.
D. Serum albumin is recommended as the sole marker of nutritional status.

The correct response is option B: Dietary intake is affected when older adults eat in social settings versus eating alone.

Medical comorbidities and a host of other factors, including economic, geographic, and psychosocial concerns, can affect dietary behaviors and thus nutritional status (Bales and Johnson 2012). Limited social contact (e.g., eating meals alone) impacts dietary intake (option B), as does inadequate assistance with shopping and preparing food. Institutionalization (e.g., in a hospital, assisted living, or nursing home) is almost always linked with increased nutritional risk (option C). Serum albumin declines slightly with age (0.8 g/L/decade after age 60 years) (option A) and is influenced by a host of pathological changes that are frequent in older adults, including chronic inflammation, advanced liver disease, heart failure, and nephrotic syndrome. Additionally, albumin is unlikely to be responsive to protein repletion in a timely manner (Omran and Morley 2000). Therefore, serum albumin is not recommended as a sole marker of nutritional status (Sullivan et al. 2002) (option D). **(pp. 629, 630)**

22.11 Which of the following is a true statement regarding weight and nutritional status in older adults?

A. Unintentional weight loss is associated with increased mortality.
B. Vitamin D deficiency is not common in older adults.
C. Weight loss of 5% of usual body weight in 180 days should trigger activating protocols for clinical assessment.
D. Nutritional status should not affect ability to taste or smell.

The correct response is option A: Unintentional weight loss is associated with increased mortality.

Results of the National Health and Nutrition Examination Survey show that average dietary intakes of older adults were generally lower than recommended for potassium, magnesium, calcium, and vitamins D and E (Moshfegh et al. 2009) (option B). Clinical nutritional deficiencies that can be identified in a physical examination include skin changes, fatigue, weakness, changes in ability to taste or smell, and gastrointestinal complaints (poor appetite, oral problems, nausea, vomiting, diarrhea, constipation); however, the single most important clinical measure of undernutrition in older adults is that of current body weight and any recent changes. According to the Long-Term Care Minimum Data Set (Blaum et al. 1995), a weight loss of 5% of usual body weight in 30 days or of 10% in 180 days is a trigger for activating clinical assessment protocols (option C). Unintentional recent weight loss is associated with increased mortality (Newman et al. 2001) (option A). It is well recognized that inadequate energy intakes and low body mass indices are linked with frailty in elderly individuals (Markson 1997). **(pp. 629, 630, 632)**

22.12 Which of the following is a true statement regarding the use of psychotropic medications in older adults?

A. Considering a patient's nutritional status is not necessary prior to starting the psychotropic.
B. Use of multiple medications is infrequent in elderly individuals.
C. The potential for drug-food interactions should be assessed.
D. Alcohol consumption does not have a bearing on the medication used.

The correct response is option C: The potential for drug-food interactions should be assessed.

Use of medications, including polypharmacy, is higher among elderly individuals than among younger adults. This greater use, combined with the physiological changes of aging, contributes to drug-related problems including drug-nutrient interactions (Knight-Klimas and Boullata 2004) (option B). A general approach to drug-nutrient interactions is recommended: Clinicians should 1) consider the patient's nutritional status (including malnutrition, nutrient deficiencies, and body weight) and current diet (including intake of vitamin, mineral, and herbal dietary supplements) (option A), 2) evaluate the potential for known drug-nutrient interactions for the medication being considered (option C) (which can be obtained from a drug-nutrient interaction reference book or a pharmacist), and 3) discontinue the offending agent and/or institute appropriate dietary modifications. Alcohol can enhance or negate medication effects and lead to adverse drug events, impaired psychomotor function, and sedation in older adults; therefore, it is important that clinicians also assess health status while investigating alcohol consumption (Moore et al. 2007; Wilson et al. 2014) (option D). **(pp. 627, 628)**

22.13 Which of the following is true regarding vitamins?

A. Pyridoxine (B_6) deficiency causes depression.
B. Prolonged cobalamin (B_{12}) deficiency causes reversible neurological damage.
C. L-Methylfolate has been used as an adjunctive therapy for selective serotonin reuptake inhibitor (SSRI) resistant depression.
D. Vitamin D does not help reduce risk of fractures.

The correct response is option C: L-Methylfolate has been used as an adjunctive therapy for selective serotonin reuptake inhibitor (SSRI) resistant depression.

Of the B vitamins, pyridoxine (B_6), cobalamin (B_{12}), and folate (B_9) are essential for serotonin production and myelin formation and have been implicated in depression. Pyridoxine deficiency is common in older adults, and low levels of pyridoxine have been correlated with depression (Bell et al. 1991; Stewart et al. 1984; Tolonen et al. 1988). However, studies of these factors have not demonstrated that low pyridoxine levels or pyridoxine deficiency causes depression (option A). Prolonged B_{12} deficiency has been shown to cause irreversible neurological damage (option B). L-Methylfolate has been used successfully as an adjunctive therapy for

SSRI-resistant depression (Papakostas et al. 2012) (option C). Strong evidence supports the benefits of supplements of calcium and vitamin D for reducing the risk of fractures (both nutrients together) and falls (vitamin D) (option D). Dietary calcium intakes are universally low in adults of all ages, which is a concern given the evidence for beneficial effects of supplemental calcium, either with or without concomitant vitamin D, on bone health and fracture risk. **(pp. 622, 628, 636)**

22.14 Which of the following nutrients is known to promote vascular disease?

A. Monounsaturated fat.
B. Polyunsaturated fats.
C. Trans-unsaturated fat.
D. Moderate alcohol intake.

The correct response is option C: Trans-unsaturated fat.

Key nutrients are known to be critical factors in determining vascular disease risk and may thus lead indirectly to late-life depression. Vascular promoters include saturated fat, trans-unsaturated fat (option C), cholesterol, high-fat dairy products, meats, and excess total energy (kcals), all of which are common components of a Western-style diet. Preventive dietary factors for vascular diseases include monounsaturated fat (option A), polyunsaturated fats (including omega-3 fatty acids) (option B), fiber, folate, ethanol (in moderation) (option D), fish, fruits, and vegetables, which are the primary components of a Mediterranean diet as well as other healthy diets. **(p. 622)**

22.15 Which of the following statements is true regarding depression in the elderly?

A. Corticotrophin-releasing factor (CRF) is known to be elevated in depressed individuals.
B. The antidepressant effect of aerobic exercise is less than that of antidepressant medications.
C. Corticotrophin-releasing factor can be used as an appetite stimulant for depressed patients.
D. Tricyclic antidepressants are often associated with weight loss.

The correct response is option A: Corticotrophin-releasing factor (CRF) is known to be elevated in depressed individuals.

Many geriatricians consider depression to be the most common cause of poor food intake and nutritional frailty among elderly individuals (Morley 2001). The loneliness and loss experienced by many elderly individuals affect both mood and dietary status, contributing to the anorexia and malnutrition of aging (Ferry et al. 2005). With regard to physical activity, the loss of energy and motivation that may accompany depression naturally makes efforts to exercise extremely difficult. Although depression can interfere with food intake by affecting general interest in daily activities, there are also possible physiological mechanisms whereby depression could lead to decreased appetite and weight loss. One potential explanation is that CRF, a potent anorectic agent (option C) known to be elevated in depressed individuals, may depress appetite (Morley 1996) (option A). Aerobic exercise has been shown to be as effective as antidepressants in treating major depression in elderly individuals (Blumenthal et al. 1999; Hamer et al. 2014) (option B). Side effects from medications can lead to changes in diet and nutritional status. For example, tricyclic antidepressants and conventional antipsychotics often lead to weight gain (option D). **(pp. 625, 626, 628)**

22.16 Which of the following is true regarding the dietary intake of nutrients for older adults?

A. Total daily energy expenditures increase with age.
B. Older adults need less dietary protein than younger adults.
C. The recommended daily water intake for healthy older adults is 1.5 L (six glasses) of water a day.
D. The recommended dietary fiber intake for older adults is 15 grams, the same as younger adults.

The correct response is option C: The recommended daily water intake for healthy older adults is 1.5 L (six glasses) of water a day.

The total daily energy requirements decline with age (option A) because of reductions in metabolic rate, loss of lean body mass, and a diminution of energy expenditure for physical activity. The current recommended daily allowance (RDA) for protein (4 kcal/g) is 0.80 g/kg/day and is the same for adults of all ages. Protein intakes decrease with age; however, even though most people's protein intake usually exceeds the RDA, there are indications that older adults may need more dietary protein than do younger adults (option B) to support good health, promote recovery from illness, and maintain functionality (Bauer et al. 2013). The recommendation for healthy older adults is about six glasses (1.5 L) of fluid per day (Lindeman et al. 2000) (option C), except during stressful situations where more is needed because of fluid loss (e.g., severely hot weather, heavy exertion). Recommended dietary fiber intakes (20–30 g/day) are almost never met by adults of any age (Clemens et al. 2012) (option D). **(632, 634, 635)**

References

Almeida OP, Norman P, Hankey G, et al: Successful mental health aging: results from a longitudinal study of older Australian men. Am J Geriatr Psychiatry 14(1):27–35, 2006 16407579

Almeida OP, Calver J, Jamrozik K, et al: Obesity and metabolic syndrome increase the risk of incident depression in older men: the health in men study. Am J Geriatr Psychiatry 17(10):889–898, 2009 19910877

Angevaren M, Aufdemkampe G, Verhaar HJ, et al: Physical activity and enhanced fitness to improve cognitive function in older people without known cognitive impairment. Cochrane Database Syst Rev (3):CD005381, 2008

Bales CW, Johnson MA: Nutrition for older adults, in Modern Nutrition in Health and Disease. Edited by Ross C, Caballero B, Cousins R, et al. Philadelphia, PA, Lippincott Williams & Wilkins, 2012, pp 744–756

Bauer J, Biolo G, Cederholm T, et al: Evidence-based recommendations for optimal dietary protein intake in older people: a position paper from the PROT-AGE Study Group. J Am Med Dir Assoc 14(8):542–559, 2013 23867520

Bell IR, Edman JS, Morrow FD, et al: B complex vitamin patterns in geriatric and young adult inpatients with major depression. J Am Geriatr Soc 39(3):252–257, 1991 2005338

Berke EM, Gottlieb LM, Moudon AV, et al: Protective association between neighborhood walkability and depression in older men. J Am Geriatr Soc 55(4):526–533, 2007 17397430

Blaum CS, Fries BE, Fiatarone MA: Factors associated with low body mass index and weight loss in nursing home residents. J Gerontol A Biol Sci Med Sci 50(3):M162–M168, 1995 7743402

Blumenthal JA, Babyak MA, Moore KA, et al: Effects of exercise training on older patients with major depression. Arch Intern Med 159(19):2349–2356, 1999 10547175

Clarke R: Homocysteine, B vitamins, and the risk of dementia. Am J Clin Nutr 85(2):329–330, 2007 17284725

Clemens R, Kranz S, Mobley AR, et al: Filling America's fiber intake gap: summary of a roundtable to probe realistic solutions with a focus on grain-based foods. J Nutr 142(7):1390S–1401S, 2012 22649260

Colcombe SJ, Erickson KI, Scalf PE, et al: Aerobic exercise training increases brain volume in aging humans. J Gerontol A Biol Sci Med Sci 61(11):1166–1170, 2006 17167157

Detsky AS, Smalley PS, Chang J: The rational clinical examination. Is this patient malnourished? JAMA 271(1):54–58, 1994 8258889

Donini LM, Savina C, Rosano A, et al: MNA predictive value in the follow-up of geriatric patients. J Nutr Health Aging 7(5):282–293, 2003 12917741

Ferry M, Siobre B, Lambertin A, et al: The SOLINUT study: analysis of the interaction between nutrition and loneliness in persons aged over 70 years. J Nutr Health Aging 9(4):261–268, 2005 15980927

Frisardi V, Solfrizzi V, Imbimbo PB, et al: Towards disease-modifying treatment of Alzheimer's disease: drugs targeting beta-amyloid. Curr Alzheimer Res 7(1):40–55, 2010 19939231

Hamer M, Lavoie KL, Bacon SL: Taking up physical activity in later life and healthy ageing: the English longitudinal study of ageing. Br J Sports Med 48(3):239–243, 2014 24276781

Knight-Klimas TC, Boullata JI: Drug-nutrient interactions in the elderly, in Handbook of Drug-Nutrient Interactions. Edited by Boullata JI, Armenti VT. Totowa, NJ, Humana Press, 2004, pp 363–410

Lampinen P, Heikkinen RL, Kauppinen M, et al: Activity as a predictor of mental well-being among older adults. Aging Mental Health 10(5):454–466, 2006 16938681

Larson EB, Wang L, Bowen JD, et al: Exercise is associated with reduced risk for incident dementia among persons 65 years of age and older. Ann Intern Med 144(2):73–81, 2006 16418406

Lindeman RD, Romero LJ, Liang HC, et al: Do elderly persons need to be encouraged to drink more fluids? J Gerontol A Biol Sci Med Sci 55(7):M361–M365, 2000 10898251

Luckey AE, Parsa CJ: Fluid and electrolytes in the aged. Arch Surg 138(10):1055–1060, 2003 14557120

Marks BL, Madden DJ, Bucur B, et al: Role of aerobic fitness and aging on cerebral white matter integrity. Ann NY Acad Sci 1097:171–174, 2007 17413020

Markson EW: Functional, social, and psychological disability as causes of loss of weight and independence in older community-living people. Clin Geriatr Med 13(4):639–652, 1997 9354746

Moore AA, Whiteman EJ, Ward KT: Risks of combined alcohol/medication use in older adults. Am J Geriatr Pharmacother 5(1):64–74, 2007 17608249

Morley JE: Anorexia in older persons: epidemiology and optimal treatment. Drugs Aging 8(2):134–155, 1996 8845587

Morley JE: Decreased food intake with aging. J Gerontol A Biol Sci Med Sci 55(Spec No 2):81–88, 2001 11730241

Moshfegh A, Goldman J, Ahuja J, et al: What We Eat in America, NHANES 2005–2006: Usual Nutrient Intakes From Food and Water Compared to 1997 Dietary Reference Intakes for Vitamin D, Calcium, Phosphorus, and Magnesium. Beltsville, MD, U.S. Department of Agriculture, Agricultural Research Service, 2009. Available at: http://www.ars.usda.gov/SP2UserFiles/Place/12355000/pdf/0506/usual_nutrient_intake_vitD_ca_phos_mg_2005-06.pdf. Accessed November 18, 2014.

Newman AB, Yanez D, Harris T, et al; Cardiovascular Study Research Group: Weight change in old age and its association with mortality. J Am Geriatr Soc 49(10):1309–1318, 2001 11890489

Omran ML, Morley JE: Assessment of protein energy malnutrition in older persons, part II: laboratory evaluation. Nutrition 16(2):131–140, 2000 10696638

Panza F, Frisardi V, Seripa D, et al: Alcohol consumption in mild cognitive impairment and dementia: harmful or neuroprotective? Int J Geriatr Psychiatry 27(12):1218–1238, 2012 22396249

Papakostas GI, Shelton RC, Zajecka JM, et al: L-methylfolate as adjunctive therapy for SSRI-resistant major depression: results of two randomized, double-blind, parallel-sequential trials. Am J Psychiatry 169(12):1267–1274, 2012 23212058

Parrott MD, Shatenstein B, Ferland G, et al: Relationship between diet quality and cognition depends on socioeconomic position in healthy older adults. J Nutr 143(11):1767–1773, 2013 23986363

Przybelski RJ, Binkley NC: Is vitamin D important for preserving cognition? A positive correlation of serum 25-hydroxyvitamin D concentration with cognitive function. Arch Biochem Biophys 460(2):202–205, 2007 17258168

Psaltopoulou T, Sergentanis TN, Panagiotakos DB, et al: Mediterranean diet, stroke, cognitive impairment, and depression: a meta-analysis. Ann Neurol 74(4):580–591, 2013 23720230

Ravona-Springer R, Moshier E, Schmeidler J, et al: Changes in glycemic control are associated with changes in cognition in nondiabetic elderly. J Alzheimers Dis 30(2):299–309, 2012 22426020

Roberts RE, Deleger S, Strawbridge WJ, et al: Prospective association between obesity and depression: evidence from the Alameda County Study. Int J Obes Relat Metab Disord 27(4):514–521, 2003 12664085

Sacks GS, Dearman K, Replogle WH, et al: Use of subjective global assessment to identify nutrition-associated complications and death in geriatric long-term care facility residents. J Am Coll Nutr 19(5):570–577, 2000 11022870

Scarmeas N, Stern Y, Tang MX, et al: Mediterranean diet and risk for Alzheimer's disease. Ann Neurol 59(6):912–921, 2006 16622828

Stewart JW, Harrison W, Quitkin F, et al: Low B6 levels in depressed outpatients. Biol Psychiatry 19(4):613–616, 1984 6733177

Sullivan DH, Bopp MM, Roberson PK: Protein-energy undernutrition and life-threatening complications among the hospitalized elderly. J Gen Intern Med 17(12):923–932, 2002 12472928

Thomson AD: Mechanisms of vitamin deficiency in chronic alcohol misusers and the development of the Wernicke-Korsakoff syndrome. Alcohol Alcohol Suppl 35(1):2–7, 2000 11304071

Tolonen M, Schrijver J, Westermarck T, et al: Vitamin B6 status of Finnish elderly. Comparison with Dutch younger adults and elderly. The effect of supplementation. J Vitam Nutr Res 58(1):73–77, 1988 3384588

West RK, Ravona-Springer R, Schmeidler J, et al: The association of duration of type 2 diabetes with cognitive performance is modulated by long-term glycemic control. Am J Geriatr Psychiatry 22(10):1055–1059, 2014 24534521

Wilson SR, Knowles SB, Huang Q, Fink A: The prevalence of harmful and hazardous alcohol consumption in older U.S. adults: data from the 2005–2008 National Health and Nutrition Examination Survey (NHANES). J Gen Intern Med 29(2):312–319, 2014 24101531

CHAPTER 23

Individual and Group Psychotherapy

23.1 Cognitive-behavioral therapy (CBT) for people with moderate to severe cognitive impairment focuses on which of the following?

A. Challenging assumptions of being a burden to family.
B. Helping to generate realistic assessment of the risk of falls.
C. Incorporating caregivers into the therapeutic process.
D. Adapting to the environment.

The correct response is option D: Adapting to the environment.

CBT is a viable treatment option for persons with cognitive impairment. In cognitive-behavioral approaches, a modification strategy for individuals with milder impairments is to target cognitive change (e.g., challenge their beliefs about being a "burden," generate realistic assessments about fall risks in those with fear of falling) (options A and B). For individuals with more moderate to severe impairment, the focus shifts to behavioral changes and adaptations to the environment (option D). Several modifications to therapy may be used to better accommodate and target cognitive impairments. One common modification is the incorporation of a caregiver in the therapy process (option C). **(p. 658)**

23.2 Which of the following is true about problem-solving therapy (PST)?

A. It comprises 4–10 sessions.
B. The therapist "assigns" problems to the patient to solve.
C. The dropout rate from PST is higher than from other interventions.
D. Sessions must be conducted in person.

The correct response is option A: It comprises 4–10 sessions.

PST is a learning-based behavioral intervention that helps patients focus on solving problems that they feel are contributing to their depression (Areán et al. 1993). In PST, patients are taught a seven-step method for solving any kind of problem. PST takes between 4 and 10 sessions (option A). Although the main goal of treatment is to teach patients to become better problem solvers, the patient chooses the problems to work on (option B) and develops and selects the solution. In a meta-analysis, there was far less dropping out from PST than from interventions such as CBT and interpersonal therapy (Cuijpers et al. 2007) (option C). This therapy is effective by telephone and videoconference (Choi et al. 2014) (option D). **(pp. 651–652)**

23.3   Which of the following is true regarding psychotherapy with older adults?

A. Psychotherapy can be beneficial for people who cannot tolerate the side effects of medication.
B. Older patients are more likely than their younger counterparts to go to a therapist's office rather than see a therapist in a primary care setting.
C. Older adults are more concerned about stigma than are younger adults.
D. Older adults are less particular about the race, ethnicity, and culture of their therapists than are their younger counterparts.

The correct response is option A: Psychotherapy can be beneficial for people who cannot tolerate the side effects of medication.

Psychotherapy, both individual and group, can be helpful alone or in conjunction with medication. It can be particularly useful for older adult psychiatric patients who cannot or will not tolerate medication (option A). In presenting therapy as a treatment option, several factors should be considered. Older adults have been shown to be less concerned than younger adults about stigma attached to seeking treatment for depression (Rokke and Scogin 1995) (option C). However, older adults prefer that mental health treatment be provided in a primary care context rather than through specialty clinics (option B). As a result of their unique sociohistorical context, they often feel more comfortable receiving care from practitioners who share the same race, ethnicity, and religion (Bartels et al. 2004; Chen et al. 2006; Gum et al. 2010; Hinrichsen 2006; Snodgrass 2009) (option D). **(pp. 649–650)**

23.4   Which of the following is the most studied psychotherapy modality for depression in older adults?

A. Psychodynamic psychotherapy.
B. Interpersonal therapy.
C. Cognitive-behavioral therapy (CBT).
D. Problem-solving therapy.

The correct response is option C: Cognitive-behavioral therapy (CBT).

In the literature on depression in older adults, CBT has been the most frequently studied psychotherapy (Gould et al. 2012; Karlin et al. 2015) (option C; options A, B, and D are incorrect). **(p. 651)**

23.5   Which of the following is true regarding substance abuse in older adults?

A. Rates of illicit drug use have not changed since 2002.
B. Prescription medications and alcohol are the most commonly abused substances.
C. Well-established treatment protocols exist for treating substance abuse in late life.
D. Older adults should always be treated alongside younger people in addiction programs.

The correct response is option B: Prescription medications and alcohol are the most commonly abused substances.

Since 2002 the rate of illicit drug use more than doubled (from 1.9% to 4.1%) (option A) among adults ages 55–59 years (Substance Abuse and Mental Health Services Administration (SAMHSA) 2011). Sadly, there has been very little focus on the development of treatments specifically for older adults (option C), despite the fact that a number of studies indicate that substance use disorder treatment needs to be age specific for the treatment to be acceptable to older adults (Satre et al. 2003, 2004; Schonfeld et al. 2000) (option D). Prescription medication misuse and alcohol abuse were most prevalent in a study of older adults by Schonfeld et al. (2010) (option B). **(pp. 655–656)**

23.6   Cognitive reappraisal is the ability to reflect on and revise previously held beliefs. Which of the following is true regarding cognitive reappraisal?

A. Cognitive reappraisal is unrelated to executive functioning.
B. Cognitive reappraisal is not a part of CBT.
C. People with even minimal diminution in cognitive reappraisal are not appropriate candidates for psychotherapy.
D. Cognitive reappraisal requires patients to attend to their thoughts, hold them in working memory, generate alternative thoughts, and then implement these alternative thoughts.

The correct response is option D: Cognitive reappraisal requires patients to attend to their thoughts, hold them in working memory, generate alternative thoughts, and then implement these alternative thoughts.

Psychotherapies, especially cognitive-behavioral therapies (option B), are thought to rely on executive functioning (option A) and memory skills (Hariri et al. 2000; Mohlman 2008; Mohlman and Gorman 2005). Cognitive reappraisal requires patients to attend to their thoughts, hold them in working memory, generate alternative ideas, and implement these alternative thoughts (option D). The presence of cognitive impairments does not necessarily disqualify a patient from consideration for psychotherapy (option C). Several successful modifications of standard psychotherapy interventions for depression and anxiety have been developed for patients with comorbid cognitive impairments. **(p. 658)**

23.7   What is the most commonly diagnosed anxiety disorder in older adults?

   A. Substance/medication-induced anxiety disorder.
   B. Agoraphobia.
   C. Generalized anxiety disorder.
   D. Panic disorder.

The correct response is option C: Generalized anxiety disorder.

Anxiety disorders are among the most prominent mental disorders of late life, with generalized anxiety being the most commonly diagnosed (option C; options A, B, and D, are incorrect). **(p. 653)**

23.8   Which of the following is true regarding relaxation training in older adults?

   A. Relaxation training should be taught in the patient's home, where he or she is most relaxed.
   B. Relaxation training can be helpful for treating mild anxiety.
   C. Relaxation training takes months to show efficacy.
   D. Efficacy is achieved relatively rapidly, but gains are not maintained.

The correct response is option B: Relaxation training can be helpful for treating mild anxiety.

Relaxation training has some advantages for treating mild anxiety in older adults (option B). General symptom improvements were maintained at 1-month follow-up (option C), and gains in treatment responders were maintained at a 1-year fol-low-up assessment (option D) (Rickard et al. 1994). Theoretically, the strategies can be delivered during a regular visit to a primary care physician (option A). **(p. 655)**

23.9   Which of the following is true regarding comorbid personality disorders and de-pressive disorders in older persons?

   A. Rates of personality disorders are lower in older adults with depression than in the general population of older adults.
   B. Older adults with depression and personality disorders are less likely to have depressive symptoms recur than are those with depression alone.
   C. Studies have shown that selective serotonin reuptake inhibitors (SSRIs) alone are the best treatment for older adults with personality disorders and depres-sion.
   D. Modified dialectical-behavioral therapy (DBT) has been shown to be effective in treating comorbid personality disorders and depressive disorders in older adults.

The correct response is option D: Modified dialectical-behavioral therapy (DBT) has been shown to be effective in treating comorbid personality disor-ders and depressive disorders in older adults.

Meta-analyses have concluded that the prevalence rate for personality disorders in older adults is between 10% and 20% (Abrams 1996; Abrams and Horowitz 1999), essentially analogous to the 13% prevalence rate for younger age groups (Torgersen et al. 2001). However, personality disorder rates are even higher (approximately 30%) among depressed older adult samples (Abrams 1996; Thompson et al. 1988) (option A). Depressed older adult patients with comorbid personality disorder are four times more likely to experience maintenance or re-emergence of depression symptoms than are those without personality disorder diagnoses (Morse and Lynch 2004) (option B). In a randomized clinical trial specifically targeting personality disorders in older adults, compared with patients in a medication-only condition (option C), participants who received DBT plus medication management reached the level of remission more quickly and showed improvements in interpersonal sensitivity and aggression (option D) (Lynch et al. 2007). **(pp. 656–657)**

23.10 Which of the following is *not* a common psychological problem addressed through interpersonal therapy (IPT) for depression?

A. Loss and grief.
B. Interpersonal disputes and conflicts.
C. Role transitions.
D. Insomnia and hypersomnia.

The correct response is option D: Insomnia and hypersomnia.

IPT focuses on four common psychosocial problems related to depression: loss and grief (option A), interpersonal disputes and conflicts (option B), role transitions (option C), and interpersonal skill deficits. Insomnia and hypersomnia (option D) are not addressed in IPT. **(p. 652)**

23.11 What percentage of older adults who might benefit from psychotherapy actually receives treatment?

A. 1%.
B. 10%.
C. 25%.
D. 50%.

The correct response is option B: 10%.

Psychotherapy has been shown to be an effective treatment for a number of mental disorders seen in older adults. However, it has been estimated that only 10% of older adults in need of psychiatric services actually receive professional care, and there has been minimal utilization of mental health services in this age group (Lebowitz et al. 1997; Weissman et al. 1981) (option B; options A, C, and D are incorrect). **(p. 649)**

23.12 Which of the following is true about reminiscence psychotherapy?

A. It takes place between one patient and one therapist.
B. There is no evidence that it has any therapeutic efficacy.
C. It is less effective than CBT.
D. It draws on a patient's personal memories and life experiences with the goal of improving self-esteem and developing a sense of social cohesiveness.

The correct response is option D: It draws on a patient's personal memories and life experiences with the goal of improving self-esteem and developing a sense of social cohesiveness.

Life review and reminiscence psychotherapies are based on the patient's reexperiencing of personal memories and significant life experiences. Reminiscence therapy showed comparable reductions in depressive symptoms as CBT in a meta-analysis performed by Pinquart et al. (2007) (option C). Reminiscence therapy is often administered in a group setting (option A) with the goal of improving one's self-esteem and sense of social cohesiveness (option D). Recent research suggests that this is an acceptable and viable intervention in treating late-life depression (Preschl et al. 2012; Serrano Selva et al. 2012) (option B). **(p. 653)**

23.13 Which of the following is true regarding cognitive-behavioral therapy (CBT) for anxiety disorders in older persons?

A. It does not help patients who cannot distinguish between medical and psychiatric symptoms.
B. It includes repeated exposure to feared stimuli.
C. It has been proven ineffective.
D. It is less effective than medication management.

The correct response is option B: It includes repeated exposure to feared stimuli.

CBT appears to be the best form of psychotherapy to manage the diagnostic and treatment issues that exist in older populations with anxiety (Ayers et al. 2007; Stanley and Novy 2000; Stanley et al. 1996, 2004; Wetherell et al. 2003) (option C). CBT for anxiety disorders focuses on modifying anxious responses to inappropriately feared stimuli. Therapy includes repeated exposure to feared stimuli (option B) to facilitate habituation and to provide corrective learning (Foa and Kozak 1986; Moscovitch et al. 2009). Cognitive modifications may include reducing the perceived danger of physical symptoms of anxiety in panic disorder (e.g., recognizing that heart rate increases do not indicate a threat of heart attack) (option A). CBT has been found to be effective for a range of anxiety symptoms (Barrowclough et al. 2001), with comparable effectiveness to medication management (Gorenstein et al. 2005) (option D). **(pp. 653–654)**

23.14 Which of the following is true regarding acceptance and commitment therapy (ACT)?

A. It aims to increase a patient's acceptance of unwanted thoughts or experiences.
B. It aims to teach patients to commit to a strategy of avoiding unwanted thoughts and experiences.
C. It consistently has higher dropout rates than more traditional therapies.
D. It targets the frequency and intensity of anxiety symptoms.

The correct response is option A: It aims to increase a patient's acceptance of unwanted thoughts or experiences.

ACT focuses on increasing cognitive flexibility, decreasing experiential avoidance, and increasing engagement with values-based actions. Rather than targeting the frequency or intensity of anxious symptoms (option D), ACT aims to increase the patient's acceptance of those experiences (option A) through learning to mindfully observe them rather than attempting to push them away (option B). A preliminary trial that demonstrated the feasibility of using ACT in older adults with anxiety disorders resulted in a lower dropout rate than conventional CBT (Wetherell et al. 2011) (option C). **(pp. 654–655)**

23.15 What is the prevalence rate of personality disorders in the overall population of older adults?

A. Less than 5%.
B. Between 5% and 10%.
C. Between 10% and 20%.
D. Between 25% and 30%.

The correct response is option C: Between 10% and 20%.

Meta-analyses have concluded that the prevalence rate for personality disorders in older adults is between 10% and 20% (Abrams 1996; Abrams and Horowitz 1999) (option C; options A, B, and D are incorrect). **(p. 656)**

References

Abrams RC: Personality disorders in the elderly. Int J Geriatr Psychiatry 11:759–763, 1996 17061248

Abrams RC, Horowitz SV: Personality disorders after age 50: a meta-analytic review of the literature, in Personality Disorders in Older Adults: Emerging Issues in Diagnosis and Treatment. Edited by Rosowsky E, Abrams RC. Mahwah, NJ, Lawrence Erlbaum, 1999, pp 55–68

Areán PA, Perri MG, Nezu AM, et al: Comparative effectiveness of social problem-solving therapy and reminiscence therapy as treatments for depression in older adults. J Consult Clin Psychol 61(6):1003–1010, 1993 8113478

Ayers CR, Sorrell JT, Thorp SR, Wetherell JL: Evidence-based psychological treatments for late-life anxiety. Psychol Aging 22(1):8–17, 2007 17385978

Barrowclough C, King P, Colville J, et al: A randomized trial of the effectiveness of cognitive-behavioral therapy and supportive counseling for anxiety symptoms in older adults. J Consult Clin Psychol 69(5):756–762, 2001 11680552

Bartels SJ, Coakley EH, Zubritsky C, et al; PRISM-E Investigators: Improving access to geriatric mental health services: a randomized trial comparing treatment engagement with integrated versus enhanced referral care for depression, anxiety, and at-risk alcohol use. Am J Psychiatry 161(8):1455–1462, 2004 15285973

Chen H, Coakley EH, Cheal K, et al: Satisfaction with mental health services in older primary care patients. Am J Geriatr Psychiatry 14(4):371–379, 2006 16582046

Choi NG, Hegel MT, Marti N, et al: Telehealth problem-solving therapy for depressed low-income homebound older adults. Am J Geriatr Psychiatry 22(3):263–271, 2014 23567376

Cuijpers P, van Straten A, Warmerdam L, et al: Problem solving therapies for depression: a meta-analysis. Eur Psychiatry 22(1):9–15, 2007 17194572

Foa EB, Kozak MJ: Emotional processing of fear: exposure to corrective information. Psychol Bull 99(1):20–35, 1986 2871574

Gorenstein EE, Kleber MS, Mohlman J, et al: Cognitive-behavioral therapy for management of anxiety and medication taper in older adults. Am J Geriatr Psychiatry 13(10):901–909, 2005 16223969

Gould RL, Coulson MC, Howard RJ: Cognitive behavioral therapy for depression in older people: a meta-analysis and meta-regression of randomized controlled trials. J Am Geriatr Soc 60(10):1817–1830, 2012 23003115

Gum AM, Iser L, Petkus A: Behavioral health service utilization and preferences of older adults receiving home-based aging services. Am J Geriatr Psychiatry 18(6):491–501, 2010 21217560

Hariri AR, Bookheimer SY, Mazziotta JC: Modulating emotional responses: effects of a neocortical network on the limbic system. Neuroreport 11(1):43–48, 2000 10683827

Hinrichsen GA: Why multicultural issues matter for practitioners working with older adults. Prof Psychol Res Pr 37(1):29–35, 2006

Karlin BE, Trockel M, Brown GK, et al: Comparison of the effectiveness of cognitive behavioral therapy for depression among older versus younger veterans: results of a national evaluation. J Gerontol B Psychol Sci Soc Sci 70(1):3–120, 2015 24218096

Lebowitz BD, Pearson JL, Schneider LS, et al: Diagnosis and treatment of depression in late life. Consensus statement update. JAMA 278(14):1186–1190, 1997 9326481

Lynch TR, Cheavens JS, Cukrowicz KC, et al: Treatment of older adults with co-morbid personality disorder and depression: a dialectical behavior therapy approach. Int J Geriatr Psychiatry 22(2):131–143, 2007 17096462

Mohlman J: More power to the executive? A preliminary test of CBT plus executive skills training for treatment of late-life GAD. Cognit Behav Pract 15:306–316, 2008

Mohlman J, Gorman JM: The role of executive functioning in CBT: a pilot study with anxious older adults. Behav Res Ther 43(4):447–465, 2005 15701356

Morse JQ, Lynch TR: A preliminary investigation of self-reported personality disorders in late life: prevalence, predictors of depressive severity, and clinical correlates. Aging Ment Health 8(4):307–315, 2004 15370047

Moscovitch DA, Antony MM, Swinson RP: Exposure-based treatments for anxiety disorders, in Oxford Handbook of Anxiety and Related Disorders. Edited by Antony MM, Stein MB. New York, Oxford University Press, 2009, pp 461–475

Pinquart M, Duberstein PR, Lyness JM: Effects of psychotherapy and other behavioral interventions on clinically depressed older adults: a meta-analysis. Aging Ment Health 11(6):645–657, 2007 18074252

Preschl B, Maercker A, Wagner B, et al: Life-review therapy with computer supplements for depression in the elderly: a randomized controlled trial. Aging Ment Health 16(8):964–974, 2012 22788983

Rickard HC, Scogin F, Keith S: A one-year follow-up of relaxation training for elders with subjective anxiety. Gerontologist 34(1):121–122, 1994 8150300

Rokke PD, Scogin F: Depression treatment preferences in younger and older adults. Journal of Clinical Geropsychology 1:243–257, 1995

Satre DD, Mertens J, Areán PA, Weisner C: Contrasting outcomes of older versus middle-aged and younger adult chemical dependency patients in a managed care program. J Stud Alcohol 64(4):520–530, 2003 12921194

Satre DD, Mertens JR, Areán PA, Weisner C: Five-year alcohol and drug treatment outcomes of older adults versus middle-aged and younger adults in a managed care program. Addiction 99(10):1286–1297, 2004 15369567

Schonfeld L, Dupree LW, Dickson-Euhrmann E, et al: Cognitive-behavioral treatment of older veterans with substance abuse problems. J Geriatr Psychiatry Neurol 13(3):124–129, 2000 11001134

Schonfeld L, King-Kallimanis BL, Duchene DM, et al: Screening and brief intervention for substance misuse among older adults: the Florida BRITE project. Am J Public Health 100(1):108–114, 2010 19443821

Serrano Selva JP, Latorre Postigo JM, Ros Segura L, et al: Life review therapy using autobiographical retrieval practice for older adults with clinical depression. Psicothema 24(2):224–229, 2012 22420349

Snodgrass J: Toward holistic care: integrating spirituality and cognitive behavioral therapy for older adults. J Relig Spirit Aging 21(3):219–236, 2009

Stanley MA, Novy DM: Cognitive-behavior therapy for generalized anxiety in late life: an evaluative overview. J Anxiety Disord 14(2):191–207, 2000 10864385

Stanley MA, Beck JG, Glassco JD: Treatment of generalized anxiety in older adults: a preliminary comparison of cognitive-behavioral and supportive approaches. Behav Ther 27:565–581, 1996

Stanley MA, Diefenbach GJ, Hopko DR: Cognitive behavioral treatment for older adults with generalized anxiety disorder. A therapist manual for primary care settings. Behav Modif 28(1):73–117, 2004 14710708

Substance Abuse and Mental Health Services Administration (SAMHSA): Results from the 2010 National Survey on Drug Use and Health: Summary of National Findings (HHS Publ No SMA-11-4658; NSDUH Series H-41). 2011. Available at: http://www.samhsa.gov/data/nsduh/2k10nsduh/2k10results.htm. Accessed June 10, 2014.

Thompson LW, Gallagher D, Czirr R: Personality disorder and outcome in the treatment of late-life depression. J Geriatr Psychiatry 21(2):133–153, 1988 3216093

Torgersen S, Kringlen E, Cramer V: The prevalence of personality disorders in a community sample. Arch Gen Psychiatry 58(6):590–596, 2001 11386989

Weissman MM, Myers JK, Thompson WD: Depression and its treatment in a US urban community—1975–1976. Arch Gen Psychiatry 38(4):417–421, 1981 6111302

Wetherell JL, Gatz M, Craske MG: Treatment of generalized anxiety disorder in older adults. J Consult Clin Psychol 71(1):31–40, 2003 12602423

Wetherell JL, Afari N, Ayers CR, et al: Acceptance and Commitment Therapy for generalized anxiety disorder in older adults: a preliminary report. Behav Ther 42(1):127–134, 2011 21292059

CHAPTER 24

Working With Families of Older Adults

24.1 What percentage of older adults with moderate to severe dementia live alone, using extensive supervision and assistance from local and long-distance family
caregivers?

A. 10%.
B. 30%.
C. 5%.
D. 50%.

The correct response is option B: 30%.

Evidence suggests that 30% of older adults with moderate to severe dementia live
alone, often with extensive supervision and assistance from local and long-distance
family caregivers (option B; options A, C, and D are incorrect). **(p. 670)**

24.2 Psychiatrists working collaboratively with social workers or nurses can help provide timely or sustained assistance for families. Which of the following specific
interventions has been shown to delay nursing home placement by more than a
year?

A. Treating substance-related or anxiety disorders in caregivers.
B. Closely monitoring for abuse, exploitation, or neglect of patients.
C. Providing individual and family counseling for spouse caregivers.
D. Providing care management and monitoring the family's capacity and toler-
ance.

**The correct response is option C: Providing individual and family counseling
for spouse caregivers.**

Psychiatrists working with family caregivers over time will monitor the quality
of family care; the mental health, capacity, and vulnerability of caregivers; and the
impact of demands of care on family relationships (Sun et al. 2013) (option D).

Psychiatrists should also be alert to abuse, exploitation, or neglect of patients, which should prompt immediate recommendations for treatment, respite, or relinquishment of caregiving responsibilities (option B). Other goals in working with family caregivers include treating their own mood, substance-related, or anxiety disorders that limit the effectiveness of care (option A). Options A, B, and D pertain to better care of older adults at home; research suggests that social workers' individual and family counseling with spouse caregivers can mobilize and sustain community and secondary family support, reduce and prevent further primary caregiver depression, preserve caregiver self-reported health, change negative appraisals of behavioral symptoms, and even delay nursing home placement by over a year compared with a control group (Mittelman et al. 1996, 2004, 2007) (option C). **(p. 672)**

24.3   Which of the following strategies may be helpful in adequately assessing, counseling, and treating dementia patients and their families in the office setting?

A. Patients with dementia should not be interviewed without a family member present.
B. Family caregivers should be allowed to talk privately with the psychiatrist to avoid having to confront the older adult about his or her symptoms and declining condition.
C. Only one family member should accompany the patient to the visit because having too many family members during the evaluation may be confusing to the patient.
D. To avoid confronting doubt or denial initially, the clinician might suggest to caregivers that they not worry about Alzheimer's disease until a diagnosis has been confirmed.

The correct response is option B: Family caregivers should be allowed to talk privately with the psychiatrist to avoid having to confront the older adult about his or her symptoms and declining condition.

Although the patient is entitled to time alone with the psychiatrist initially (option A), time alone with family informants is invaluable to the psychiatrist as he or she assesses the effects of functional loss and other family stressors. Most family caregivers prefer to talk privately with the psychiatrist to avoid confronting the older adult about his or her symptoms and declining condition (option B). It may be helpful to have two family members accompany the patient for an evaluation (option C). One family member can distract or sit with the older adult while another speaks privately with the psychiatrist. Initially, communication with patients and their family members will likely be in response to the common emotional reactions to learning that there is a diagnosis of degenerative dementia. Rather than confront their doubt or denial, the clinician might suggest to them that they behave as if the diagnosis of Alzheimer's disease had been confirmed while awaiting confirmation based on symptoms or progression of the disease (option D). **(p. 674)**

24.4 When providing information and education for older spouses who are caregivers, which of the following principles should be kept in mind?

A. Older spouses in first marriages are generally more comfortable facing threatening health information together rather than apart.
B. They do not appreciate the psychiatrist asking about what else is going on in their lives because they may see this as unrelated to the care of their loved one.
C. Subtle or vague suggestions that they need to take care of themselves can help families who are overwhelmed by caregiving responsibilities.
D. When dealing with a combative patient, asking the family about guns in the house early on may be interpreted as an invasion of privacy.

The correct response is option A: Older spouses in first marriages are generally more comfortable facing threatening health information together rather than apart.

Older spouses in first marriages are generally more comfortable facing threatening health information together, and one spouse may be put off by attempts to separate him or her from the impaired spouse (option A). Providing the same information to both spouses at the same time helps older couples preserve their couple identity and accept the psychiatric recommendations as a mutual and shared adaptive challenge. Families of older adults expect to be asked what they have tried in coping with their relative's impairment, and these families appreciate the psychiatrist's asking about what else is going on in their lives (option B). Families also appreciate preventive self-care reminders from psychiatrists, but vague suggestions that caregivers need to take care of themselves often frustrate overwhelmed families that have few resources (option C). Families of older adults want psychiatrists to tailor information and education relevant to their immediate, pressing concerns. For example, a family concerned about the combative behavior of an older adult may be helped by a psychiatrist who responds, "First, let's get the guns out of the house" (Lynch et al. 2008) (option D). **(pp. 675–676)**

24.5 Which of the following is true in assessing family caregivers of older adults with dementia?

A. Family caregivers who report being frustrated, overwhelmed, edgy, or exhausted will acknowledge having depression and anxiety.
B. Older husband caregivers may be particularly at risk of increased alcohol use in response to care demands.
C. Poor nutrition should prompt a suggestion to have all meals at home in order to adequately meet the patient's nutritional needs.
D. If the family belongs to an ethnic minority group, the psychiatrist should monitor for legal protections or fully sanctioned empowerment to make care decisions.

The correct response is option B: Older husband caregivers may be particularly at risk of increased alcohol use in response to care demands.

Older husband caregivers may be particularly at risk of increased alcohol use in response to care demands (option B). The psychiatrist should probe further if the caregiver hints about increased use of alcohol or psychoactive medications in response to stress. Many family caregivers report being frustrated, overwhelmed, edgy, or exhausted but will deny having depression, anxiety, or psychiatric symptoms (option A). A person caring for his or her partner may be frustrated by the other's loss of interest in cooking. A suggestion to try regular meals at a familiar restaurant may conserve the couple's energy and better meet their nutritional and social needs (option C). In many regions of the country, gay, lesbian, bisexual, and transgender communities still do not have legal protections or fully sanctioned empowerment to make care decisions for their partners or families (option D). **(p. 677)**

24.6   Which intervention is most effective for families of older adults?

A. Unimodal strategies concentrating resources on family counseling.
B. Didactic educational approaches.
C. Participation in support groups.
D. Problem-solving and/or active participatory skill-building strategies.

The correct response is option D: Problem-solving and/or active participatory skill-building strategies.

The most effective interventions for family caregivers emphasize problem-solving and/or active participatory skill-building strategies for behavior change (option D) over purely didactic educational approaches (option B). Combining individual and family counseling, family education, support group participation, and care management is associated with decreased caregiver burden and depression (option A). Referrals to support groups should be balanced, and participation should not be oversold (option C). Benefits of participation in support groups are derived from experiential similarity, consumer information, coping and survivor models, expressive or advocacy outlets, and (for some participants) the creation of substitute family or social outlets. However, one support group does not fit all. Black individuals frequently do not feel the need to talk about family business among strangers but may respond to a church-based group on family care. **(pp. 678–679)**

24.7   Which of the following is the most common symptom reported by caregivers of patients with Alzheimer's disease?

A. Fatigue.
B. Irritability.
C. Anxiety.
D. Insomnia.

The correct response is option C: Anxiety.

Depression and anxiety (option C) are the most frequently reported psychiatric symptoms among caregivers of Alzheimer's disease patients. Fatigue (option A) and exhaustion are also common issues. Encouraging rest, respite, exercise, and energy economies can be helpful for family members. Many family caregivers report being frustrated, overwhelmed, edgy, or exhausted but will deny having depression, anxiety, or psychiatric symptoms (options B and D). **(pp. 671, 675, 677)**

24.8   When considering educational strategies for families, what should be done during the initial evaluation?

A. Offer as much information regarding diagnosis and treatment as possible.
B. Talk about potential problems in the future, such as psychosis.
C. Provide the family with a complete list of suggestions and referrals.
D. Avoid overwhelming families with too many treatment suggestions or too much information.

The correct response is option D: Avoid overwhelming families with too many treatment suggestions or too much information.

Many families are too overwhelmed at a first psychiatric evaluation to absorb information or instructions. Overwhelming families with too many treatment suggestions or referrals is just as likely to lead to poor compliance as is changing multiple medication regimens all at once (option D; options A, B, and C are incorrect). Information should be presented in hopeful terms, such as "Treating your depression should have positive effects on your partner's mood as well" or "Many families surprise themselves with their resilience." **(p. 680)**

24.9   When working with dementia patients and their families, which of the following general principles is not accurate?

A. Denial is a common defense of family caregivers.
B. Overutilization of services and overreporting of burden occur frequently.
C. Successful family caregivers are flexible in adjusting expectations of themselves, the older adult, and other family members.
D. A primary caregiver at home is generally preferred.

The correct response is option B: Overutilization of services and overreporting of burden occur frequently.

A primary caregiver at home is efficient and preferred (option D). Primary caregivers, however, need breaks, respite, backup people, and services to supplement their personalized care. Even in ideal situations, contingency plans are necessary (Derence 2005; Lund et al. 2009). More underutilization of services and underreporting of burden occur than overutilization and overreporting (option B). Denial is a common defense of family caregivers (option A). Some people need to deny the inevitable outcome (e.g., loss of a beloved spouse or partner, eventual placement of a parent in a nursing home) to provide hopeful, consistent daily care. Successful family caregivers are flexible in adjusting expectations of themselves, the older adult, other family members, and professionals as they work to fit the needs and capacities of all (option C). **(pp. 671–672)**

24.10 Which one of the following is not a correct key message for family caregivers?

A. Be willing to listen to the older adult and know that it will get easier.
B. It is tempting for distant relatives to second-guess or criticize.
C. The older adult is not unhappy or upset because of what you have done.
D. Considering what is best for your family involves compromise among competing needs, loyalties, and commitments.

The correct response is option A: Be willing to listen to the older adult and know that it will get easier.

The caregiver should be willing to listen to the older adult but should know that it will not necessarily get easier, although things will change (option A). Options B, C, and D are correct key messages for family caregivers. **(Table 24–1, "Key messages for family caregivers," p. 681)**

References

Derence K: Dementia-specific respite: the key to effective caregiver support. N C Med J 66(1):48–51, 2005 15786679

Lund D, Utz R, Casarta M, et al: Examining what caregivers do during respite time to make respite more effective. J Appl Gerontol 28(1):109–131, 2009

Lynch CA, Moran M, Lawlor BA: Firearms and dementia: a smoking gun? Int J Geriatr Psychiatry 23(1):1–6, 2008 18081001

Mittelman MS, Ferris SH, Shulman E, et al: A family intervention to delay nursing home placement of patients with Alzheimer disease. A randomized controlled trial. JAMA 276(21):1725–1731, 1996 8940320

Mittelman MS, Roth DL, Haley WE, Zarit SH: Effects of a caregiver intervention on negative caregiver appraisals of behavior problems in patients with Alzheimer's disease: results of a randomized trial. J Gerontol B Psychol Sci Soc Sci 59(1):27–34, 2004 14722336

Mittelman MS, Roth DL, Clay OJ, Haley WE: Preserving health of Alzheimer caregivers: impact of a spouse caregiver intervention. Am J Geriatr Psychiatry 15(9):780–789, 2007 17804831

Sun F, Durkin DW, Hilgeman MM, et al: Predicting desire for institutional placement among racially diverse dementia family caregivers: the role of quality of care. Gerontologist 53(3):418–429, 2013 22961466

CHAPTER 25

Clinical Psychiatry in the Nursing Home

25.1   Which of the following is true regarding nursing home admission in patients with dementia?

A. Performance of activities of daily living (ADLs) does not have an impact on nursing home admission.
B. Disturbances of behavior are among the most common reasons for nursing home admission.
C. Dementia with Lewy bodies is highly prevalent among nursing home populations.
D. Depression is the most common psychiatric diagnosis among nursing home residents.

The correct response is option B: Disturbances of behavior are among the most common reasons for nursing home admission.

Disturbances of behavior, in addition to impaired ability to perform ADLs, have been identified as the most common reasons that patients with dementia are admitted to nursing homes (Steele et al. 1990) (option B; option A is incorrect), and disruptive behaviors frequently complicate care after admission (Cohen-Mansfield et al. 1989; Teeter et al. 1976; Zimmer et al. 1984). A study of 714 residents in three private nursing facilities found a 7.7% prevalence rate of Parkinson's disease and a 3.7% prevalence rate of Parkinson disease dementia (Hoegh et al. 2013). The prevalence rates of dementia with Lewy bodies and frontotemporal dementia have not been specifically ascertained in nursing home populations (option C). Among community-dwelling elders in the United States and Europe, depression increases the risk of nursing home admission (Ahmed et al. 2007; Harris and Cooper 2006; Onder et al. 2007), and this association remains after controlling for age, physical illness, and functional status (Harris 2007). Among nursing homes residents, depressive disorders represent the second most common psychiatric diagnosis, after dementia (option D). **(pp. 691–693)**

25.2 Which of the following has *not* been shown to be associated with depression among nursing home residents?

A. Diabetes.
B. Increase in pain complaints.
C. Risk of delirium.
D. Unchanged nutritional status.

The correct response is option D: Unchanged nutritional status.

Evidence for morbidity associated with depression comes from studies that showed an increase in pain complaints among residents with depression (Mc-Cusker et al. 2014; Parmelee et al. 1991) (option B), an association between depression and biochemical markers of subnutrition (Katz et al. 1993) (option D), and independent associations of delirium (option C) and diabetes (option A) with depression (McCusker et al. 2014). **(p. 694)**

25.3 Which of the following has been associated with poor antidepressant treatment response in nursing home residents?

A. Absence of cognitive impairment.
B. Depressive symptoms associated with vascular risk factors and executive dysfunction.
C. Preserved self-care abilities.
D. High serum levels of albumin.

The correct response is option B: Depressive symptoms associated with vascular risk factors and executive dysfunction.

Poor antidepressant treatment responses have been amply demonstrated in very old outpatients whose depressive symptoms are associated with vascular risk factors and executive dysfunction (Sneed et al. 2007, 2008) (option B). A treatment study by Katz et al. (1990) demonstrated that measures of self-care deficits and serum levels of albumin were highly intercorrelated and that both predicted a lack of response to treatment with nortriptyline. Therefore, although this study demonstrated that major depression is a specific, treatable disorder—even in long-term-care patients with medical comorbidity—there is also evidence in this setting for a treatment-relevant subtype of depression characterized by high levels of disability (option C) and low levels of serum albumin (option D). Several studies of nursing home residents have demonstrated poorer response to treatment with noradrenergic and serotonergic antidepressant drugs in very old residents with comorbid cognitive impairment or dementia (Magai et al. 2000; Oslin et al. 2000; Rosen et al. 2000; Streim et al. 2000; Trappler and Cohen 1996, 1998) (option A). **(pp. 694–695)**

25.4 Which of the following nonpharmacological interventions emphasizes a multi-component psychosocial approach?

A. Snoezelen rooms.
B. Namaste Care.
C. VA Community Living Centers program.
D. Standardized nonpharmacological interventions.

The correct response is option C: VA Community Living Centers program.

The largest intervention trial of nonpharmacological interventions to date has been conducted in the VA Community Living Centers, which are residential nursing facilities that include the provision of dementia care for veterans (Karlin et al. 2014). Program elements included a psychologist serving as the primary interventionist and behavioral coordinator, working closely with facility staff to develop and implement a behavioral intervention plan to address challenging behaviors associated with dementia. The multicomponent psychosocial approach was based on a model developed by Teri et al. (2005) for training direct care workers in assisted living residences (option C). Namaste Care, a program developed for nursing home residents with advanced dementia, emphasizes the calming effects of touch as well as sound, smell, and taste (Fullarton and Volicer 2013; Simard and Volicer 2010) (option B). Snoezelen rooms provide stimulation to meet patients' multisensory needs (Berg et al. 2010; van Weert et al. 2005) (option A). A randomized placebo-controlled trial of nonpharmacological individualized interventions to address unmet needs demonstrated significant declines in total, physical nonaggressive, and verbal agitation (Cohen-Mansfield et al. 2012) (option D). **(pp. 695–696)**

25.5 Which of the following is an institutional and systemic factor associated with physical restraint use?

A. Insufficient staffing.
B. Agitation and behavior problems.
C. Presence of monitoring or treatment devices.
D. Need to promote body alignment.

The correct response is option A: Insufficient staffing.

Institutional and systemic factors associated with restraint use include pressure to avoid litigation, staff attitudes, insufficient staffing (option A), and the availability of restraint devices. Patient factors predicting the use of restraints, in addition to agitation and behavior problems (option B), include age, cognitive impairment, risk of injuries to self (e.g., from falls) or others (e.g., from combative behavior), physical frailty, the presence of monitoring or treatment devices (option C), and the need to promote body alignment (option D). **(p. 718)**

25.6 Which of the following best describes the purpose of a second-stage assessment at the time of admission to a nursing home?

A. To evaluate the patient for dementia.
B. To provide acute psychiatric treatment after admission to a nursing home rather than a psychiatric facility.
C. To make a specific psychiatric diagnosis.
D. To allow for appropriate admission to nursing homes of patients who have a severe psychiatric disorder.

The correct response is option C: To make a specific psychiatric diagnosis.

When an initial first-stage screening reveals that a serious mental disorder (other than dementia) might be present, a second-stage assessment that includes a psychiatric evaluation must be made to ascertain whether the patient has a mental disorder, to make a specific psychiatric diagnosis (option C), and to determine whether there is a need for acute psychiatric care that precludes adequate or appropriate treatment in a nursing home (option B). Patients found to have dementia on the initial screen are exempt from the preadmission psychiatric evaluation (option A). Thus, preadmission screening is intended 1) to prevent inappropriate admission to nursing homes of patients who do not have dementia but who have severe psychiatric disorders (option D) and 2) to help ensure that patients with disabilities due to treatable psychiatric disorders are not placed in long-term-care facilities before they receive the benefits of adequate psychiatric treatment. **(p. 720)**

25.7 Which of the following is true regarding the surveyor guidelines based on the Centers of Medicare and Medicaid Services regulations related to quality of care?

A. The guidelines address psychotropic medication use only.
B. The guidelines have not been updated since original publication.
C. The guidelines do not address the provision of care for residents with mental health problems.
D. The guidelines address upper limits for daily dosages and acceptable indications for medications.

The correct response is option D: The guidelines address upper limits for daily dosages and acceptable indications for medications.

Regulations related to quality of care require that residents not receive "unnecessary drugs" and that antipsychotic medications not be given "unless these are necessary to treat a specific condition as diagnosed and documented in the clinical record" (Health Care Financing Administration 1991, p. 48,910). The surveyor guidelines based on these regulations further limit the use of antipsychotic medications, antianxiety agents, sedative-hypnotics, and related medications (Centers for Medicare and Medicaid Services 2014). For each of these classes, the guidelines specify a list of acceptable indications, upper limits for daily dosages (option D), requirements for monitoring treatment and adverse effects, and time frames for attempting dosage reductions and discontinuation. These guidelines are periodically updated to reflect new clinical knowledge and the availability of new drugs approved by the U.S. Food and Drug Administration, with a recent revision posted to the Centers for Medicare and Medicaid Services (CMS) Web site in 2014 (Centers for Medicare and Medicaid Services 2014) (option B). In addition to addressing the use of psychotropic drugs, the interpretive guidelines also outline conditions for the use of physical restraints (option A). Although much of the emphasis of the federal regulations is on eliminating inappropriate treatment, requirements also call for the provision of necessary and appropriate care for residents with mental health problems (option C). **(pp. 721–722)**

25.8   Which of the following is true regarding the Nursing Home Quality Initiative?

A. The information is available only to health care providers.
B. It includes only long-stay quality measures.
C. Antipsychotic medication administration is not addressed.
D. Information is posted on the Medicare.gov Web site.

The correct response is option D: Information is posted on the Medicare.gov Web site.

In 2002, CMS introduced the Nursing Home Quality Initiative, which derives quality measures from regularly reported Minimum Data Set data and posts these on the Medicare.gov Web site in a program called Nursing Home Compare (Medicare.gov 2014) (option D). This publicly accessible Web site (option A) enables health care consumers to compare the quality of care delivered by individual facilities in the same region or across the nation. At the time this book chapter was written, five short-stay quality measures and 13 long-stay quality measures were posted (option B). These measures include the percentage of residents experiencing moderate to severe pain, falls with injuries, depressive symptoms, weight loss, increased need for help with ADLs, physical restraint, and receipt of antipsychotic medication (option C). **(p. 722)**

25.9   Which of the following is true regarding short-stay residents at nursing homes?

A. Addressing their depression and anxiety is not a primary objective of mental health care during their stay.
B. They are more likely than long-term-care patients to have a primary diagnosis of stroke.
C. They are more likely than long-term-care patients to have ambulatory dysfunction.
D. They are less likely than long-term-care patients to be admitted directly from an acute care hospital.

The correct response is option B: They are more likely than long-term-care patients to have a primary diagnosis of stroke.

In general, short-stay residents—patients who, after relatively brief stays in nursing homes, are discharged to the community or die—differ from long-term-care patients in that they are younger; more likely to be admitted directly from an acute care hospital (option D); less likely to have irreversible cognitive impairment, incontinence, or ambulatory dysfunction (option C); and more likely to have a primary diagnosis of hip fracture, stroke (option B), or cancer. The objectives of mental health care for short-stay patients are related not so much to managing behavior problems associated with dementia as to helping patients cope with disease and disability, to searching for delirium and reversible causes of cognitive impairment, and to treating disorders such as depression and anxiety that can be impediments to rehabilitation and recovery (option A). **(p. 727)**

25.10 Which of the following is a component of the intrinsic system of mental health care in nursing homes?

A. Optimizing the ways staff and residents interact.
B. Evaluating the interactions between medical and mental health problems.
C. Establishing psychiatric diagnoses.
D. Administering specific treatments for mental disorders.

The correct response is option A: Optimizing the ways staff and residents interact.

The intrinsic system of mental health care in nursing homes can be conceptualized as including a wide range of components: design of the environment; implementation of psychosocial programs; formulation of institutional policies and procedures for assessment, care delivery, monitoring, and quality improvement; and optimization of the ways in which staff and residents interact (option A). The intrinsic system for mental health services as just described is necessary but not sufficient to meet the needs of nursing home residents. In addition, the services of mental health professionals are important in evaluating the interactions between medical and mental health problems (option B), in establishing psychiatric diagnoses (option C), and in planning and administering specific treatments for mental disorders (option D). **(pp. 731–732)**

References

Ahmed A, Lefante CM, Alam N: Depression and nursing home admission among hospitalized older adults with coronary artery disease: a propensity score analysis. Am J Geriatr Cardiol 16(2):76–83, 2007 17380615

Berg A, Sadowski K, Beyrodt M, et al: Snoezelen, structured reminiscence therapy and 10-minutes activation in long term care residents with dementia (WISDE): study protocol of a cluster randomized controlled trial. BMC Geriatr 10:5, 2010 20113526

Centers for Medicare and Medicaid Services: State Operations Manual, Appendix PP: Guidance to Surveyors for Long Term Care Facilities. Baltimore, MD, Centers for Medicare and Medicaid, Rev 107, 04-04-14. Baltimore, MD, Centers for Medicare and Medicaid. 2014. Available at: https://www.cms.gov/Regulations-and-Guidance/Guidance/Manuals/downloads/som107ap_pp_guidelines_ltcf.pdf. Accessed June 12, 2014.

Cohen-Mansfield J, Marx MS, Rosenthal AS: A description of agitation in a nursing home. J Gerontol 44(3):M77–M84, 1989 2715584

Cohen-Mansfield J, Thein K, Marx MS, et al: Efficacy of nonpharmacologic interventions for agitation in advanced dementia: a randomized, placebo-controlled trial. J Clin Psychiatry 73(9):1255–1261, 2012 23059151

Fullarton J, Volicer L: Reductions of antipsychotic and hypnotic medications in Namaste Care. J Am Med Dir Assoc 14(9):708–709, 2013 23890761

Harris Y: Depression as a risk factor for nursing home admission among older individuals. J Am Med Dir Assoc 8(1):14–20, 2007 17210498

Harris Y, Cooper JK: Depressive symptoms in older people predict nursing home admission. J Am Geriatr Soc 54(4):593–597, 2006 16686868

Health Care Financing Administration: Medicare and Medicaid: requirements for long-term care facilities—HCFA. Final rule. Fed Regist 56:48865–48921, 1991

Hoegh M, Ibrahim AK, Chibnall J, et al: Prevalence of Parkinson disease and Parkinson disease dementia in community nursing homes. Am J Geriatr Psychiatry 21(6):529–535, 2013 23567411

Karlin BE, Visnic S, McGee JS, Teri L: Results from the multisite implementation of STAR-VA: a multicomponent psychosocial intervention for managing challenging dementia-related behaviors of veterans. Psychol Serv 11(2):200–208, 2014 23937081

Katz IR, Simpson GM, Curlik SM, et al: Pharmacologic treatment of major depression for elderly patients in residential care settings. J Clin Psychiatry 51 (suppl):41–47, discussion 48, 1990

Katz IR, Beaston-Wimmer P, Parmelee P, et al: Failure to thrive in the elderly: exploration of the concept and delineation of psychiatric components. J Geriatr Psychiatry Neurol 6(3):161–169, 1993 8397760

Magai C, Kennedy G, Cohen CI, Gomberg D: A controlled clinical trial of sertraline in the treatment of depression in nursing home patients with late-stage Alzheimer's disease. Am J Geriatr Psychiatry 8(1):66–74, 2000 10648297

McCusker J, Cole MG, Voyer P, et al: Observer-rated depression in long-term care: frequency and risk factors. Arch Gerontol Geriatr 58(3):332–338, 2014 24345307

Medicare.gov: The Official U.S. Government Site for Medicare, Nursing Home Compare. 2014. Available at: http://www.medicare.gov/nursinghomecompare/search.html?AspxAutoDetect Cookie-Support=1. Accessed January 5, 2015.

Onder G, Liperoti R, Soldato M, et al: Depression and risk of nursing home admission among older adults in home care in Europe: results from the Aged in Home Care (AdHOC) study. J Clin Psychiatry 68(9):1392–1398, 2007 17915978

Oslin DW, Streim JE, Katz IR, et al: Heuristic comparison of sertraline with nortriptyline for the treatment of depression in frail elderly patients. Am J Geriatr Psychiatry 8(2):141–149, 2000 10804075

Parmelee PA, Katz IR, Lawton MP: The relation of pain to depression among institutionalized aged. J Gerontol 46(1):15–21, 1991 1986040

Rosen J, Mulsant BH, Pollock BG: Sertraline in the treatment of minor depression in nursing home residents: a pilot study. Int J Geriatr Psychiatry 15(2):177–180, 2000 10679849

Simard J, Volicer L: Effects of Namaste Care on residents who do not benefit from usual activities. Am J Alzheimers Dis Other Demen 25(1):46–50, 2010 19332652

Sneed JR, Roose SP, Keilp JG, et al: Response inhibition predicts poor antidepressant treatment response in very old depressed patients. Am J Geriatr Psychiatry 15(7):553–563, 2007 17586780

Sneed JR, Keilp JG, Brickman AM, Roose SP: The specificity of neuropsychological impairment in predicting antidepressant non-response in the very old depressed. Int J Geriatr Psychiatry 23(3):319–323, 2008 17726720

Steele C, Rovner B, Chase GA, Folstein M: Psychiatric symptoms and nursing home placement of patients with Alzheimer's disease. Am J Psychiatry 147(8):1049–1051, 1990 2375439

Streim JE, Oslin DW, Katz IR, et al: Drug treatment of depression in frail elderly nursing home residents. Am J Geriatr Psychiatry 8(2):150–159, 2000 10804076

Teeter RB, Garetz FK, Miller WR, Heiland WF: Psychiatric disturbances of aged patients in skilled nursing homes. Am J Psychiatry 133(12):1430–1434, 1976 985657

Teri L, Huda P, Gibbons L, et al: STAR: a dementia-specific training program for staff in assisted living residences. Gerontologist 45(5):686–693, 2005 16199404

Trappler B, Cohen CI: Using fluoxetine in "very old" depressed nursing home residents. Am J Geriatr Psychiatry 4:258–262, 1996

Trappler B, Cohen CI: Use of SSRIs in "very old" depressed nursing home residents. Am J Geriatr Psychiatry 6(1):83–89, 1998 9469218

van Weert JC, van Dulmen AM, Spreeuwenberg PM, et al: Behavioral and mood effects of snoezelen integrated into 24-hour dementia care. J Am Geriatr Soc 53(1):24–33, 2005 15667372

Zimmer JG, Watson N, Treat A: Behavioral problems among patients in skilled nursing facilities. Am J Public Health 74(10):1118–1121, 1984 6476166

CPSIA information can be obtained
at www.ICGtesting.com
Printed in the USA
LVOW03s0726250516

489797LV00003B/3/P